Oral Surgery for the General Dentist

Guest Editors

HARRY DYM, DDS
ORRETT E. OGLE, DDS

DENTAL CLINICS OF NORTH AMERICA

www.dental.theclinics.com

January 2012 • Volume 56 • Number 1

SAUNDERS an imprint of ELSEVIER, Inc.

W.B. SAUNDERS COMPANY
A Division of Elsevier Inc.

1600 John F. Kennedy Boulevard • Suite 1800 • Philadelphia, Pennsylvania 19103-2899

http://www.dental.theclinics.com

DENTAL CLINICS OF NORTH AMERICA Volume 56, Number 1
January 2012 ISSN 0011-8532, ISBN 978-1-4557-1032-4

Editor: Yonah Korngold; y.korngold@elsevier.com
Developmental Editor: Donald Mumford

Dental Clinics of North America (ISSN 0011-8532) is published quarterly by Elsevier Inc., 360 Park Avenue South, New York, NY 10010-1710. Months of issue are January, April, July, and October. Business and Editorial Offices: 1600 John F. Kennedy Boulevard, Suite 1800, Philadelphia, PA 19103-2899. Periodicals postage paid at New York, NY and additional mailing offices. Subscription prices are $259.00 per year (domestic individuals), $447.00 per year (domestic institutions), $122.00 per year (domestic students/residents), $310.00 per year (Canadian individuals), $563.00 per year (Canadian institutions), $375.00 per year (international individuals), $563.00 per year (international institutions), and $184.00 per year (international and Canadian students/residents). International air speed delivery is included in all *Clinics* subscription prices. All prices are subject to change without notice. **POSTMASTER:** Send address changes to *Dental Clinics of North America*, Elsevier Health Sciences Division, Subscription Customer Service, 3251 Riverport Lane, Maryland Heights, MO 63043. **Customer Service (orders, claims, online, change of address): Elsevier Health Sciences Division, Subscription Customer Service, 3251 Riverport Lane, Maryland Heights, MO 63043. Tel: 1-800-654-2452 (U.S. and Canada). Fax: 314-447-8029. E-mail: journalscustomer service-usa@elsevier.com (for print support); journalsonlinesupport-usa@elsevier.com (for online support).**

Reprints. For copies of 100 or more, of articles in this publication, please contact the Commercial Reprints Department, Elsevier Inc., 360 Park Avenue South, New York, NY 10010-1710. Tel.: 212-633-3812; Fax: 212-462-1935; E-mail: reprints@elsevier.com.

The *Dental Clinics of North America* is covered in *MEDLINE/PubMed (Index Medicus), Current Contents/Clinical Medicine, ISI/BIOMED* and *Clinahl.*

Printed and bound by CPI Group (UK) Ltd, Croydon, CR0 4YY

Transferred to digital print 2012

Contributors

GUEST EDITORS

HARRY DYM, DDS
Chairman of Department of Dentistry/Oral and Maxillofacial Surgery, The Brooklyn
Hospital Center, Brooklyn; Clinical Professor, Oral and Maxillofacial Surgery, Columbia
University, College of Dental Medicine, New York; Attending, Oral and Maxillofacial
Surgery, Woodhull Medical and Mental Health Center; Attending, Oral and Maxillofacial
Surgery, New York Harbor Healthcare System, The Brooklyn VA Campus, Brooklyn,
New York

ORRETT E. OGLE, DDS
Director, Residency Training Program, Oral and Maxillofacial Surgery, Woodhull Hospital,
Brooklyn; Associate Clinical Professor, Department of Oral Surgery, School of Dental
Medicine, Columbia University, New York; Chief, Program Director, Oral and Maxillofacial
Surgery, Department of Dentistry; Department of Oral and Maxillofacial Surgery,
Woodhull Medical and Mental Health Center, Brooklyn, New York

AUTHORS

SHELLY ABRAMOWICZ, DMD, MPH
Instructor, Department of Oral and Maxillofacial Surgery, Harvard School of Dental
Medicine; Attending Surgeon, Department of Plastic and Oral Surgery, Children's Hospital
Boston, Boston, Massachusetts

M. TODD BRANDT, DDS, MD
Blue Ridge Oral and Maxillofacial Surgery, Fishersville, Virginia

MICHAEL H. CHAN, DDS
Director of Oral and Maxillofacial Surgery, Oral and Maxillofacial Surgery/Dental Service,
Department of Veterans Affairs, New York Harbor Healthcare Systems (Brooklyn
Campus); Attending, Department of Oral and Maxillofacial Surgery, The Brooklyn Hospital
Center, Brooklyn, New York

EARL CLARKSON, DDS
Program Director, Department of Dentistry/Oral and Maxillofacial Surgery, The Brooklyn
Hospital Center, Brooklyn, New York

SEAN W. DIGMAN, DDS
Department Chair, Oral and Maxillofacial Surgery Residency, Department of Oral and
Maxillofacial Surgery, David Grant USAF Medical Center, Travis AFB, California

LADI DOONQUAH, MD, DDS
Associate Lecturer, Faculty of Medical Sciences, University of the West Indies;
Consultant Facio-Maxillary Surgeon, Department of Surgery, University Hospital of the
West Indies, Mona, Kingston, Jamaica

HARRY DYM, DDS
Chairman of Department of Dentistry/Oral and Maxillofacial Surgery, The Brooklyn
Hospital Center, Brooklyn; Clinical Professor, Oral and Maxillofacial Surgery, Columbia
University, College of Dental Medicine, New York; Attending, Oral and Maxillofacial
Surgery, Woodhull Medical and Mental Health Center; Attending, Oral and Maxillofacial
Surgery, New York Harbor Healthcare System, The Brooklyn VA Campus, Brooklyn,
New York

MARK C. FLETCHER, DMD, MD
Private Practice, Avon; Clinical Instructor; Division of Oral and Maxillofacial Surgery,
University of Connecticut School of Dental Medicine, Farmington; Attending, Hartford
Hospital and Connecticut Children's Medical Center, Hartford, Connecticut

JAMES GREEN, DMD
Senior Resident, Department of Dentistry/Oral and Maxillofacial Surgery, The Brooklyn
Hospital, Brooklyn, New York

MARC B. HERTZ, DDS, MD
Attending, Oral & Maxillofacial Surgery, Department of Oral Surgery, Woodhull Medical
and Mental Health Center, Brooklyn; Attending, Oral & Maxillofacial Surgery, Department
of Dentistry, New York Downtown Hospital, New York; Private Practice, Brooklyn,
New York

DAVID HUANG, DDS
Department of Dentistry/Oral and Maxillofacial Surgery, The Brooklyn Hospital, Brooklyn,
New York

HOWARD ISRAEL, DDS
Professor of Clinical Surgery, Division of Oral and Maxillofacial Surgery, Weill-Cornell
Medical College, Cornell University, New York, New York

W. SCOTT JENKINS, DMD, MD
Jenkins and Morrow, PLLC, Lexington, Kentucky

AMANDIP KAMOH, DDS
Chief Resident, Oral and Maxillofacial Surgery, Woodhull Medical & Mental Health Center,
Brooklyn; Oral and Maxillofacial Surgery, Buffalo, New York

STUART E. LIEBLICH, DMD
Associate Clinical Professor, Oral and Maxillofacial Surgery, University of Connecticut
Health Center, Farmington; Private Practice, Avon Oral and Maxillofacial Surgery, Avon,
Connecticut

GHAZAL MAHJOUBI, DMD
Departments of Dentistry and Oral and Maxillofacial Surgery, Woodhull Medical and
Mental Health Center, Brooklyn, New York

ANIKA D. MITCHELL, BBMedSci, MBBS
Junior Resident, Faculty of Medical Sciences, University of the West Indies; Medical
Officer, Department of Surgery, University Hospital of the West Indies, Mona, Kingston,
Jamaica

LEVON NIKOYAN, DDS
Resident, Department of Oral and Maxillofacial Surgery, Woodhull Medical and Mental
Center, Brooklyn, New York

ORRETT E. OGLE, DDS
Director, Residency Training Program, Oral and Maxillofacial Surgery, Woodhull Hospital, Brooklyn; Associate Clinical Professor, Department of Oral Surgery, School of Dental Medicine, Columbia University, New York; Chief, Program Director, Oral and Maxillofacial Surgery, Department of Dentistry; Department of Oral and Maxillofacial Surgery, Woodhull Medical and Mental Health Center, Brooklyn, New York

STEPHEN PETRANKER, MD, MBA
Chief, Department of Anesthesia, Woodhull Medical and Mental Center, Brooklyn, New York

JOSEPH E. PIERSE, DMD, MA
Oral & Maxillofacial Surgery Resident, Prosthodontist, Department of Dentistry/ Oral & Maxillofacial Surgery, The Brooklyn Hospital Center, Brooklyn, New York

JOSEPH F. SPERA, DMD
Diplomate, American Board of Oral and Maxillofacial Surgeons; Fellow, American Association of Oral and Maxillofacial Surgeons; Member, American Academy of Cosmetic Surgery; Private Practice, Oral, Maxillofacial and Facial Cosmetic Surgery; Staff, Resident Training and Education, Department of Oral and Maxillofacial Surgery and Hospital Dentistry, Christiana Care Health System, Wilmington, Delaware; Department of Oral and Maxillofacial Surgery, Thomas Jefferson University Hospital, Philadelphia, Pennsylvania

AVICHAI STERN, DDS
Attending, Department of Dentistry/Oral and Maxillofacial Surgery, The Brooklyn Hospital, Brooklyn, New York

JASON SWANTEK, DDS
Chief Resident, Oral and Maxillofacial Surgery, Woodhull Medical & Mental Health Center, Brooklyn, New York; Oral and Maxillofacial Surgery, Palatine, Illinois

JONATHAN TAGLIARENI, DDS
Resident, Department of Dentistry/Oral and Maxillofacial Surgery, The Brooklyn Hospital, Brooklyn, New York

ADAM WEISS, DDS
Senior Resident, Division of Oral and Maxillofacial Surgery, The Brooklyn Hospital Center, Brooklyn, New York

JOSHUA C. WOLF, DDS
Resident, Department of Oral and Maxillofacial Surgery, The Brooklyn Hospital Center, Brooklyn, New York

Contents

Preface   **xiii**

Harry Dym and Orrett E. Ogle

Dedication   **xv**

Anxiety Control in the Dental Patient   **1**

Orrett E. Ogle and Marc B. Hertz

> Oral sedation with benzodiazepines and anxiolysis with nitrous oxide are 2 effective methods to help alleviate anxiety and fear of dental procedures. Many patients would prefer to have their dentistry performed with sedation if it were offered to them. This article presents a detailed discussion on minimal sedation that should give the reader a good understanding of this valuable aspect of clinical care.

Hemostasis in Oral Surgery   **17**

Amandip Kamoh and Jason Swantek

> The control of hemorrhage is a key component for the clinician to understand before performing oral surgical procedures. Hemostasis may be obtained primarily by local hemostatic measures. If hemostasis is not achieved with this modality, various hemostatic agents exist, which may be used as adjuncts to obtain hemostasis. Preoperative, perioperative, and postoperative methodologies toward hemostasis in oral surgery have been presented.

Oral Surgery for Patients on Anticoagulant Therapy: Current Thoughts on Patient Management   **25**

Ladi Doonquah and Anika D. Mitchell

> Minor oral surgical procedures make up a significant part of the daily practice of dentistry. With the increased sophistication of medical technology and medications there is increased likelihood of performing surgery on patients who are being treated for conditions that require some type of anticoagulant therapy. These patients are at an increased risk for perioperative bleeding or thrombotic complications if anticoagulation is discontinued or the dosage is adjusted. Therefore, a fine balance needs to be obtained and adequate preparation of these patients is the key to establishing this balance. This article reviews suggested approaches to the management of such patients.

Biopsy Techniques and Diagnoses & Treatment of Mucocutaneous Lesions   **43**

Michael H. Chan and Joshua C. Wolf

> Oral mucosal lesions are commonly encountered in clinical practice. One study reported that they occurred in approximately 27.9% of patients aged 17 years and older and in 10.3% of children aged 2 to 17 years. The diagnosis and treatment of mucosal diseases should be an integral part of the general practitioner's practice. According to an American Dental

Association survey conducted in 2007, 44% of biopsies were performed by a general practictioner. Understanding of the fundamentals of diagnosing mucocutaneous lesions requires a sound knowledge of their origin and clinical course, and of biopsy methods using contemporary diagnostic tools and techniques.

Diagnosis and Management of Common Postextraction Complications   75

Joseph E. Pierse, Harry Dym, and Earl Clarkson

Extraction of impacted teeth is one of the most common surgical procedures performed by oral and maxillofacial surgeons. Every surgical procedure results in some degree of postoperative bleeding and inflammation, typically manifesting as pain and edema. Although the complex physiology of the human body is beyond the scope of this article, the educated clinician should have an understanding of the time line associated with these processes so as to determine whether a patient's complaint of postoperative bleeding, pain, or swelling represents a normal response to surgical trauma or an aberrant reaction.

Management of Acute Postoperative Pain after Oral Surgery   95

Mark C. Fletcher and Joseph F. Spera

This article provides a brief review of the acute pain mechanism as it relates to the effects of a surgical insult. A brief understanding of the physiologic modulation of acute pain establishes a rational framework for the concept of preemptive and postoperative analgesia. A brief review of commonly used analgesic agents is presented. Research in pain management and new drug development is ongoing as new concepts in neurophysiology and pharmacology are being elucidated.

Risk Management in the Dental Office   113

Harry Dym

This article is devoted to risk-management strategies regarding oral surgical procedures in the general dental office. Lawsuits are more likely to be filed following poor outcomes related to oral surgical procedures rather than after operative or prosthetic dental procedures. The article is not meant to discourage practitioners from performing oral surgical procedures if they have the experience, training, and appropriate skill set to complete the planned procedure. Rather, it advises clinicians as to the steps one can take to limit the chances of litigation from occurring, and avoid the emotionally and painful time-consuming process associated with a malpractice lawsuit.

Endodontic Surgery   121

Stuart E. Lieblich

Conventional endodontic therapy is successful approximately 80–85% of the time. Many of these failures will occur after one year. The presence of continued pain, drainage, mobility or an increasing size of a radiolucent area are some of the indications to treat the case surgically. Since many of these cases may have had final restorations placed by the dentist, the salvage of these cases is of importance to the patient. Advances in periapical surgery have included the use of ultrasonic root end preparation. With the use of these piezoelectric devices, a more controlled apical preparation can be achieved. Additionally, isthmus areas between canals can be appropriately prepared and sealed. The precision afforded with these devices reduces the chances for a malpositioned fill and a more successful outcome.

Local Anesthesia: Agents, Techniques, and Complications   133

Orrett E. Ogle and Ghazal Mahjoubi

This article outlines the different classes of local anesthetics available for dental procedures. It also gives an overview of the mechanism of action and metabolism of each different class of local anesthetic. Furthermore, it discusses indications and contraindications of each local anesthetic and the proper dosage of each. The techniques for the administration of local anesthetics with the relevant anatomy are explained. An overview is given of the possible complications that can occur because of local anesthetic use and their possible treatment options.

Diagnosis and Treatment of Temporomandibular Disorders   149

Harry Dym and Howard Israel

Current concepts and recommended treatment for temporomandibular disorders (TMDs) and temporomandibular joint pain and dysfunction have evolved over time. This article attempts to distill the current information for this often confusing topic into relevant clinical issues that will allow the general dental practitioner to be better able to diagnose and interpret clinical findings, and institute a therapeutic regimen that will provide needed relief to patients suffering from TMD dysfunction. Current management methods, both surgical and nonsurgical, are reviewed and discussed.

Preoperative Evaluation of the Surgical Patient   163

Stephen Petranker, Levon Nikoyan, and Orrett E. Ogle

A thorough preoperative evaluation to identify correctable medical abnormalities and understand the residual risk is mandatory for all patients undergoing any surgical procedure, including oral surgery. Routine preoperative evaluation will vary among patients, depending on age and general health. This article addresses the preoperative evaluation of surgical patients in general, and the evaluation for general anesthesia in the operating room.

Pediatric Dentoalveolar Surgery   183

Sean W. Digman and Shelly Abramowicz

Dentoalveolar surgery in children presents general dentists with unique challenges not encountered in adults. The long-term effects that treatments have on these children must always be taken into consideration. A clear understanding of the growth and development of pediatric patients is necessary to correctly identify dental abnormalities.

Alveolar Bone Grafting and Reconstruction Procedures Prior to Implant Placement   209

Harry Dym, David Huang, and Avichai Stern

Before implant placement, adequate bone must be present; this is a fundamental step in treatment planning for implants. Understanding the basics of bone grafting and reconstruction techniques is critical for successful implant placement. Alveolar bone grafting can be very intimidating when first attempted. With careful instruction, education, and practice, grafting can be accomplished by many practitioners. Different methods incorporate similar surgical principles while leading to the development of more advanced grafting techniques.

Sinus Lift Procedures: An Overview of Current Techniques   219

Avichai Stern and James Green

For more than 30 years the maxillary sinus augmentation graft has been a mainstay of implant-directed maxillary reconstruction. The purpose of this article is to review the fundamentals of maxillary sinus reconstruction including anatomy and physiology of the sinus, indications for surgery, preoperative evaluation, surgical techniques, and management of complications. While there are some relative contraindications for the procedure, there are almost no absolute contraindications. With preparation, education, and experience, the maxillary sinus augmentation/elevation graft is a procedure that greatly benefits the patient, with a predictable outcome.

Review of Antibiotics and Indications for Prophylaxis   235

Adam Weiss and Harry Dym

Antibiotic prophylaxis to prevent infective endocarditis has been controversial through the years, with various changes made to recommendations provided to treating physicians and dentists. The dentist must always use his or her best judgment when applying any guideline. However, it is important to remember that the guidelines may be cited in any malpractice litigation as evidence of the standard of care. Early diagnosis with prompt treatment with effective antimicrobial therapy is the best way to lower the mortality and morbidity. When prescribing antibiotics, the clinician must realize that the overprescription of antibiotics has led to resistance to antibiotic regimens and the rise of antibiotic-resistant bacteria.

Exodontia: Tips and Techniques for Better Outcomes   245

Harry Dym and Adam Weiss

This article reviews and highlights exodontia tips as well as new techniques to make simple and complex exodontia more predictable and efficient with improved patient outcomes. A discussion of a powered periotome that has been developed to aid in the atraumatic extraction of teeth and another new device, the piezosurgery, increasingly used for outpatient oral surgery procedures are included. Physics forceps, a new type of exodontia forceps, is also discussed in this article.

Surgical Management of Cosmetic Mucogingival Defects   267

Harry Dym and Jonathan M. Tagliareni

Mucogingival conditions are deviations from the normal anatomic relationship between the gingival margin and the mucogingival junction. Mucogingival surgery is plastic surgery designed to correct defects in the gingiva surrounding the teeth. Common mucogingival conditions are recession, absence, or reduction of keratinized tissue, and probing depths extending beyond the mucogingival junction. Surgical techniques used to augment cosmetic mucogingival defects include the free gingival autograft, the subepithelial connective tissue graft, rotational flaps, lateral sliding flaps, coronally repositioned flaps, and the use of acellular dermal matrix grafts.

Suturing Principles for the Dentoalveolar Surgeon   281

M. Todd Brandt and W. Scott Jenkins

Dentists should be aware of the characteristics of suture material, and the technique used should provide effectiveness and ease. Dentists who routinely perform dentoalveolar surgery should have at least 1 type of absorbable and 1 type of nonabsorbable suture readily available within their operatory supply. This article focuses on the physical properties of suture materials and their tissue reactivity, and it reviews various suturing techniques used in contemporary dentoalveolar surgery. Familiarity with the concepts presented in this article, and continuous practice of the surgical skills presented, enhances surgical acumen and allows for improved healing, increased postoperative comfort, and successful surgery.

Index   305

FORTHCOMING ISSUES

April 2012
Sleep Medicine and Dentistry
Ron Attanasio, DDS, and
Dennis R. Bailey, DDS,
Guest Editors

July 2012
Regenerative Endodontics
Sami Chogle, DDS,
Guest Editor

October 2012
Primary Care and Dentistry
Ira B. Lamster, DDS, MMSc,
Guest Editor

RECENT ISSUES

October 2011
Dental Implants
Ole T. Jensen, DDS, MS, *Guest Editor*

July 2011
**Technological Advances in Dentistry
and Oral Surgery**
Harry Dym, DDS, and
Orrett E. Ogle, DDS,
Guest Editors

April 2011
**Esthetic and Cosmetic Dentistry for Modern
Dental Practice: Update 2011**
John R. Calamia, DMD,
Richard D. Trushkowsky, DDS, and
Mark S. Wolff, DDS, PhD, *Guest Editors*

RELATED INTEREST

Oral and Maxillofacial Surgery Clinics of North America,
August 2011 (Vol. 23, No. 3)
Complications in Dentoalveolar Surgery
Dennis-Duke R. Yamashita, DDS, and James P. McAndrews, DDS, *Guest Editors*

THE CLINICS ARE NOW AVAILABLE ONLINE!

Access your subscription at:
www.theclinics.com

Preface

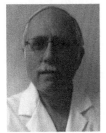 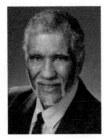

Harry Dym, DDS   Orrett E. Ogle, DDS
Guest Editors

An increased percentage of dental school graduates are now pursuing a one- or two-year program of study in a general dentistry hospital residency training program. This is often due to strictly personal desires to increase their level of experience or in many cases because of state regulations (New York State) required for state licensure; this additional training coupled with economic realities has had an impact on how they view their scope of practice and their role as health care community providers. General dentists in America now rightfully view themselves as the primary oral health care practitioner, similar to the family physician, and, as such, feel that, based on their education and training, can and should be able to provide a high level of patient care in multiple areas. Gone are the days when general dentists only drilled, filled, and billed, leaving other areas of practice, such as oral surgery, endodontics, periodontics, etc, for the local specialist.

In this issue of *Dental Clinics of North America*, edited and written by Harry Dym and Orrett Ogle, we hope to bring many of the latest techniques and philosophies relating to oral medicine and oral surgical procedures in a lucid and clear fashion to the general dentist community. It is our firm belief that only through continued and ongoing comprehensive education can our profession grow and continue to be held in high regard by both the public and our medical colleagues. We trust that all practitioners will realize their own level of abilities and seek oral and maxillofacial surgical consultation when they feel the case is more complex and beyond their comfort zone.

We have written an issue dedicated to a variety of areas in oral surgery that we feel there is a clinical need and public demand for. This volume covers multiple areas in oral surgery from complex exodontia to oral medicine, and regenerative bone procedures, to a discussion of new insights in the treatment of temoporomandibular disorders. The editors are in agreement that our invited authors have all contributed excellent work, worthy of this prestigious series; we are certain this volume will prove useful to all clinically active dentists.

Once again I (Harry Dym) am privileged to be joined by my dear colleague of over three decades, Orrett Ogle, in this joint venture. I continue to marvel at his surgical ability, his love for resident education, and his level of human caring and concern. This issue has also been predominantly a joint venture between two hospital teaching programs—The Brooklyn Hospital Center and the Woodhull Medical Center. We have

Dent Clin N Am 56 (2012) xiii–xiv
doi:10.1016/j.cden.2011.10.001
0011-8532/12/$ – see front matter

been involved with both institutions and their residency training programs for about thirty years and continue to grow in our own level of experience as a result.

The authors would like to thank Elsevier and our editor, Don Mumford, for their contribution to dental education. We feel strongly that this series, *Dental Clinics of North America*, plays a vital role in the timely dissemination of topical and current dental/medical information to the dental and oral surgical community.

We would be remiss if we did not take this time to acknowledge people who have played and continue to play meaningful roles in our professional and personal lives and without whom our lives would be diminished:

1. Peter M. Sherman, DDS, Chairman of Dentistry and Oral Surgery at the Woodhull Medical Center.
2. Richard Becker, MD, CEO and President of The Brooklyn Hospital Center.
3. Earl Clarkson, DDS, Director of Oral and Maxillofacial Surgery at The Brooklyn Hospital Center and Senior Attending at Woodhull Medical Center.
4. Gary Stephens, MD, Chief Medical Officer of The Brooklyn Hospital Center.
5. Paul Albertson, Executive Vice-President and Chief Operating Officer of The Brooklyn Hospital Center.
6. Benson Yeh, MD, Vice-President Academic Affairs and Designated Institutional Officer of The Brooklyn Hospital Center.
7. Carlos Naudon, Chairman of the Board of Trustees of The Brooklyn Hospital Center.
8. Joe Guaracino, Chief Financial Officer of The Brooklyn Hospital Center.
9. George Harris and The Lucious N. Littauer Foundation.
10. Freidy Dym, my wife and best friend of thirty-three years, who has supported my academic pursuits with gusto and love (Harry Dym).
11. Yehoshua, Hindy, Daniel, Akiva, Noah, Malka, Shoshana, Shira—my children and grandchildren, who make it all worthwhile (Harry Dym).
12. Stanley Bodner, PhD, a clinical psychologist, scholar, and true friend for decades, possessed of great insight into the human condition (Harry Dym).
13. Rabbi Isaac Sadowsky, a man possessed of great spirituality and humility, who has been a teacher and mentor to me for 15 years (Harry Dym).
14. Finally to my administrative staff Felipe DeJesus, Gloria Stallings, and Jennifer Nimako for doing a thousand things and helping my residency training programs run efficiently (Harry Dym).

Harry Dym, DDS
Department of Dentistry/Oral and Maxillofacial Surgery
The Brooklyn Hospital Center
121 DeKalb Avenue
Brooklyn, NY 11201, USA

Orrett E. Ogle, DDS
Oral and Maxillofacial Surgery, Department of Dentistry
Woodhull Medical and Mental Health Center
760 Broadway
Brooklyn, NY 11206, USA

E-mail addresses:
hdymdds@yahoo.com (H. Dym)
Orrett.Ogle@WoodhullHC.NYCHHC.org (O.E. Ogle)

Dedication

Dr Harry Dym wishes to dedicate this volume to his father-in-law, Solomon Rosner. Although Rosner passed away a few short years ago, his outstanding qualities, which he imbued into his entire family, are still very much alive and vibrant. His passion for life, his respect of honor and education, and his devotion to family and friends remain his everlasting legacy and his inheritance.

Dent Clin N Am 56 (2012) xv
doi:10.1016/j.cden.2011.10.002
0011-8532/12/$ – see front matter © 2012 Elsevier Inc. All rights reserved.

Anxiety Control in the Dental Patient

Orrett E. Ogle, DDS[a],*, Marc B. Hertz, DDS, MD[b,c,d]

KEYWORDS

- Oral sedation • Nitrous oxide • Oral benzodiazepines
- Triazolam • Halcion • Anxiolysis

It is estimated that as many as 75% of adults in the United States experience some degree of dental fear ranging from mild to severe[1] and that approximately 5% to 10% are so fearful of dental treatment that they avoid any dental care.[2] Most of these 5% to 10% seek dental care only when they have severe pain or swelling that may result in invasive interventions. This situation often leads to a cruel cycle in which their avoidance causes them to need extensively invasive procedures, which further reinforces their fear of dentistry.

In a European (Netherlands) study to estimate the point prevalence of dental fear and dental phobia relative to 10 other common fears, the prevalence of dental fear ranked fourth, at 24.3%, which was lower than fear of snakes (34.8%), heights (30.8%), and physical injuries (27.2%). Among phobias, dental phobia was the most common (3.7%), followed by height phobia (3.1%) and spider phobia (2.7%).[3] The American Dental Association (ADA) estimated that 35 to 50 million adults have so much anxiety about dental visits that they worry, postpone, or avoid seeing their dentist.

The fear of dentistry is real, profound, and difficult to overcome. Sedation offers a method of alleviating the fear, and for some it is the only way they will have their dental needs treated. From a national telephone survey it was estimated that almost 23 million people would be willing to go to the dentist more frequently if general anesthesia and conscious sedation were more readily available.[4] The more invasive the procedure (such as oral surgery or endodontics), the more fearful people are. The anticipated invasiveness of the procedure dramatically increases the demand for

The authors have nothing to disclose.

[a] Oral and Maxillofacial Surgery, Department of Dentistry, Woodhull Medical and Mental Health Center, 760 Broadway, Brooklyn, NY 11206, USA
[b] Department of Oral Surgery, Woodhull Medical and Mental Health Center, 760 Broadway, Brooklyn, NY 11206, USA
[c] Department of Dentistry, New York Downtown Hospital, 170 William Street, New York, NY 10038, USA
[d] Private Practice, 2026 Ocean Avenue, Brooklyn, NY 11230, USA
* Corresponding author.
E-mail address: orrett.ogle@woodhullhc.nychhc.org

anesthesia or sedation services, with preference rising from 2% for a routine dental cleaning to 47% for a tooth extraction, 55% for an endodontic procedure, and 68% for periodontal surgery.[5] The evidence therefore indicates that there is both a need and a demand for sedation services in general dental practice. This article addresses sedation methods in dentistry using inhalation (nitrous oxide [N_2O], sometimes referred to as relative analgesia) and oral sedation. Intravenous (IV) sedation, which must meet the standards for general anesthesia, is not covered because most general dentists usually do not have the necessary advanced training in IV sedation.

Sedation is used for the reduction of anxiety, irritability, or agitation by the administration of sedative drugs to facilitate the planned dental procedure. The purpose is to allow the dentist to work more effectively and to help the patient become as relaxed and comfortable as possible. The American Society of Anesthesiologists defines the continuum of sedation as follows[6]:

- Minimal sedation: normal response to verbal stimuli
- Moderate sedation: purposeful response to verbal/tactile stimulation (this is usually referred to as conscious sedation)
- Deep sedation: purposeful response to repeated or painful stimulation
- General anesthesia: unarousable even with painful stimulus.

Sedation as used in this article is minimal sedation, a minimally depressed level of consciousness produced by a pharmacologic method that retains the patient's ability to independently and continually maintain an airway and respond normally to tactile stimulation and verbal command. Although cognitive function and coordination may be modestly impaired, ventilatory and cardiovascular functions are unaffected.

STATE LAWS

Most US states require some combination of formal training and standard-of-care equipment plus a permit issued by the state dental board before dentists can provide sedation to their patients. Some states also have different permits for different levels of sedation. Most of the states have linked their requirements to the recommendations of the ADA's anesthesia and sedation guidelines,[7] which recommend special training for minimal and moderate sedation ranging from 16 hours (minimal sedation) to 24 hours (moderate oral sedation) to 60 hours (IV moderate sedation) of didactic classroom instruction.[8] The ADA guidelines also require that dentists observe or document a certain number of clinical patient experiences or cases depending on the route of administration used to achieve sedation.[8] **Table 1** lists the educational requirements for all 50 states and the District of Columbia.

The use of N_2O is not as regulated nor are there clearly established educational requirements as there are with oral and IV sedation. The ADA guidelines mentioned earlier do not apply if the intent is to provide only anxiolysis (a lightly altered mood in which there is a decrease or elimination of anxiety), in which the N_2O is carefully titrated to induce anxiolysis rather than sedation. Many states do not clearly address the issue or they adopt the ADA's policy on anxiolysis. It seems that most states permit the unregulated use of N_2O by licensed dentists, even although some states may require a permit.

Most states do not have separate requirements for pediatric and adult patients. In addition, the American Academy of Pediatric Dentistry's guidelines say nothing about the educational requirements necessary before dentists can provide anesthesia to their pediatric patients. The Georgia State Board of Dentistry is changing its sedation rules; in Georgia 120 hours of training would be required before anyone who is not a pediatric dentist could sedate a child.[9]

Oral sedation weekend courses do not give one adequate training to sedate children; you need to be formally trained.

PREOPERATIVE EVALUATION

The preoperative evaluation is an important interaction between the dentist and the patient. This process allows the dentist to carefully evaluate the patient's overall health status, determine risk factors for sedation, educate the patient, and discuss the procedure in detail. Most general dental procedures are uncomplicated, and extensive patient evaluation is unnecessary. However, of utmost importance is a detailed medical history. The aim of the history is to identify issues that demand attention and caution. Items that must be addressed are:

1. Abnormalities of the major organ systems: cardiovascular, pulmonary, renal, hepatic, and endocrine (**Table 2**)
2. Drug allergies, latex allergy, current medications, and potential drug interactions
3. History of stroke or transient ischemic attack (TIA) (certain oral sedation methods may trigger a TIA)
4. Neuromuscular disorders (such as muscular dystrophy)
5. History of tobacco, alcohol, or substance use or abuse
6. Pregnancy
7. Previous adverse experience with sedation/analgesia as well as general anesthesia.

Based on the medical history the patient can then be stratified using the classification of the American Society of Anesthesiology (ASA) (**Box 1**).

Only ASA 1 and ASA 2 patients are acceptable for sedation.

MONITORING

Patients receiving oral sedation must be monitored before, during, and after their procedure. The monitoring must be continuous during the dental procedure and up to the time of discharge. During the procedure, monitoring detects early signs of patient distress such as alterations in oxygenation, pulse, and blood pressure. Hospital-type monitoring equipment is not necessary but continuous monitoring of pulse oximetry, heart rate, and blood pressure is mandatory. A pulse oximeter measures oxygen saturation and enhances the assessment of respiratory status while the individual is sedated. The most common and the most serious adverse outcome of conscious sedation is respiratory compromise and its related consequences. It is therefore imperative that special attention be paid to the airway. Any decrease in the pulse oximetry less than 96% should be addressed immediately. True desaturation is defined as a pulse oximeter reading of SpO_2 less than 95% while the patient is quiet and still. However, with oral sedation apnea is rarely seen with normal dosing in the absence of airway obstruction. When it does occur, it is easily managed with stimulation, positive pressure ventilation, and supplemental oxygen administration.

Oral sedation is intended to produce only a minimally depressed level of consciousness, and this level of consciousness must be monitored continuously. Responses to verbal commands during the procedure serve as the guide to the patient's level of consciousness. An appropriate level of consciousness implies that the patient can control their own airway and take deep breaths as necessary. After administration

Table 1
Educational requirements for administration of sedation

States	Educational Regulations
Alabama, Oregon	16 h of instructive classroom training and obtain a permit
Alaska; Connecticut; DC; Hawaii; Illinois; Indiana; Kentucky; Minnesota; Nebraska; Oklahoma; Utah	Board of Dental Examiners does not currently require formal training before providing oral conscious sedation to dental patients; any licensed dentist can administer oral sedation
Arkansas; Georgia; Massachusetts.	24 h of instructive classroom training with 10 clinical patient experiences, and obtain a permit; advanced cardiac life support (ACLS) certification is also required
Arizona	30 h of instructive classroom training with 5 clinical patient experiences and obtain a permit
California	General practice, pediatric, or periodontal residency; or 25-hour board-approved course with 1 live adult patient; for a pediatric permit: 1 live pediatric patient experience is required
Colorado	16 h of instructive classroom training in the administration of minimal sedation techniques and must include management of complications and emergencies; no state permit
Delaware; Florida; Iowa; Michigan[a]; Nevada; South Dakota; Vermont; Wyoming	60-hour IV sedation course, administer 20 clinical patient cases, and obtain a permit before providing oral or IV conscious sedation
Idaho; West Virginia	18 h of instructive classroom training with 20 clinical patient experiences, and obtain a permit. ACLS certification is also required
Kansas; New Mexico; New York; Virginia; Wisconsin	18 h of instructive classroom training, observe 20 clinical patient experiences, and obtain a permit
Louisiana	16 h of instructive classroom training, a component on handling emergencies, and obtain a permit. ACLS certification is required

State	Requirements
Maine; New Hampshire; North Carolina[b]	24 h of instructive classroom training, document 3 live patient experiences, and obtain a permit. ACLS certification is also required
Maryland; Tennessee	24 h of instructive classroom training with 20 clinical patient experiences, and obtain a permit. ACLS certification is also required
Mississippi	22 h of instructive classroom training with 15 clinical patient experiences, and obtain a permit. ACLS certification is required
Missouri	A comprehensive training program in oral conscious sedation; at least 15 additional hours of continuing education pertaining to medical emergencies, anesthesia complications, and patient management; ACLS can be substituted for the 15 additional hours but is not required
Montana	40-hour IV sedation course, administer 20 clinical patient cases, and obtain a permit
New Jersey	40 h of university-based didactic training and obtain a permit
South Carolina	18 h of instructive classroom training with 20 clinical patient experiences; adult patients only; state permit not required
Texas	2-d university-based training course and obtain a permit
Washington	14–21 h of instructive classroom; no state permit needed

[a] Permit not required in Michigan.
[b] Except in North Carolina.

Table 2
Selected medical conditions and implications for ASA 1 and ASA 2 patients

Medical Condition	Considerations
Diabetes mellitus	The patient's blood glucose level should be controlled, and insulin doses should be adjusted as needed
Hypertension	Adequate anxiolysis or sedation and good local anesthesia are important in alleviating unwanted stress and anxiety, which could increase the intraprocedure blood pressure
Hepatitis	Sedatives, lidocaine, and amide-linked local anesthetics should be used with caution
Sleep apnea	Ancillary oxygen should be used via a nasal prong. Conscious sedation may exacerbate sleep apnea
CVA	Monitoring the blood pressure is essential, and if it increases significantly the procedure must be terminated
Hyperthyroidism	May increase cardiac sensitivity to epinephrine
Ischemic coronary artery disease or stable angina	May need sublingual nitroglycerin, which should be readily available
Psychiatric disorders	Check medications and avoid drug interactions or oversedation

Oral sedation is safe and for ASA 1 or 2 patients there are not many cautions. Cautions include psychosis, impaired lung, kidney or liver function, and advanced age. Age by itself is not a factor, but the presence of comorbid conditions must be determined. Heart disease is generally not a contraindication but patients should not have any functional limitations and must be ASA 1 or 2.

of the sedative medication, response of the patient to verbal commands may be delayed, and responses are frequently slowed or slurred. At times, light tactile stimulation may be required to get the patient's attention. However, once aroused the patient should respond appropriately to verbal commands. Level of consciousness should be assessed every 15 minutes.

ORAL SEDATION: AGENTS AND TECHNIQUES

For adult and teenage patients the agents used most frequently for oral sedation are triazolam (Halcion) and diazepam (Valium). For any effect to take place, these drugs must be absorbed into the blood stream and delivered to the site of action, usually believed to be in the central nervous system, in sufficient quantities to be effective. The time from ingestion to sedation is therefore important.

Triazolam (marketed under the name Halcion) is a benzodiazepine derivative drug that is primarily only used as a sedative. In addition to its hypnotic properties triazolam also possesses, anterograde amnesia, anxiolytic, sedative, and anticonvulsant properties. Because of its fast onset of action and short half-life (approximately 2–4 hours) it has become a useful agent for oral sedation in dentistry.

Box 1
ASA physical classification

- Class 1: normal healthy patient
- Class 2: a patient with a systemic disease that is well controlled and with no functional limitations
- Class 3: a patient with a systemic disease that is not well controlled, or having more than 1 systemic disease, or with some function limitation
- Class 4: a patient with severe systemic disease that is a threat to life and functionally incapacitating
- Class 5: a moribund patient who is not expected to survive 24 hours with or without surgery
- Class 6: a brain-dead patient whose organs are being harvested

---

Drug Facts

The main pharmacologic effects of triazolam are the enhancement of the neurotransmitter γ-aminobutyric acid (GABA) at the $GABA_A$ receptor. It is lipophilic and is metabolized in the liver via microsomal oxidation or glucuronidation pathways and does not generate active metabolites. It has little effect on the circulatory or respiratory system, and several studies have shown no changes in blood pressure, pulse, or percentage of oxygen saturation and only a slight change in respiratory rate.

Triazolam belongs to the pregnancy category X of the US Food and Drug Administration (FDA). This categorization means that it is known to have the potential to cause birth defects. Common side effects include coordination problems, dizziness, drowsiness, headache, light-headedness, nausea/vomiting, and nervousness. However, reports of adverse drug reactions are rare, and tend to be mild.

Contraindications

There are a few absolute contraindications to the use of triazolam; the main contraindications are hypersensitive to triazolam or other benzodiazepine drugs, patients with myasthenia gravis, patients with glaucoma, pregnant women, lactating mothers, and psychiatric patients.

Office protocol

- No alcohol or other sedatives should be consumed for 24 hours before the appointment.
- There should be no chance of young women being pregnant.
- The patient must have an adult escort to take them home after the appointment.
- They cannot drive, operate machinery, or undertake any activity that could be hazardous.
- No alcohol or other sedatives should be taken for 24 hours after the appointment.
- Use the nil-by-mouth guidelines listed in **Table 3**.
- The patient comes to the office 1 hour before the start of their dental procedure.
- Dosages range from 0.125 mg to 0.5 mg is administered (usually 0.25 mg).
- Have the patient observed by a trained staff member with instructions to alert the dentist if there are any problems or if the patient is snoring.
- If there is no sedation evident after 30 minutes, administer half the original dose.
- If even slight sedation is noted at 30 minutes, the patient has adequate sedation for the procedure. As the patient becomes drowsy, they should be casually walked to the treatment area. 75% of patients have amnesia from this point

Table 3
NPO guidelines for the typical dental office patients (babies are not included)

Ingested Material	Minimum Fasting Time (h)
Regular meal[a]	8–10 h
Light meal[b]	6 h
Clear liquids[c]	2 h
Nonhuman milk[d]	6–8 h

[a] Meals that include fried or fatty foods or meat. Both the amount and type of foods ingested must be considered when determining an appropriate fasting period.
[b] A light meal typically consists of toast and clear liquids.
[c] Examples of clear liquids include water, fruit juices without pulp, carbonated beverages, clear tea, and black coffee.
[d] Nonhuman milk is considered solid in terms of gastric emptying time. The amount ingested must be considered when determining an appropriate fasting period.

that lasts for 2 to 3 hours. It is common to this technique that the level of sedation may not seem adequate, but there is sufficient amnesia to allow them to forget most if not all of the appointment.

- If N₂O-oxygen is to be used, it should be titrated to effect via a scavenged nasal hood system.
- Place blood pressure cuff and pulse oximetry probe.
- Administer local anesthesia slowly with a small-gauge needle at about 1 hour after administration of the initial sedative drug and wait for it to become effective.
- If a patient snores they may be oversedated and should be aroused by verbal commands or a gentle nudge.
- Try to limit the dental procedure to 1 hour.
- Keep the patient in the dental office until they are able to walk with a stable gait unassisted; have an adult take the patient home.

Diazepam (sold under the trade name Valium), like triazolam, belongs to the benzodiazepine family and is a long-acting classic benzodiazepine. It is often considered the prototypical benzodiazepine and the grandfather of the drug class. As a rule of thumb, in higher doses diazepam acts as a sedative and may promote sleep, whereas in lower doses, it simply reduces anxiety without sedation. Diazepam possesses anxiolytic, anticonvulsant, sedative, hypnotic, skeletal muscle relaxant, and amnestic properties. It can be used in dentistry to reduce tension and anxiety and induce retrograde amnesia.

The pharmacologic action of diazepam enhances the effect of the neurotransmitter GABA by binding to the benzodiazepine site on the GABA_A receptor, leading to central nervous system depression. The GABA_A receptor is an inhibitory channel that, when activated, decreases neuronal activity and causes inhibitory processes in the cerebral cortex that have anxiolytic effects. When diazepam is administered orally, it is rapidly absorbed and has a fast onset of action (usually within 20–40 minutes). The bioavailability after oral administration is 100%, and peak plasma levels occur between 30 minutes and 90 minutes after administration. It undergoes oxidative metabolism by demethylation and hydroxylation as well as glucuronidation in the liver as part of the cytochrome P450 enzyme system. Diazepam has several pharmacologically active metabolites. The main active metabolite of diazepam is desmethyldiazepam (also known as nordazepam or nordiazepam). Other minor active metabolites are temazepam and oxazapam. Because of these active metabolites, diazepam has a biphasic half-life of about 1 to 3 days and 2 to 7 days for the active metabolite desmethyldiazepam,[10] which may result in prolonged action, causing daytime drowsiness and hangover for up to 48 hours. Advantages of diazepam are a rapid onset of action and high efficacy rates, and like most benzodiazepines it also has a low toxicity in overdose. Diazepam by itself is safe, even in large doses.[11]

Contraindications

Use of diazepam should be avoided in individuals with the following conditions: ataxia, acute narrow-angle glaucoma, severe liver deficiencies, severe sleep apnea, myasthenia gravis, and anyone with hypersensitivity or allergy to any drug in the benzodiazepine class.

Office protocol
Same as outlined earlier.

- Dosages range from 5 mg to 10 mg (usually 5 mg, but 10 mg would also be acceptable for well-built men).
- Because of its long half-life (80 hours) the dosage should not be repeated.

EMERGENCY AND REVERSAL

As a group, benzodiazepines are the safest and most effective sedatives. Need for reversal has never been reported with standard oral doses of benzodiazepines in adults. The most common signs of overdosage are drowsiness, confusion, hallucination, and reduced reflexes. There are minimal effects on respiration, pulse, and blood pressure unless the overdosage is extreme.

Management

Keep patient stimulated, decrease lighting if confused, and start IV. Stimulation should be the major component of managing the overdose.

- Flumazenil (Romazacon) 0.2 mg IV as initial dose; repeat 0.2 mg every 1-minute interval to a maximum of 1 mg.
- A single intraoral injection of flumazenil (0.2 mg) cannot immediately reverse oversedation with triazolam. A larger dose might be effective.[12,13] There may be incomplete reversal by a single intraoral injection of flumazenil and the reversal may not persist. As a competitive receptor antagonist, flumazenil binds to the same site as the agonist triazolam. Although the clinical duration of triazolam administered as a single dose is comparable with that of flumazenil, research has shown that incremental dosing of this short-acting benzodiazepine results in long-lasting sedation that is dose-dependent[13] and is not reversed with a single dose of flumazenil.
- Caffeine: 5 to 7 mg/kg for maximal effect. 50 to 100 mg produces a temporary increase in mental clarity and energy level and reduces drowsiness. Sources of caffeine are brewed coffee (a 6-oz [177-mL] cup is about 150 mg); Caffedrine capsules and NoDoz tablets (100 mg each); and Dexatrim and other diet pills have about 200 mg of caffeine in each pill.
- Give methylphenidate (Ritalin) 10 mg immediate-release tablet in severe somnolence. Repeat in 30 minutes if somnolence is prolonged. However, this strategy may increase hallucinations, precipitating Tourette-type syndrome. The half-life of Ritalin is 2 to 4 hours.

Aside from overdosage, emergencies occurring during sedation almost always involve airway or respiratory compromise. An Ambu bag should always be available for assisting breathing, or some other device to administer positive pressure. The deeper the sedation, the higher the risk. The most common cause of airway obstruction is occlusion of the posterior oropharynx with the tongue. Simply lifting the chin to extend the head, stimulating the patient and telling them to breath most often resolves this issue. If the patient is very somnolent then supplementary oxygen may be given via a nasal hood.

ORAL SEDATION IN CHILDREN

Only an appropriately trained and permitted dentist should administer oral sedation to children in an office setting. Sedation for children carries significant potential for adverse outcomes, and nearly all states require special training before a dentist can sedate a child. To be considered for oral sedation in the dental office setting, children should be only ASA 1 or ASA 2.

The most serious adverse outcome of pediatric conscious sedation is respiratory compromise, which can lead to hypoxemia and predispose the child to a range of deleterious conditions. Because of this possibility, it is imperative that during the medical history special attention is paid to the respiratory system. The most common acute medical condition affecting young children is the common cold (upper respiratory infection). The hypersecretion and edema associated with an upper respiratory tract infection can dramatically diminish the ability of the child to keep their airway clear, especially if they have received a sedative. In addition, N_2O -oxygen administered via a nasal hood has little effect on the child with nasal congestion. In this instance, treatment should be deferred for 2 weeks from the cessation of symptoms.[14] Apart from medical conditions, there are other issues that may not make the child a good candidate for oral sedation. The child's cooperative ability and willingness to take prescribed oral medication must be carefully assessed. Nausea and vomiting after oral intake of drug may occur and the sedation may be ineffective. To maintain safety and maximize the use of sedation time, the dentist should be able to complete the necessary dental treatment in less than 1 hour because sedation maybe effective for only 45 to 60 minutes.

Midazolam is the ideal oral sedative for children. It is twice as potent as diazepam and is water soluble, making it easy to mix with juices for oral administration. Midazolam is also available premixed with cherry syrup. Unlike diazepam, midazolam has little if any hangover effect and its short half-life allows for a full recovery before discharge.

Midazolam (Versed) is a short-acting benzodiazepine and possesses most of the properties of the other benzodiazepines. It is available as midazolam hydrochloride syrup for oral administration to pediatric patients for sedation, anxiolysis, and amnesia and is intended for use only in monitored settings. Immediate availability of resuscitative drugs and age-appropriate and size-appropriate equipment for bag/valve/mask ventilation and personnel trained in their use should be assured. The dentist who uses this medication in pediatric patients must also be aware that the response to sedative agents in each child is variable and that regardless of the intended level of sedation a patient may move easily from light to deep sedation, with potential loss of protective reflexes.

The recommended dose for pediatric patients is a single dose of 0.25 to 0.5 mg/kg, depending on the desired effect, up to a maximum dose of 20 mg. In general, it is recommended that the dose be individualized and modified based on patient age, level of pretreatment anxiety, and the level of sedation required. The younger (6 months to 6 years of age) and less cooperative patients may require a higher than usual dose up to 1 mg/kg. A dose of 0.25 mg/kg may suffice for older (6 to <16 years of age) or cooperative patients, especially if the anticipated intensity and duration of sedation are less critical,[15] Nil-by-mouth guidelines and office protocol are the same as that for triazalam (see **Table 3**).

CONTROVERSIES

1. One problem associated with oral sedation is that it is not predictable. Basically, you do not know how well the drug is absorbed from the stomach, and sedation becomes a hit-or-miss issue.
2. Although it is popular, we do not recommend the use of triazolam in children because it is more potent than either midazolam or diazepam and it has not yet been approved by the FDA for use as a sedative. When used by dentists as an oral sedative it has been used off label.
3. Titration or layered dosing of oral medication is a popular technique. However, its safety has been questioned. Many dentists with anesthesia training believe the practice to be too unpredictable and unsafe.

Oral medication can take up to 2 hours to absorb. A patient could swallow a pill, and the dentist, not seeing the effects of the drug an hour or 2 later, may deliver a second pill; meanwhile, the first pill is being absorbed and the patient has ingested twice the amount he or she needs.

N₂O ANALGESIA

N_2O has been used for anesthesia in dentistry since 1844, when Horace Wells first used it as a method of pain control on 12 to 15 dental patients in his office in Hartford, Connecticut. Today, N_2O is used as an anxiolytic (as an adjunct to local anesthetic), and when combined with oxygen it is possibly the safest sedative in dentistry. It is not subject to US Drug Enforcement Administration regulations but many states have laws regulating its sale, possession, and nonmedical use on human subjects. Most states do not have anything in their laws or regulations that would limit a dentist's use of N_2O, if the intent is not to achieve deep sedation, conscious sedation, or general anesthesia but only anxiolysis. (West Virginia requires a class 2 certificate authorizing the dentist to induce anxiolysis, and in North Dakota a permit for minimal sedation must be obtained if N_2O inhalation analgesia is to be used in combination with an enteral dosing.) Although unregulated and safe, the practitioner administering N_2O should be trained in the use of appropriate emergency response.

N_2O is a nonflammable, colorless, and virtually odorless gas with a faint, sweet smell. It is absorbed rapidly, allowing for both rapid onset and recovery (2–3 minutes). It has a minimum alveolar concentration of 105% and a blood/gas partition coefficient of 0.46. N_2O does not combine with hemoglobin, but is carried free in the blood and excreted unchanged through the lungs. It is an effective analgesic/anxiolytic agent, causing central nervous system depression and euphoria with little effect on the respiratory system.[16]

The ADA recognizes N_2O/oxygen inhalation as a safe and effective technique to reduce anxiety and produce analgesia/anxiolysis in the dental patient. N_2O has only minor anesthetic properties and must be used with a local anesthetic to suppress the pain caused by dental work. Analgesia/anxiolysis is defined as diminution or elimination of pain and anxiety in a conscious patient.[17] The patient should respond normally to verbal commands. All vital signs should be stable, there is no significant risk of losing protective reflexes, and the patient is able to return to preprocedure mobility and mental clarity.

Pharmacology

The pharmacologic mechanism of action of N_2O is not fully known. However, it has been shown to directly modulate a broad range of ligand-gated ion channels, and this likely plays a major role in many of its effects.[18] The analgesic effect of N_2O seems to be initiated by neuronal release of endogenous opioid peptides with subsequent activation of opioid receptors and descending $GABA_A$ receptors and noradrenergic pathways that modulate nociceptive processing at the spinal level. The anxiolytic effect involves activation of the $GABA_A$ receptor either directly or indirectly through the benzodiazepine binding site. N_2O may act to imitate nitric oxide in the central nervous system as well, and this may relate to its analgesic and anxiolytic properties.[19] There is evidence that the relaxation and relief from anxiety during inhalation of N_2O is a specific anxiolytic effect that is independent of the analgesic action of N_2O. The anesthetic, hallucinogenic, and euphoriant effects are likely caused predominantly or fully via inhibition of N-methyl-D-aspartate receptor-mediated currents.[18,19]

Analgesia

To achieve analgesia/anxiolysis without unconsciousness, subanesthetic concentrations of N_2O are used. N_2O is normally administered via a nasal hood as a mixture with 30% to 50% gas and 70% to 50% oxygen. The objectives of N_2O/oxygen inhalation include:

1. Reduction or elimination of anxiety
2. Reduction of untoward reaction to dental treatment
3. Raising of the pain reaction threshold
4. Increasing the tolerance for longer appointments
5. To potentiate the effect of another sedative.

Disadvantages of N_2O/oxygen inhalation may include:
1. Lack of potency and it is dependent largely on psychological reassurance.
2. The patient must be able to breathe through the nose (the efficacy of N_2O may be diminished or absent in patients experiencing a cold or some other acute respiratory condition that prevents them from breathing through their nose. Appointments for patients in this situation are best rescheduled).
3. The nasal hood interferes with injection to the anterior maxillary region.
4. There is a risk of N_2O pollution and potential occupational exposure health hazards.

N_2O is minimally metabolized in humans (with a rate of 0.004%) and retains its potency when exhaled into the room by the patient. It can therefore pose a prolonged and toxic exposure hazard to the clinic staff if the room is poorly ventilated. Long-term exposure can cause reproductive side effects, vitamin B_{12} deficiency, and numbness. When N_2O is administered, a continuous-flow fresh-air ventilation system or nitrous scavenger system must be used to prevent a waste-gas build-up. The National Institute for Occupational Safety and Health (NIOSH) recommends that workers' exposure to N_2O should be controlled during the administration of anesthetic gas in medical, dental, and veterinary operators.[20] NIOSH recommend a time-weighted average concentration of 50 ppm when N_2O is used in dental offices.[21] In an effort to reduce the occupational health hazards associated with N_2O, the American Academy of Pediatric Dentistry recommended that exposure to ambient N_2O be minimized through the use of effective scavenging systems and periodic evaluation and maintenance of the delivery and scavenging systems.[22] Scavenger systems in dental operatories are not efficient in capturing N_2O because the system is not closed and during oral dental operations gas escapes through the opened mouth. There are commercially available devices to monitor the level of N_2O in the operatory or how much an individual has been exposed to. N_2O. One such device specifically mentioned by the Labor Department is the Landauer N_2O monitor (Landauer Inc, Glenwood, IL, USA). It is a diffusion-type air-monitoring badge assembly worn in the breathing zone by personnel. However, it is not clear if this device is still available to dentists.

Indications and Patient Selection

Because of its safety, and because the gas can easily be turned off, dosage can be accurately titrated and because of the rapidity of recovery, patients with ASA 1, ASA 2, or ASA 3 would be acceptable candidates for N_2O analgesia. Patients diagnosed with cardiovascular disease benefit greatly from the use of N_2O during dental procedures. It provides anxiolysis, increases the pain threshold, and supplies a surplus of oxygen. This situation reduces the myocardial workload, avoiding myocardial ischemia, which in turn averts acute cardiovascular events. In addition, N_2O causes vasodilatation, decreasing the likelihood of a perioperative hypertensive episode.

In apprehensive patients sedation and analgesia with N_2O increases the acceptance of the local anesthesia required for dental procedures to painlessly proceed. Apprehension is diminished, perception of the injection is altered, and administration of the local anesthetic is remarkably tolerated. N_2O is especially helpful when administering local anesthesia proximal to an infected region, achieving regional anesthesia in a more pleasant and less traumatic manner. Moreover, N_2O is an invaluable tool when either administering an intrapulpal injection before extraction of a hot tooth or in the pursuit of gaining access to the pulp chamber for endodontic purposes.

Contraindications for use of N_2O/oxygen inhalation may include:
1. Some chronic obstructive pulmonary diseases patients
2. Severely emotionally disturbed or drug-related dependencies, particularly marijuana
3. First trimester of pregnancy.

Caution should be used and medical consultation probably should be requested with patients presenting with:
Severe obstructive pulmonary disease
Congestive heart failure, class 3
Sickle cell disease[23]
Acute otitis media, recent tympanic membrane graft.[24]

TECHNIQUE

1. Fasting is not required, but it is a good idea to recommend that only a light meal be consumed in the 2 hours before the administration of N_2O.
2. Record blood pressure and pulse.
3. Selection an appropriately sized nasal hood. Claustrophobic patients may find the nasal hood confining and unpleasant. Many of the available nasal hoods are sometimes too narrow for some African American patients. A larger hood may be more comfortable.
4. Turn on the gas with 100% oxygen flowing before placing the nasal hood. A flow rate of 5 to 6 L/min generally is acceptable to most patients but sometimes higher flow rates may be required. Too slow a flow rate gives the patient a feeling of suffocation. The flow rate can be adjusted after observation of the reservoir bag.

5. Allow the patient to breath the 100% oxygen for 2 to 4 minutes before turning on the N_2O. Titrate the N_2O in 10% intervals to desired level (30% or 50% nitrous). N_2O provides pain control up to 25%. After 25% it begins to produce light anesthesia. Do not exceed a 50:50 N_2O/O_2 mixture.
6. When the patient begins to feel tingling or is sedated, administer local anesthesia. The N_2O level should be kept high during the administration of local anesthesia. Once the patient is numb, the N_2O concentration can be decreased. If the individual becomes excited, then reduce the concentration of the nitrous. Some patients may feel that they are losing control and demand that the gas be turned off.
7. During treatment, the patient respiration and level of consciousness should be continually visually monitored.
8. Once the procedure is terminated, turn off the N_2O flow and allow the patient to breath 100% oxygen for 3 to 5 minutes. Because N_2O is 34 times more soluble than nitrogen in blood, diffusion hypoxia may occur.
9. The patient must return to pretreatment responsiveness before discharge.

Equipment

Modern portable N_2O inhalation sedation units provide continuous flow of N_2O that is titratable from 0% to 70%. They consist of either 2 or 4 yoked E-sized cylinders with an equal quantity of light blue N_2O and green O_2 gas cylinders on the apparatus. A full O_2 gas cylinder has a pressure of approximately 2000 psi visible on the O_2 pressure gauge, whereas a full N_2O gas cylinder reads approximately 750 psi on the N_2O pressure gauge. Nevertheless, while the N_2O is being depleted, this psi reading remains the same. The psi reading drastically decreases when close to 90% of N_2O has been exhausted. Central storage systems are commonly used in offices that administer N_2O more frequently. They have larger compressed gas cylinders (size G for N_2O and size H for O_2), which are remotely located from the operatory. In these systems, multiple treatment rooms share their source of N_2O/O_2 supply via copper piping connections that originate in the central storage area. Both systems incorporate a flow meter, a reservoir bag, an O_2 flush button, and a scavenging nasal hood. The flow meter displays the rate of flow of both gases. The reservoir bag contains spare gas that can be inhaled by the patient should additional volume for respiration be required. It can also be used to visually monitor respirations and manually assist ventilations. The function of the O_2 flush button is to deliver a high volume of 100% O_2 in emergency situations. The scavenging nasal hood is composed of 2 masks and has 4 connecting tubes entering it. One set delivers the N_2O/O_2 to the inner mask and the other two, which are exclusively within the outer mask, are connected to the vacuum system, which caries the exhaled gases away. This set-up minimizes occupational exposure to N_2O and prevents its chronic inhalation by dental personal.

Several safety features exist to prevent mishaps during use of N_2O/O_2. The pin index safety system on the yoke and cylinders precludes the wrong cylinders from being attached to the yoke. The color coding of cylinders prevents confusing 1 type of gas cylinder with another. Swapping of the low-pressure tubing is prohibited by the diameter index safety system. The O_2 fail-safe terminates the delivery of N_2O when the O_2 cylinder is nearing an empty state. In response to the activation of the O_2 fail-safe, the opening of the emergency air inlet valve permits the patient to inhale atmospheric air. In addition, there exists a specific minimum oxygen liter flow rate (usually 3.0 L/min) necessary before the flow of N_2O is allowed to commence. Likewise, there is a minimum O_2 percentage rate (30%) that must be delivered to the patient.

An emergency cart (kit) must be readily accessible. It should include equipment to resuscitate a nonbreathing, unconscious patient and provide continuous support until trained emergency personnel arrive. A positive pressure oxygen delivery system capable of administering more than 90% oxygen at a 10 L/min flow for at least 60 minutes (650 L, E cylinder) must be available. The dentist and at least 1 other staff member should be certified in basic life support.

SUMMARY

The fear of dentistry is real, profound, and is difficult to overcome. Sedation offers a method of alleviating the fear, and for some it is the only way they have their dental needs treated. Oral sedation with benzodiazepines and anxiolysis with N_2O are 2 effective methods to help alleviate anxiety and fear of dental procedures. Many patients would prefer to have their dentistry performed with sedation if it were offered to them. This article presents a detailed discussion on minimal sedation that should give the reader a good understanding of this valuable aspect of clinical care.

REFERENCES

1. Kleinknecht RA, Thorndike RM, McGlynn FD, et al. Factor analysis of the dental fear survey with cross-validation. J Am Dent Assoc 1984;108(1):59–61.
2. Gatchel RJ, Ingersoll BD, Bowman L, et al. The prevalence of dental fear and avoidance: a recent survey study. J Am Dent Assoc 1983;107(4):609–10.
3. Oosterink FM, de Jongh A, Hoogstraten J. Prevalence of dental fear and phobia relative to other fear and phobia subtypes. Eur J Oral Sci 2009;117:135–43.
4. Dionne R, Gordon S, McCullagh L, et al. Assessing the need for anesthesia and sedation in the general population. J Am Dent Assoc 1998;129(2):167–73.
5. Chanpong B, Haas DA, Locker D. Need and demand for sedation or general anesthesia in dentistry: a national survey of the Canadian population. Anesth Prog 2005;52(1):3–11.
6. Continuum of Depth of Sedation: definition of general anesthesia and levels of sedation/analgesia. Approved October 27, 2004. American Society of Anesthesiologists; October 21, 2009.
7. ADA Policy Statement: the use of sedation and general anesthesia by dentists (PDF); guidelines for the use of sedation and general anesthesia by dentists. Available at: http://www.ada.org/2946.aspx. Accessed May 2011.
8. ADA.org: guidelines for teaching pain control and sedation to dentist and dental students. Available at: www.ada.org/sections/about/pdfs/anxiety_guidelines.pdf. Accessed May 2011.
9. Available at: http://www.agd.org/publications/articles/?ArtID=7020. Accessed May 2011.
10. Riss J, Cloyd J, Gates J, et al. Benzodiazepines in epilepsy: pharmacology and pharmacokinetics. Acta Neurol Scand 2008;118(2):69–86.
11. Greenblatt DJ, Woo E, Allen MD, et al. Rapid recovery from massive diazepam overdose. JAMA 1978;240(17):1872–4.
12. Hosaka K, Jackson D, Pickrell JE, et al. Flumazenil reversal of sublingual triazolam–a randomized controlled clinical trial. J Am Dent Assoc 2009;140(5):559–66.
13. Jackson DL, Milgrom P, Heacox GA, et al. Pharmacokinetics and clinical effects of multi-dose sublingual triazolam in healthy volunteers. J Clin Psychopharmacol 2006;26(1):4–8.
14. Tait AR, Knight PR. The effect of general anesthesia on upper respiratory infections in children. Anesthesiology 1987;67:930–5.

15. Rx List – The internet drug index. Available at: http://www.rxlist.com/midazolam_hydrochloride_syrup-drug.htm. Accessed May 2011.
16. Paterson SA, Tahmassebi JF. Pediatric dentistry in the new millennium: use of inhalation sedation in pediatric dentistry. Dent Update 2003;30(7):350–8.
17. American Society of Anesthesiologists. Practice guidelines for sedation and analgesia by nonanesthesiologists: an updated report by the American Society of Anesthesiologists task force on sedation and analgesia by nonanesthesiologists. Anesthesiology 2002;96:1004–17.
18. Yamakura T, Harris RA. Effects of gaseous anesthetics nitrous oxide and xenon on ligand-gated ion channels. Comparison with isoflurane and ethanol. Anesthesiology 2000;93(4):1095–101.
19. Emmanouil DE, Quock RM. Advances in understanding the actions of nitrous oxide. Anesth Prog 2007;54(1):9–18.
20. Criteria for a recommended standard: occupational exposure to waste anesthetic gases and vapors. Cincinnati (OH): US Department of Health, Education, and Welfare, Public Health Service, Center for Disease Control, National Institute for Occupational Safety and Health, DHEW (NIOSH) Publication No. 77B140; 1984.
21. National Institute for Occupational Safety and Health. Recommendations for Occupational Safety and Health–Compendium of Policy Documents and Statements (DHHS/NIOSH Pub. No. 92–100). Cincinnati (OH): NIOSH; 1992.
22. American Academy of Pediatric Dentistry. Policy on minimizing occupational health hazards associated with nitrous oxide. Pediatr Dent 2008;30(Suppl 7): 64, 65.
23. Ogundipe O, Pearson MW, Slater NG, et al. Sickle cell disease and nitrous oxide-induced neuropathy. Clin Lab Haematol 1999;21(6):409–12.
24. Fish BM, Banerjee AR, Jennings CR, et al. Effect of anaesthetic agents on tympanometry and middle-ear effusions. J Laryngol Otol 2000;114(5):336–8.

Hemostasis in Oral Surgery

Amandip Kamoh, DDS[a,b,*], Jason Swantek, DDS[a,c]

KEYWORDS
- Hemostasis • Hemostic agents • Hemorrhage control

Bleeding during oral surgical procedures can be bothersome to the operator and time-consuming to control. It may also compromise visibility and possibly the procedure itself. This article will cover the area of hemorrhage control in surgery. The topic can be divided into three main areas:

1. Preoperative assessment and identification of risk factors of bleeding
2. Intraoperative control of bleeding
3. Management of postoperative bleeding.

PREOPERATIVE ASSESSMENT

There are many confounding factors that can ultimately potentiate perioperative bleeding as well as create difficulty in controlling bleeding. Therefore, it is essential to obtain a comprehensive medical history that also entails all medications in the patient's regimen. A thorough medical history is the best screening technique to identify potential bleeding issues.

When managing the anticoagulated patient, one must consider preoperative, intraoperative, and postoperative measures.

Preoperatively, if the patient is on anticoagulant therapy, one may need to break up exodontia into multiple visits to decrease the amount of bleeding encountered.[1] Timing of the appointment has to be taken into consideration with patients who are at high risk for bleeding postoperatively; early morning appointments allow for patients to return to the clinic, if bleeding persists despite all measures. In medically compromised patients, laboratory values such as international normalized ratio (INR), prothrombin time (PT), and platelet count may be of critical value.

The authors have nothing to disclose.
[a] Oral and Maxillofacial Surgery, Woodhull Medical & Mental Health Center, Brooklyn, NY, USA
[b] Oral & Maxillofacial Surgery, 65 Spring Meadow Drive #5, Williamsville, NY 14221, USA
[c] Oral and Maxillofacial Surgery, 254 Brookdale Lane North, Palatine, IL 60067, USA
* Corresponding author. Oral and Maxillofacial Surgery, 65 Spring Meadow Drive #5, Williamsville, NY 14221.
E-mail address: akamohdds@gmail.com

Many patients' daily regimen consists of anticoagulant therapy such as aspirin, clopidogrel, warfarin, and heparin for underlying comorbidities. Therefore the clinician should be well versed in hemorrhage control after oral surgery. Although some practitioners advocate the discontinuation of anticoagulants before an oral surgical procedure, it is usually unnecessary. For the majority of these cases, local hemostatic measures are effective in managing postoperative bleeding. Stopping the anticoagulant can have deleterious effects and likely poses a greater risk to the patient. It has been assumed that stopping warfarin for short periods of time presents a negligible risk to the patient. However, it has been reported that discontinuing anticoagulation medication before a dental procedure gives a 1% incidence of serious thromboembolic complication.[2] Local hemostatic measures generally suffice when managing patients on daily low doses of anticoagulants. More likely than not, the risk of discontinuing anticoagulants is higher than the risk of perioperative bleeding.

All antiplatelet medications affect clotting by inhibiting platelet aggregation, but they do so by a variety of different mechanisms. Aspirin irreversibly acetylates cyclooxygenase, inhibiting the production of thromboxane A_2, which results in decreased platelet aggregation. Clopidogrel selectively inhibits adenosine diphosphate (ADP)-induced platelet aggregation. Aspirin begins irreversibly inhibiting platelet aggregation within 1 hour of ingestion, and clopidogrel begins within 2 hours; this lasts for the life of the platelets (7–10 days). The formation of new platelets helps overcome this inhibitory effect; complete recovery of platelet aggregation may occur in 50% of cases by day 3 and in 80% of cases by day 4. Aspirin and clopidogrel work synergistically to inhibit platelet aggregation. Aspirin can double the baseline bleeding time, but this may still be within the normal range. Clopidogrel is considered a more potent antiplatelet agent and can prolong the bleeding time by 1.5 to 3 times normal. Combined use of aspirin and clopidogrel produces additive and possible synergistic effects as the two block complementary pathways in the platelet aggregation cascade. It is generally accepted that the cardioprotective benefits of low-dose aspirin outweigh the potential for untoward bleeding episodes in at-risk patients with cardiovascular disease. Nonsteroidal anti-inflammatory drugs (NSAIDs) other than aspirin have a reversible effect on platelet aggregation, and platelet function is restored once the drug is cleared from the circulation. Minor surgical procedures can be safely performed without altering the antiplatelet medication dose.[3] When more than 2 or 3 teeth need to be extracted, it is generally advisable to do this in multiple visits rather than have the patient stop the anticoagulants.

Bleeding disorders can be broken up into disorders of intrinsic and extrinsic coagulation pathways. The intrinsic pathway involves factors VIII, IX, XI, XII, which all affect the activated partial thromboplastin time (aPTT). The extrinsic pathway involves factor VII, which will affect the PT. The intrinsic and extrinsic pathways both lead up to the common pathway, where factor X is activated to factor Xa. If there are any anomalies along factors in either the intrinsic or extrinsic paths, the formation of the fibrin clot can be compromised. Laboratory tests such as PTT and PT can help lead toward determining which pathway is affected, while bleeding time values will provide information concerning platelet functionality.

There are many congenital disorders that may have an impact on hemostasis-such as hemophilia, von Willebrand Disease, and others. Hemophilia is a rare bleeding disorder that can range from mild to severe, depending on how much clotting factor is present in the blood. Hemophilia is classified as type A or type B, based on which type of clotting factor is lacking,factor VIII in type A and factor IX in type B. Von Willebrand disease is a inherited condition that results when the blood lacks von Willebrand factor, a protein that helps the blood to clot and also carries another clotting protein, factor VIII. There are also many acquired bleeding disorders can be caused by certain factor deficiencies secondary to liver disease or vitamin K deficiency. These patients are typically closely monitored by their primary care physicians or hematologists; therefore more information can be obtained by contacting the appropriate provider.

Spolarichs' study showed that many surgical patients fail to inform their surgeons of their use of herbal medications in preoperative interviews; therefore it is even more important to question patients specifically about herbal supplement usage.[4] Herbal supplements such as ephedra, ginger, garlic, gingko biloba, ginseng, dong quai, St John's wort, licorice, and kava kava can all have possible perioperative complications such as prolonged bleeding. Pribitkin and Boger[5] documented garlic's inhibitory effect on platelet aggregation in people, which occurs within 5 days of oral administration. Ginger is a potent inhibitor of thromboxane synthetase and can theoretically prolong bleeding times with long-term use. Ginkgo has been noted to have a potent inhibitory effect on platelet activating factor and consequently on platelet aggregation. Dong quai has been known to prolong PT and aPTT, and it may interact with the effects of warfarin. Licorice inhibits platelet aggregation and contains coumarin. Kava has been shown in vitro to cause platelet dysfunction through inhibition of thromboxane synthesis. It is recommended that herbal supplements be discontinued 2 weeks before patients undergo invasive surgical procedures.

Preoperatively, the surgeon should assess the bleeding risk of the patient as well as the bleeding risk of the surgery. For example, extracting multiple teeth in a single visit greatly increases the risk of perioperative bleeding.[6] Patients with severe periodontal disease or gingival inflammation are also placed at a higher risk of perioperative bleeding. This surgical plan might involve scaling and root planing and chlorhexidine gluconate mouth rinse 2 weeks before an elective procedure. Once the bleeding risk is assessed, the surgeon can then formulate an intraoperative and postoperative plan.

INTRAOPERATIVE CONTROL OF BLEEDING

Management of bleeding has many key components that start with good surgical technique as well as anesthetic support. The less bleeding the surgeon encounters, the better visibility he or she will have. Typically, the control of bleeding starts before the incision is made with the injection of a vasoconstrictor. Intraoperatively, the surgeon may use various topical hemostatic agents to assist in the control of bleeding.

VASOCONSTRICTOR

The control of bleeding should start prior to incision with the infiltration of vasoconstrictor into the surgical site. Epinephrine is the most commonly used vasoconstrictor, which is usually combined with a local anesthetic.[7] In a patient with significant cardiovascular disease, 0.04 mg (2 carpules of epinephrine 1:100,000) is the maximum dosage. In the healthy patient, the maximum dosage of epinephrine is 0.2 mg (11 carpules of epinephrine 1:100,000).[8] After the injection of epinephrine, a decrease in gingival blood flow should be apparent in approximately 5 minutes.[9]

INTRAOPERATIVE CONSIDERATIONS

Intraoperatively, the surgeon must take into consideration planning of the incision as well as surgical anatomy in the prevention of bleeding. The incision should be designed so that the site will be closed over bony support. This allows the application of pressure directly to the surgical site in the event of uncontrolled bleeding. The incision should also be large enough to allow adequate access to the surgical site. A small flap has a great risk of inadvertent tearing, which is a large risk factor for bleeding. The mucosa and periosteum should be sharply incised and elevated in an atraumatic manner. The surgeon should also avoid vascular structures such as the mental vessels, greater palatine artery, inferior alveolar artery and vein, and the lingual artery and vein.

If perioperative bleeding occurs, the mainstay of hemostasis is the application of pressure to the surgical site. If the bleeding arises from an extraction site, pressure can be applied to the site by packing the socket and having the patient bite forcefully on a piece of gauze dressing. Pressure should be maintained for at least 3 to 5 minutes to allow the formation of a blood clot. The gauze should be removed slowly so as to not dislodge the clot. Another form of mechanical surgical hemostasis is suturing. Suturing cannot only be used to obtain primary closure of the surgical site, but also to apply continuous pressure to the site, allowing hemostasis to occur. A nonresorbable, multifilament suture is recommended in these situations, since it has a high tensile strength. A figure-of-eight suture over an extraction site is common in combination with other hemostatic agents to provide pressure within the walls of the extraction socket. Placement of multiple interrupted sutures is also recommended. Although a running suture is quicker to place than multiple interrupted sutures, if the running suture fails, then the site is at risk for bleeding over the whole area that the suture was covering.

Electrocautery and chemical cautery are also options in achieving hemostasis. These techniques work best if a site of brisk bleeding can be visualized and isolated. Although cauterization is a great option, one must be cognizant of avoiding damage to surrounding vital structures.

HEMOSTATIC AGENTS

Several topical hemostatic agents are currently available for use in oral and maxillofacial surgery. The ideal hemostatic agent should be effective, safe to use within the body, and affordable. They can be divided into two categories: active and passive hemostatic agents. Passive hemostatic agents provide a framework where platelets can aggregate so that a stable clot can form. Active hemostatic agents have biologic activity and directly participate in the coagulation cascade to induce a clot.

Gelfoam (Pfizer, New York, NY, USA) is a porous, pliable, absorbable gelatin sponge that is prepared from purified pork skin gelatin. This product has properties that allow it to absorb about 40 times its weight in blood, and it can expand to 200% of its initial volume. When applied to a site, Gelfoam provides a mechanical matrix, which facilitates clotting. The spongy physical properties of the gelatin sponge hasten clot formation and provide structural support to the forming clot. Gelfoam has very little tissue reaction and liquefies in the oral cavity within a week, fully absorbing within 4 to 6 weeks. Although it is not necessary, thrombin can be applied to the Gelfoam before use to aid in hemostasis.

Surgicel (Ethicon, Somerville, NJ, USA) is oxidized regenerated cellulose, derived from plant-based alpha-cellulose. Surgicel has acidic properties due to a low pH, and it achieves hemostasis via denaturation of blood proteins, mechanical activation of the clotting cascade, and local vasoconstriction. This product is thought to be relatively bacteriostatic when compared with other hemostatic agents, due to a low pH. The acidic environment Surgicel creates can be harmful to any adjacent vital structures like the inferior alveolar nerve. Loescher and Robinson[10] reported that Surgicel can cause temporary sensory disturbances. Absorption of Surgicel will occur in approximately 4 to 8 weeks.

Tranexamic acid is an antifibrinolytic agent that completely inhibits the activation of plasminogen to plasmin, preventing the degradation of fibrin. In oral surgery, tranexamic acid solution is most commonly given as a mouthwash postoperatively to prevent bleeding. Ramstrom and colleagues[11] demonstrated a significant reduction in postoperative bleeding in the anticoagulated patient when a 4.8% solution of tranexamic acid mouthwash was used postoperatively, 10 mL 4 times daily, for 7 days. Studies have not shown any significant decrease in hemorrhage control when tranexamic acid is used intraoperatively (irrigation, soaked gauze). An intraoperative tranexamic acid injection can also be used as a hemostatic measure. Choi and colleagues[12] showed that total blood loss during maxillary surgery was significantly reduced when a bolus of tranexamic acid was given preoperatively. Aminocaproic acid solution, although less potent than tranexamic acid, is an antifibrinolytic agent that is more widely available in the United States and can be used as an alternative.

Chitosan-based products are a new generation of hemostatic medical products that have been shown to achieve early hemostasis as well as improve postoperative healing. Chitosan is a naturally occurring, biocompatible, electropositively charged polysaccharide that is derived from shrimp shell chitin. This charge attracts the negatively charged red blood cells forming an extremely viscous clot, which seals the wound and causes hemostasis. The formation of a clot occurs independently of the intrinsic or extrinsic clotting pathways and is effective for patients on anticoagulant medications. Although these products are derived from shellfish, no reactions have been found in skin testing using chitosan on shellfish-sensitive patients. HemCon Medical Technologies, Incorporated (Portland, OR, USA) currently manufactures many chitosan-based products including dental dressings. A recent study showed that hemostasis was achieved in less than 1 minute in patients where HemCon dental dressing was used, which was significantly faster than the control average hemostasis time, 9.5 minutes. Approximately 32% of HemCon dental dressing-treated sites had significantly better healing compared with the control sites.[13]

MANAGEMENT OF POSTOPERATIVE BLEEDING

Patient education, especially patients at a high risk of postoperative bleeding, is essential in the immediate postoperative period. The patient must be made aware that bleeding or minor oozing may persist for up to 24 hours after an extraction. If the patient is on anticoagulant medication, this may prolong the bleeding. The importance of pressure dressing postoperatively is also invaluable and needs to be stressed to the patient. All postoperative instructions should include the following: avoid rinsing the mouth vigorously or spitting for 24 hours; avoid disturbing the socket with foreign objects, and most importantly apply pressure over the socket firmly for 20 minutes. If bleeding starts at any time postoperatively, the patient can be instructed to reapply pressure over the surgical site for 20 minutes with either a gauze dressing or a damp tea bag.

Management of the postoperatively bleeding patient can provide a challenge to the practitioner. Postoperative hemorrhage in the anticoagulated patient is most likely to occur within 6 days.[14] The use of the surgical techniques and agents described previously as well as good anesthetic support will be invaluable. The application of pressure to the surgical site can slow or halt the bleeding while an assessment of the patient is made. First, it is prudent to assess the amount of blood loss the patient has had since the surgery. Although hemorrhagic shock resulting from an intraoral surgical site is rare, it cannot be forgotten. If the patient displays any signs of shock (tachycardia, hypotension, cold/clammy skin, lethargy), then a rapid response should be initiated with immediate intravenous fluid replacement to replenish the intravascular volume and reestablish tissue perfusion.

Drug interactions are often overlooked in a postoperative bleeding incidence. A thorough review of the patient's medications is necessary, especially if the patient has started a new medication (antibiotic, pain medicine) since the surgery. For example, warfarin has increased effects and a greater potential for bleeding when combined with macrolides (erythromycin, azithromycin), sulfa-containing drugs, NSAIDs, and quinolones. Immediate discontinuation of the interacting drug must be considered in the treatment plan for hemostasis.

The intraoperative control of bleeding techniques described previously can be used in the postoperatively bleeding patient. Often when the postoperative bleeding patient presents, the surgical site is not only bleeding but often contains a large amount of granulation tissue. The best means of hemorrhage control is to thoroughly irrigate the surgical site and remove all visible granulation tissue under local anesthesia before suturing. Although one may be inclined to use vasoconstrictor in these situations, this should be avoided. Administering a vasoconstrictor (ie, epinephrine) will help cease bleeding in the surgical site; however, the problem at hand is only being masked. Once the epinephrine is eliminated from the surgical field about 2 hours later, bleeding will most likely resume.

SUMMARY

Management of a bleeding surgical site can be very disconcerting to the inexperienced practitioner. Preoperatively assessing a patient's risk of perioperative bleeding will allow the surgeon to be more prepared when an incident occurs. The use of good surgical technique, proper anesthetic support, mechanical hemostasis techniques, and topical hemostatic agents will allow the practitioner to work more efficiently.

REFERENCES

1. Brennan MT, Wynn RL, Miller CS. Aspirin and bleeding in dentistry: an update and recommendations. Oral Surg Oral Med Oral Pathol Oral Radiol Endod 2007;104(3):316–23.
2. Christine R, editor. North West Medicines Information Centre. Surgical management of the primary care dental patient on antiplatelet medication. Available at: http://www.dundee.ac.uk/tuith/Static/info/antiplatelet.pdf. Accessed June 23, 2011.
3. Servin F. Low-dose aspirin and clopidogrel: how to act in patients scheduled for day surgery. Curr Opin Anaesthesiol 2007;20(6):531–4.
4. Spolarich AE, Andrews L. An examination of the bleeding complications associated with herbal supplements, antiplatelet, and anticoagulant medications. J Dent Hyg 2007;81(3):67.
5. Pribitkin ED, Boger G. Herbal therapy: what every facial plastic surgeon must know. Arch Facial Plast Surg 2001;3(2):127–32.
6. Tessier D, Bash D. A surgeon's guide to herbal supplements. J Surg Res 2003;114(1):30–6.
7. Wahl MJ. Dental surgery in anticoagulated patients. Arch Intern Med 1998;158:1610–6.
8. Dym H, Ogle OE. Atlas of minor oral surgery. 1st edition. Philadelphia (PA): WB Saunders Company; 2000.
9. Dodson TB, Bays RA, Paul RE, et al. The effect of local anesthesia with vasoconstrictor on gingival blood flow during a Lefort I osteotomy. J Oral Maxillofac Surg 1996;54(7):810–4.
10. Loescher AR, Robinson PP. The effect of surgical medicaments on peripheral nerve function. Br J Oral Maxillofac Surg 1998;36(5):327–32.

11. Ramström G, Sindet-Pedersen S, Hall G, et al. Prevention of postsurgical bleeding in oral surgery using tranexamic acid without dose modification of oral anticoagulants. J Oral Maxillofac Surg 1993;51(11):1211–6.

12. Choi WS, Irwin MG, Samman N. The effect of tranexamic acid on blood loss during orthognathic surgery: a randomized controlled trial. J Oral Maxillofac Surg 2009;67(1):125–33.

13. Malmquist JP, Clemens SC, Oien HJ, et al. Hemostasis of oral surgery wounds with the HemCon dental dressing. J Oral Maxillofac Surg 2008;66(5):1177–83.

14. Morimoto Y, Niwa H, Minematsu K, et al. Risk factors affecting postoperative hemorrhage after tooth extraction in patients receiving oral antithrombotic therapy. J Oral Maxillofac Surg 2011;69(6):1550–6.

Oral Surgery for Patients on Anticoagulant Therapy: Current Thoughts on Patient Management

Ladi Doonquah, MD, DDS[a,b,*], Anika D. Mitchell, BBMedSci, MBBS[a,b]

KEYWORDS

• Hemostasis • Anticoagulation therapy • Minor oral surgery

Medical advances have led to an increase in life expectancy; however, there has also been a greater prevalence of many chronic illnesses. This has resulted in more patients who present to dental offices on anticoagulant medications. There are a variety of discordant approaches to the treatment of surgical patients on anticoagulant therapy, despite many new studies that purport to provide a guide forward.[1–6] Some have presented new guidelines that attempt a strict algorithmic approach to patient management. Wahl,[7] in a major review of the literature, suggested that most patients undergoing minor oral surgery did not need to stop or decrease their warfarin or antiplatelet drugs, whereas Todd[3] suggested a more individually tailored approach. This article reviews the different aspects of this ever-present challenge and provides our perspective and guidelines to assist with the management of these patients.

ASSESSMENT

A thorough medical and dental history is critical to the identification of patients who may be on some type of hemostasis-altering medication. The dentist must be familiar with the types of diseases and conditions that necessitate the alteration of coagulation mechanisms and the different laboratory tests that are used to assess the coagulation status in these patients.[7–9] Consultation and coordination of care with the patient's

Financial disclosures/conflict of interest: None.
[a] Faculty of Medical Sciences, University of the West Indies, Mona, Kingston 7, Jamaica
[b] Department of Surgery, University Hospital of the West Indies, Mona, Kingston 7, Jamaica
* Corresponding author. Faculty of Medical Sciences, University of the West Indies, Mona, Kingston 7, Jamaica.
E-mail address: ldoonquah@hotmail.com

primary care physician and any other appropriate medical specialist is important to the successful management of the surgical intervention.[10–12] This, however, does not supplant the primary role of the dentist being the leader of the team taking care of these patients, once the dentist assumes the role of the patient's surgeon. In addition there should be an awareness of the different laboratory tests and their implications in the management of patients on oral anticoagulation therapy (OAT).

INVESTIGATIONS

The laboratory investigations that are useful in the evaluation and preparation of the patient include a complete blood count (CBC), prothrombin time (PT), activated partial thromboplastin time (aPTT), international normalized ratio (INR), and, in some cases, bleeding time. The CBC involves quantitative evaluation of hemoglobin (g/dL) and platelets (**Table 1**).

The quantitative levels of platelets may be normal, but platelet function maybe reduced because of medications, such as aspirin, or clinical conditions, such as uremia. The vascular phase of hemostasis and platelet function is evaluated with the bleeding time. This is a test where a 1-mm slit is made in the skin and blotted with filter paper and timed to determine when bleeding stops. The normal time should be 7 to 9 minutes. However, this test is now less commonly used in standard workup of patients, and some studies have shown that there is little predictive outcome with respect to postoperative bleeding in patients having minor oral surgery.[13] A prolonged bleeding time offers more information with regard to bleeding risk, although a normal test cannot exclude the possibility.

The coagulation tests that are commonly used in practice to monitor bleeding risk and anticoagulant therapy are prothrombin time (PT), activated partial thromboplastin time (aPTT), and thrombin time (TT).[14,15] aPTT is a measure of the intrinsic pathway of coagulation used in the monitoring of heparin therapy and is usually abnormal in patients with hemophillia.[14] Values are compared with a control and should be within 7 seconds of the control. Values usually range from 25 to 35 seconds. It is usually pro-longed if a patient has less than approximately 30% of normal activity. PT measures the integrity of the extrinsic coagulation pathway (**Fig. 1**). This test is used to monitor

Table 1
Complete blood count components

Test	Normal Ranges		Clinical Significance	Clinical Presentation
	Male	Female		
Red blood cells	4.7–6.1 million cells/μL	4.2–5.4 million cells/μL	Anemia. If present can represent chronic blood loss, which may mean bleeding diathesis.	Fatigability, pallor, tachycardia
Hematocrit	40.7%–50.3%	36.1%–44.3%	As above	As above
Hemoglobin	13.8–17.2 g/dL	12.1–15.1 g/dL	As above	As above
Platelets	150 to 400 × 10⁹/L		Thrombocytopenia. Rule out platelet destruction, eg, HIT	Petechiae, purpura, ecchymosis

Abbreviation: HIT, heparin-induced thrombocytopenia.

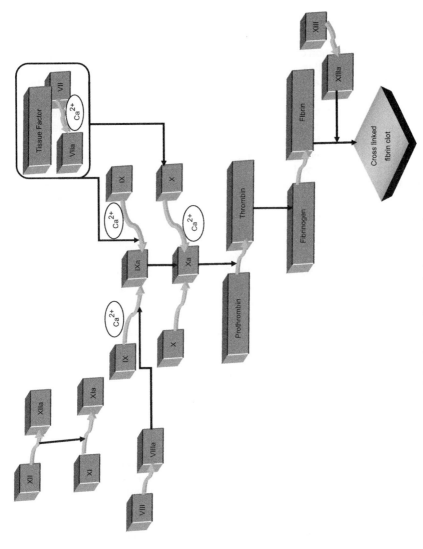

Fig. 1. Coagulation cascade and the involvement of the clotting factors in hemostasis.

warfarin therapy. Values should be compared with a control value, but normal usually range from 12 to 15 seconds. TT is a less frequently used blood test and is used to assess fibrin production. The INR measures the ratio of the patient's PT to a normal sample that is designed to standardize the differences among laboratories.[15] It is also used to monitor warfarin therapy and the extrinsic coagulation pathway. The normal range is 0.8 to 1.2 and the therapeutic range for anticoagulation is 2.0 to 4.0.[16]

ANTICOAGULANTS

Hemostasis is the arrest of bleeding either by physiologic processes involving vaso-constriction and activation of the coagulation cascade or by surgical processes. Medications that interrupt this process can be grouped into 2 primary categories: anticoagulants that interrupt the coagulation cascade and antiplatelet factors (**Fig. 2**). There is an increased risk of bleeding with the use of all anticoagulants, but some more so than others. The type of medical condition and the attendant use of anticoagulants can be used to assess bleeding risk and hence it is important for the practicing dentist to be familiar with this area of medicine.[17–19]

Warfarin is an oral anticoagulant that was discovered in Wisconsin more than 80 years ago. It was initially used as a rat poison but was discovered to have human applications as a result of a failed suicide attempt by an American sailor in 1955. It works by inhibiting vitamin K–dependant coagulation factors and its effect is dose dependant. The half-life is 36 hours and its full effect takes 72 to 96 hours. The anticoagulation efficacy is measured by the PT and INR. A target INR range of 2.0 to 4.0 is used for most patients. It is metabolized in the liver and excreted via the kidneys. Various medications can potentiate or decrease the effect of the drug, and a thorough knowledge of these medications is important. **Table 2** lists some of these medications. Warfarin is metabolized in the liver via a similar mechanism as many other drugs; therefore, when it is administered simultaneously with some medications, it may result in either an increase or decrease in the blood concentration of warfarin, thus affecting the efficacy of its action (see **Table 2**). Warfarin has also been shown to interact with many herbal medications.[20,21] Drugs that are highly protein bound will displace warfarin and increase its blood concentration, leading to an increase in the INR.

Heparin was discovered in 1916 and is usually derived from porcine mucosa. It is a parenteral drug that inhibits thrombin and factor Xa. Administration is intravenous (IV) or subcutaneous (SC) and it primarily affects the intrinsic coagulation pathway. It has a short half-life of approximately 1 hour and is mainly administered via IV infusion or intermittent SC injection. The anticoagulation effects of this drug are monitored via measuring the aPTT, which should be 1.5 to 2.0 times the normal. Platelets should also be reviewed because of the risk of the rare side effects of heparin-induced thrombo-cytopenia (HIT) and heparin-induced thrombocytopenia and thrombosis (HITT). These usually occur within the first 10 days of starting heparin therapy but can occur up to many weeks after it has been discontinued. Heparin is more commonly used in the hospital setting rather than for outpatient management.

Depolymerization of heparin produces low molecular-weight heparin (LMWH). LMWH requires less monitoring than heparin and hence is often used in outpatient management for patients who require relatively short-term anticoagulation (**Table 3**). LMWH is also used for in-hospital patient care for therapeutic or prophylactic treatment of conditions such as deep vein thrombosis (DVT).[22] LMWH is available for SC or IV use only. Warfarin is known to have its clinical and practical limitations so ultra-low molecular-weight heparins are currently being developed; for example, semuloparin and bemiparin.[23]

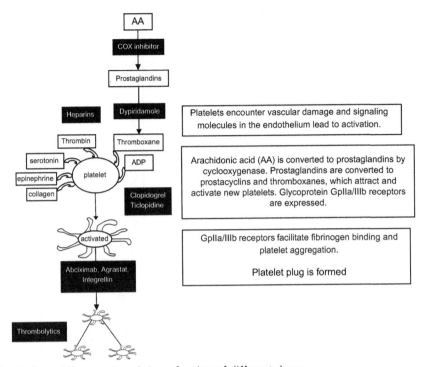

Fig. 2. Normal hemostasis and sites of action of different drugs.

Fondaparinux is a selective Factor Xa inhibitor that is administered SC. This class of drug is chemically similar to LMWH and does not require monitoring of the drug action during use.[24]

Antiplatelet Medications

There are various antiplatelet medications that are used to aid anticoagulation. Some are used both therapeutically and for prophylaxis, for example, aspirin. There are others that are used primarily for therapeutic purposes. These may be given together with aspirin or as single-dose therapy. Knowledge of how they work and the implications for their withdrawal from therapy is imperative in the proper surgical management of patients on OAT.

Table 2
Warfarin enhancers and inhibitors

Enhancers	Inhibitors
Metronidazole – antibiotic	Barbituates
Macrolide antibiotics – eg, erythromycin, clarithromycin, least affected by azythromycin	Carbamazepine
Phenytoin	Cholestyramine
Sulfamethoxazole – component of the antibiotic Bactrim	Rifampin
Ciprofloxacin	Thiazide diuretics
Ginkgo biloba, Ginseng	Vitamin K

Table 3
Anticoagulants

Anticoagulants	Mechanism of Action	Use/Indication
Unfractionated Heparin	Inhibits antithrombin III and factors IXa, Xa, XIa, XIIa, and thrombin Inhibits heparin cofactor	Prophylaxis and treatment of thromboembolic diseases (DVT, pulmonary embolus, atrial fibrillation with emboli and dialysis. Monitored via aPTT.
Low molecular-weight heparin (enoxaparin, dalteparin, tinzaperin)	Inhibit factor Xa and thrombin	As above. Acute MI and adjuncts to coronary percutaneous intervention. Monitoring is not required but can be done by assay for anti-factor Xa activity.
Selective factor Xa inhibitors (indirect) (Fondaparinux)	Inhibits factor Xa by binding to antithrombin III	Main indication for use is DVT prophylaxis but is also used for the treatment of DVT and thromboembolism. No need to monitor anticoagulant effects.
Direct thrombin inhibitors (lepirudin, argatroban, dabigatran-oral administration)	Inactivate thrombin	Acute coronary syndrome with or without percutaneous intervention, atrial fibrillation, acute ischemic stroke, treatment and prophylaxis of DVT. Monitor with aPTT.
Warfarin	Inhibits hepatic synthesis of the vitamin K–dependent coagulation factors II, VII, IX, and X and the anticoagulant proteins C and S.	Mechanical valves, chronic atrial fibrillation, deep venous thrombosis, pulmonary embolism, and dilated cardiomyopathy. Monitored with PT and INR.
Antiplatelet drugs Aspirin Clopidogrel (Plavix), Prasugrel (Effient), Ticlopidine (Ticlid) Cilostazol (Pletal) Abciximab (ReoPro), Eptifibatide (Integrilin), Tirofiban (Aggrastat) Dipyridamole (Persantine)	Cyclo-oxygenase inhibitors. ADP receptor inhibitors. Phosphodiesterase inhibitor. Glycoprotein IIB/IIIA inhibitors (intravenous use only). Adenosine reuptake inhibitors.	Treatment and prevention of arterial thrombi. see **Fig. 3**

Abbreviations: ADP, adenosine diphosphate; aPTT, activated partial thromboplastin time; DVT, deep vein thrombosis; INR, international normalized ratio; MI, myocardial infarction; PT, prothrombin time.

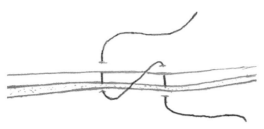

Fig. 3. Diagram of figure of 8 suture.

Aspirin is one of the most commonly encountered medications in a patient's drug history. The active ingredient is acetylsalicylic acid. It is used in the treatment of a myriad of conditions and functions as an analgesic, anti-inflammatory, antipyretic, and antiplatelet medication. It belongs to the group of medications known as nonsteroidal anti-inflammatory drugs. It irreversibly inhibits platelet action, unlike other drugs in the group. The PT, aPTT, and platelet count are usually normal in patients on aspirin therapy but the bleeding time may be prolonged.

Clopidogrel irreversibly inhibits the adenosine diphosphate receptors on platelets and thus inhibits aggregation and clot formation. It is an alternative drug for persons who require anticoagulation who are unable to tolerate aspirin therapy.

The more common antiplatelet medications enjoy widespread use in the population. Both dental and medical clinicians still encourage stoppage of these drugs from 7 to 10 days before surgery. Although there is a paucity of prospective studies on cessation of antiplatelet drugs as compared with cessation of warfarin, the few that are available support continuation for minor oral surgery.[25] One such study, by Partridge and colleagues[26] published in 2008, compares a group of 27 patients on various antiplatelet medications with a control group of 23. They found no difference in postoperative bleeding. This sample size is small and none of the patients were noted to be on dual antiplatelet therapy, which limits how much that can be extrapolated from the study. Other retrospective reports have been in congruence with Partridge and colleagues'[26] therefore, for minor limited oral surgery procedures, the literature supports maintenance of therapy.[25]

An overview of a patient's drug history is not only important for the primary anticoagulant medications but also for those with secondary anticoagulation effects. These may increase the risk of bleeding and include drugs such as simvastatin used in the management of hypercholesterolemia.[27]

Conditions That May Require Anticoagulant Therapy

Knowledge of the various disease states that often require patients to be on anticoagulants is the first step in managing these patients. The most common ones are patients with mechanical cardiac valves, atrial fibrillation, DVT, pulmonary embolism, peripheral vascular disease (PVD), myocardial infarction, and ischemic strokes, among others.

Patients who present to the dental office with these or similar conditions should undergo further evaluation to ascertain the degree of anticoagulation. The patient's primary care physician should be contacted to discuss the relative need for maintaining anticoagulants during minor oral surgery. It is important to keep in mind that many physicians will make recommendations based on general surgical patients, and must be informed of the differences as they relate to oral surgery.[28–33] There have been a number of studies in the past few decades that have documented the ability to achieve hemostasis in patients who do not have cessation of therapy.[1,2,26] Malmquist and colleagues[34] noted that there was no significant difference in hemostasis in a group of patients on oral anticoagulants who used hemocon dental dressing and the control group. Hence, there is a pronounced shift toward doing minor surgical procedures while maintaining some degree of anticoagulation therapy.

Despite this trend, there are those who argue for a more cautious approach, indicating that the problems of postoperative bleeding are not insignificant. Todd, in an article in 2003,[35] further states that the instances of serious complications as a result of withholding oral anticoagulants are not as frequent as was once thought and that some may have been attributable to prolonged withdrawal of warfarin beyond what is normally recommended. He goes on to advocate guided withdrawal for moderate-risk to high-risk patients and those undergoing more extensive oral surgery, with bridging therapy for some patients based on their risk profile.

Of the previously listed conditions that require some alteration of coagulation, the major ones that require full anticoagulation therapy are patients with mechanical cardiac valves, atrial fibrillation, pulmonary embolism, and those with a history of a recent DVT or ischemic stroke. The possible life-threatening complications that may result from cessation of therapy in these patients would dictate consideration of local hemostatic measures for minor surgical procedures while having them remain on anticoagulation treatment or doing the procedures in a hospital setting.

As has been previously stated, the historical standard of care for managing patients on oral anticoagulant therapy was to stop the medication for a number of days before surgery and check the INR. If it was close to the normal range, then surgery was performed.[7] Patients who were considered high risk and who could not be kept on these medications were hospitalized and switched to heparin, which has a shorter duration of action. The surgery was performed after briefly stopping the heparin. Once hemostasis was ensured, heparin was restarted and later switched to the oral anticoagulant. This is logistically more difficult and costly and involves hospitalization. Now, however, there are a greater variety of approaches to treat these patients, further contributing to the controversy that persists on how best to manage them.[1,2,26,36–40]

There are 5 different approaches that can be used for patients who are fully anticoagulated that require minor oral surgery, which we will classify as categories 1 to 5:

1. Cessation of OAT
2. Cessation of OAT with bridging IV heparin therapy
3. Cessation of OAT with bridging low molecular-weight SC heparin therapy
4. Decrease in dosage of OAT
5. Maintenance of OAT.

The first method is the traditional way in which we have handled these individuals. Warfarin is stopped 3 to 5 days before surgery, a PT and INR are done and, if normal or near normal, the agreed upon surgery is performed. This would be done for patients who are considered low risks for thromboembolic phenomena as determined by their medical history in conjunction with their physician.

The second method is for high-risk patients, for example those with mechanical valves, recent ischemic stroke, or a recent episode of pulmonary embolism. These patients would be hospitalized and slowly switched to IV heparin over 3 to 5 days, and remain fully anticoagulated until a few hours before surgery, whereupon the heparin would be stopped. After the prescribed surgery is completed and hemostasis is achieved, IV heparin would be restarted and later that day OAT would also be restarted. Once the warfarin has achieved full anticoagulation, the IV heparin would stop.

The third method is for patients with medium surgical risk. This method has become more popular with the advent of LMWH drugs that are longer acting.[41] OAT is stopped 3 to 5 days before surgery while LMWH is started. Upon completion of surgery, warfarin is started that same evening and LMWH is stopped when PT and INR indicate adequate anticoagulation.[42]

The fourth method involves decrease of the dosage of warfarin to get the INR in a range of 2.0 to 2.5. Once that has been attained, the surgery is performed and the dosage is increased back to normal that same evening, provided adequate hemostasis is present.

The final method involves no alteration of OAT. The INR is still done on the day of surgery. If it is between 2.0 and 4.0, the surgery is performed using adequate local hemostatic measures, such as placement of cellulose sponges, packs, suturing, and hemostatic liquids. These patients should be followed closely for up to 5 days after the procedure. Patients at high risk for thromboembolism would fall into this category.

With all methods, the patient's physician should be aware of the plan. It is imperative to have in place a variety of local hemostatic agents for use, a readily available oral surgical specialist back-up and close follow-up measures in place. It is important to remember that patients who are on anticoagulant therapy, who have surgery and are noted to have adequate hemostasis at the conclusion of the procedure, can have bleeding issues up to 10 days after surgery.[43] This is not an infrequent occurrence, so follow-up surveillance must be in place.

Patients Who Are Fully on OAT

Over the past 10 years there has been a trend toward the fifth method, maintaining anticoagulant therapy for patients who are having minor surgical procedures, such as minor oral surgery.[1,2,26,36–40] This is so because, as has been previously mentioned, cessation of therapy in high-risk patients has been linked to an increased incidence of strokes and cardiac events.[43–45] An additional consideration is that there has been a shift toward doing more procedures, even on seriously ill patients, outside of a hospital setting. There has also been a plethora of better hemostatic agents that have been developed for local control of bleeding that have enabled this move.[31,46] To better understand these agents and the mechanism of action, it is important to review the coagulation cascade and how different medications affect the various reactions (see **Fig. 1**).

HEMOSTATIC AGENTS FOR LOCAL USE
Cellulose (Surgicel, Ethicon, Somerville, NJ; ActCel Coreva, Westlake Village, CA)

Oxidized cellulose provides an absorbable physical matrix for clotting initiation. This compound has a low pH and may cause inflammation and necrosis.

Gelatin Foams (Gelfoam, Pfizer, New York, NY; Surgifoam, Ethicon, Somerville, NJ)

Gelatin foams provide a clotting framework and effectively arrest small-vessel bleeding. Larger arterial bleeds may dislodge the foam. It is manufactured as a film, sponge, or powder that is mixed to form a paste. The use of gelatin foams in minor oral surgeries, in particular dental extractions, has been shown to reduce postoperative bleeding.[47]

Ostene (Ceremed Inc, Los Angeles, CA)

This is a bone waxlike preparation of water-soluble alkylene oxide copolymers. It is inert and eliminated from the body unchanged within 48 hours. Because of its elimination from the body, it is not associated with lack of osseous union, infections, or inflammatory reactions.

HemCon Dental Dressing (HemCon Medical Technologies Inc, Portland, OR)

This substance is made from chitosan, which is an N-acetyl glucosamine polysaccharide derived from the chitin in shrimp shells. It is in a sponge form and is hemostatic and also bacteriostatic.

Microfibrillar Collagen (Avitene Davol, Warwick, UK; Instat Ethicon 360, Somerville, NJ)

Microfibrillar collagen is a hemostatic agent that attracts platelets that adhere to its fibrils and undergo activation. This triggers aggregation of the platelets into thrombi in the interstices of the fibrous mass, initiating the formation of a physiologic platelet plug.

Sutures

Suturing allows for approximation of edges and local compression as a means of achieving hemostasis. The figure of 8 suture (**Fig. 3**) technique can be used when there is no obvious vessel to tie at the site of soft tissue bleeds.

Hemostatic Solutions

Styptics are locally applied agents that stop bleeding by contracting tissue to seal injured blood vessels. Aluminum solutions are an example of these.

Tannic Acid

Tannic acid is a commercial compound that is similar to the plant polyphenol tannin, which is a well-established hemostatic agent that effectively stops bleeding from mucous membranes via vasoconstriction.

Tranexamic Acid 4.8% Oral Rinse

Tranexamic acid 4.8% oral rinse is an antifibrinolytic agent that stabilizes clots and facilitates clot formation by competitively inhibiting plasminogen, the enzyme responsible for activating plasmin. The main role of plasmin in the body is clot degradation or fibrinolysis, hence tranexamic acid noncompetitively inhibits plasmin and stabilizes clot formation. Oral tranexamic acid has been shown to be beneficial in the management of patients with both inherited and acquired bleeding diatheses undergoing minor oral surgeries.[48–52] It can also be useful as a prophylactic mouthwash in patients who are on anticoagulant medications who require oral surgery.

Fibrin Glue

Made up of fibrinogen and thrombin, fibrin glue makes a fibrin clot where applied to arrest bleeding.

SURGICAL CONSIDERATIONS

The surgical procedures that can be safely performed on patients on OAT or other congenital hematologic conditions[53–56] range from minor oral surgery, such as simple and surgical extractions, deep scaling, apicoectomy, small biopsies, periodontal surgery, and dental implants, to major surgery, such as resection of tumors, repair of facial fractures, jaw osteotomies, and craniofacial surgery.[11,36–40] The critical decision that has to be made is to use the appropriate method for each patient based on risk profile and the surgery that is required. Another important factor is to classify the extent of surgery that is contemplated. We have proposed a list that has a wide variety of procedures, grouped into 4 categories, but is short enough to aid in this endeavor (**Table 4**).

Consideration should be given to reduce the extent of surgery for patients who have to be maintained on full OAT and who are at high risk for thromboembolism, as these patients will have an increased tendency to bleed if surgery is prolonged.[12,57]

Ward and Smith,[58] in a survey of Michigan oral surgeons, proposed a risk stratification based on extent of surgery as it relates to dentoalveolar surgery only, ranging from low risk to high risk. Low risk consisted of 1 to 5 simple extractions; moderate risk was 6 to 10 simple extractions or 1 impacted tooth or alveolectomy for one quadrant; high risk was more than 10 simple extractions or 2 or more impacted teeth or alveolectomy for 2 or more quadrants or tori removal.

Most of the respondents maintained OAT for low and moderate surgical-risk categories.[58] The other categories were subjected to some form of cessation or decrease in dosage of their warfarin intake. Morimoto and colleagues,[43] in a study involving 382 patients on OAT who had different types of extractions by one surgeon, reported a 3.9 % postsurgical hemorrhage rate. The bleeding was controlled mainly by local measures, but some patients had a decrease in warfarin dosage and administration of vitamin K to enable final control. A further significant finding was the statistically significant increase in bleeding complications in patients who had surgical extractions and those who had infections at the time of surgery. This and other studies further reinforce the importance of proper preoperative surgical risk assessment for patients who have surgery while on maintenance therapy.[3,7,35,58–61]

Surgery, when performed, should be as atraumatic as possible, being careful to handle the tissues gently and to place sutures appropriately. Figure of 8 sutures should be considered for extraction sites even when adherent type hemostatic agents such as HemoCon dental dressing is used.[34] A variety of local hemostatic agents, such as gelfoam or surgicel, and hemostatic liquids should be available. The presence of an electrocautery machine along with the ability to fabricate an acrylic splint to place over the bleeding area is advisable. Granulation tissue in extraction sockets should be removed before placement of hemostatic agents, as the granulation tissue is a frequent source of postextraction bleeding. It is imperative that the postoperative medications that are given to patients do not in the short term potentiate the anticoagulant effects of warfarin. Some medications that are known to do this are the NSAIDs and to a lesser extent the cyclo-oxygenase (COX)-2 inhibitors. There are also certain antibiotics, such as macrolide antibiotics and metronidazole, that are

Table 4
Surgical risk stratification for patients taking anticoagulants

Category	Surgical Risk	Procedures
1	Low	<5 simple extractions, soft tissue biopsy <1 cm in size
2	Intermediate	5–10 simple extractions, soft tissue biopsy 1.0–2.5 cm, simple implant placement
3	Moderate	Impacted wisdom teeth, >10 simple extractions, full mouth extractions, removal of tori, multiple implant placement, osseous biopsy, alveolectomy/alveoplasty
4	High	Repair of facial fractures, facial osteotomies, bone grafts

known to enhance the effects of warfarin. These also should not be prescribed postoperatively. See **Table 2.**

Finally, close extended postprocedure monitoring is vital. There should be no hesitation to seek specialist help once postoperative bleeding occurs.

DISCUSSION

Numerous reports and reviews continue to be published extolling the safety of doing minor oral surgery without altering the dose of oral anticoagulants that patients are placed on by their physicians. Despite these studies, several published surveys reveal that a significant segment of medical and dental clinicians still persist in recommending short-term withdrawal of oral anticoagulant and antiplatelet medications before limited dentoalveolar surgery.[3,35,58] This puts the patient at increased risk of suffering a thromboembolic episode. This reticence is probably in part attributable to other studies that document increased perioperative and postoperative bleeding in patients having major abdominal, thoracic, cardiac, orthopedic, and neurosurgical procedures.

There is a marked difference, however, between minor oral surgery and major surgery that is not factored in when the findings of these studies are extrapolated. Minor dentoalveolar surgery involves anatomic sites that are usually bordered by osseous margins on at least 2 sides and maybe as much as 5, rendering them more amenable to pressure and placement of hemostatic agents. There are fewer adjacent soft tissue sites that can be a further source of bleeding. There are no large closed off cavities, like what exists in the abdomen, chest, or brain, that can sequester large amounts of collecting blood. The oral cavity is also readily accessible for monitoring by the patient and their clinician, allowing earlier detection of excessive bleeding. All of these factors allow for effective local control of bleeding from minor dentoalveolar surgery.[62-64]

However, postoperative bleeding can be a significant management problem and source of inconvenience for the patient, even if it is not life threatening. In fact, some studies document postoperative bleeding after minor oral surgery occurring up to 10 days after surgery.[41] Therefore, we think that a more tailored approach based on the individual patient is more prudent.

The area of antithrombotic therapy is constantly evolving. There are newer medications that are being tested that will be more advantageous for bridge therapy than the current medications.[23,40] There are also a variety of new and novel hemostatic agents that have been put on the market and some that are still in the early stages of clinical trials that will revolutionize this area.[31,65]

In a recent article, Ansell[41] outlined a variety of new oral antithrombotic agents that perform their actions in a manner different from warfarin. Specifically, they block the formation of factors IIa and Xa and are called oral antithrombins. Many are currently in phase III trials. There are others, such as the oral direct antithrombin drug, dabigatran etexilate (Pradaxa, Boehringer Ingelheim, Ridgefield CT, USA), that are currently in use for patients with atrial fibrillation. Dabigatran etexilate has been shown to be very effective in reducing the incidence of stroke in these patients.

The main advantages of this class of drugs, however, are the rapid onset of action, relative short duration compared with warfarin, predictable therapeutic efficacy, and vastly reduced medication interactions. These drugs also do not need to be monitored via different laboratory tests like PT and INR, hence they have a much greater safety profile.[57] If these and other similar medications fulfill their promise, then it will be a simple task to manage patients on oral anticoagulation therapy when they require oral surgical procedures.

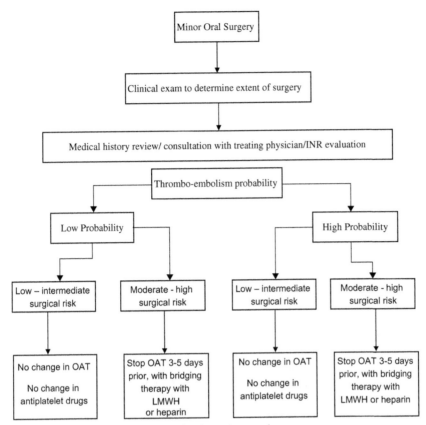

Fig. 4. Algorithm for patients on OAT having minor oral surgery.

SUMMARY

The surgical management of patients on oral anticoagulant therapy remains a challenging area for dentists. This is so because dental practitioners, who are not usually faced with life-threatening decisions on a regular basis, confront that very situation whenever these patients present for treatment. The line of demarcation between a good outcome and potential disaster is quite thin. The literature has diverse views on the management of these patients and there are few large-scale, truly randomized prospective studies in our literature on this topic.

We have therefore outlined our perspective on this topic, and have put forth strategies that have worked in our institution and that are generally supported by the latest studies. Specifically, that patients must first be assessed by their primary physician and dentist to determine their thromboembolic risk. Then their surgical needs should be evaluated and stratified. Once this is done, then a joint treatment plan based on our algorithm (**Fig. 4**) but tailored to suit the individual patient is developed and performed. Proper follow-up and back-up facilities should be in place. Patients who are at moderate to high risk of thromboembolism and patients who require moderate to high levels of surgical intervention should be referred to an oral and maxillofacial surgeon.

The basis of prudent management for these patients, however, remains rooted on the 5 planks listed earlier: (1) status of their medical condition, (2) proper laboratory assessment of their coagulation profile before surgery, (3) accurate categorization of their thromboembolic profile, (4) appropriate surgical risk stratification and effective local control, and (5) close extended postoperative monitoring.

REFERENCES

1. Nematullah A, Alabousi A, Blanas N, et al. Dental surgery for patients on antico-agulant therapy with warfarin: a systematic review and meta-analysis. J Can Dent Assoc 2009;75(1):41 a-41i.
2. Blinder D, Manor Y, Martinowitz U, et al. Dental extractions in patients maintained on oral anticoagulant therapy: comparison of INR value with occurrence of post-operative bleeding. Int J Oral Maxillofac Surg 2001;30:518.
3. Todd DW. Anticoagulant therapy: consideration of modification in conjunction with minor surgery. J Oral Maxillofac Surg 2003;61:1117–8.
4. Ansell JE. The perioperative management of warfarin therapy. Arch Intern Med 2003;163:881–3.
5. Bajkin BV, Todorovic LM. Safety of local anaesthesia in dental patients taking oral anticoagulants: is it still controversial? Br J Oral Maxillofac Surg 2010 Dec 2. DOI:10.1016/j.bjoms.2010.11.002.
6. Al-Mubarak S, Ali N, Rass M, et al. Evaluation of dental extractions, suturing and INR on postoperative bleeding of patients maintained on oral anticoagulant therapy. Br Dent J 2007;203:E15.
7. Wahl MJ. Dental surgery in anticoagulated patients. Arch Intern Med 1998;158: 1610–6.
8. Smith NL, Psaty BM, Furberg CD, et al. Temporal trends in the use of anticoagu-lants among older adults with atrial fibrillation. Arch Intern Med 1999;159:1574–8.
9. Ruigómeza A, Johanssonbc S, Wallanderbd M, et al. Incidence of chronic atrial fibrillation in general practice and its treatment pattern. J Clin Epidemiol 2002;55: 358–63.
10. Waldrep AC Jr, McKelvey LE. Oral surgery for patients on anticoagulant therapy. J Oral Surg 1968;26:374–80.
11. Mehta DK. Dental surgery in the anticoagulated patient. Br Dent J 2003;194:530.
12. Dunn AS, Turpie AG. Perioperative management of patients receiving oral antico-agulants: a systematic review. Arch Intern Med 2003;163(8):901–8.
13. Thomas S, Katbab H, abu Fanas SH. Do preoperative cutaneous bleeding time tests predict the outcome of intraoral surgical bleeding? Int Dent J 2010;60:305–10.
14. Greenberg MS, Miller MF, Lynch MA. Partial thromboplastin time as a predictor of blood loss in oral surgery patients receiving coumarin anticoagulants. J Am Dent Assoc 1972;84:583–7.
15. McBane RD II, Felty CL, Hartgers ML, et al. Importance of device evaluation for point of care prothrombin time international normalized ratio testing programs. Mayo Clin Proc 2005;80:181–6.
16. Raber N. Coagulation tests. In: Walker HK, Hall WD, Hurst JW, editors. Clinical methods: the history, physical, and laboratory examinations. 3rd edition. Boston: Butterworths; 1990. p. 739–42.
17. Kuijer P, Hutten BA, Prins MH, et al. Prediction of the risk of bleeding during anti-coagulant treatment for venous thromboembolism. Arch Intern Med 1999;159: 457–60.
18. Lip GY, Frison L, Halperin JL, et al. Comparative validation of a novel risk score for predicting bleeding risk in anticoagulated patients with atrial fibrillation. J Am Coll Cardiol 2011;57:173–80.

19. Pisters R, Lane DA, Nieuwlaat R, et al. A novel user-friendly score (HAS-BLED) to assess 1-year risk of major bleeding in patients with atrial fibrillation. Chest 2010; 138:1093–100.
20. Berman F. Herb-drug interactions. Lancet 2000;355:134–8.
21. Mar C, Bent S. An evidence-based review of the 10 most commonly used herbs. West J Med 1999;17:168–71.
22. Fareed J, Adiguzel C, Thethi I. Differentiation of parenteral anticoagulants in the prevention and treatment of venous thromboembolism. Thromb J 2011;9(1):5. DOI:10.1186/1477-9560-9-5.
23. Hirsh J, Shaughnessy SG, Halperin JL, et al. Heparin and low-molecular-weight heparin mechanisms of action, pharmacokinetics, dosing, monitoring, efficacy, and safety. Chest 2001;119:64S–94S.
24. Bauer K. New anticoagulants. Curr Opin Hematol 2008;15:509–15.
25. Madan G, Madan S, Madan G, et al. Minor oral surgery without stopping daily low-dose aspirin therapy: a study of 51 patients. J Oral Maxillofac Surg 2005; 63:1262–5.
26. Partridge CG, Campbell JH, Alvarado F. The effect of platelet-altering medications on bleeding from minor oral surgery procedures. J Oral Maxillofac Surg 2008;66:93–7.
27. Krysiak R, Zmuda W, Okopień B. The effect of ezetimibe and simvastatin on hemostasis in patients with isolated hypercholesterolemia. Fundam Clin Pharmacol 2011. DOI:10.1111/j.1472-8206.2011.00932.x.
28. Wahl MJ. Myths of dental surgery in patients receiving anticoagulant therapy. J Am Dent Assoc 2000;131:77–81.
29. Hirsh J, Fuster V, Ansel J, et al. American Heart Association/ American College of Cardiology Foundation guide to warfarin therapy. Circulation 2003;107: 1692–711.
30. Baglin TP, Keeling DM, Watson HG. Guidelines on oral anticoagulation. Br J Haematol 2006;132:277–85.
31. Kearon C, Kahn SR, Agnelli G, et al. Antithrombotic therapy for venous thromboembolic disease: American College of Chest Physicians evidence-based clinical practice guidelines (8th edition). Chest 2008;133:454S–545S.
32. Marietta M, Bertesi M, Simoni L, et al. A simple and safe nomogram for the management of oral anticoagulation prior to minor surgery. Clin Lab Haematol 2003;25:127–30.
33. Milligan PE, Banet GA, Gage BF. Perioperative reduction of the warfarin dose. Am J Med 2003;115:741–2.
34. Malmquist JP, Clemens SC, Oien HJ, et al. Hemostasis of oral surgery wounds with the HemCon dental dressing. J Oral Maxillofac Surg 2008;66:1177–83.
35. Todd DW. Anticoagulated patients and oral surgery. Arch Intern Med 2003;163: 1242.
36. Gibbons AJ, Evans IL, Sayers MS, et al. Warfarin and extractions. Br Dent J 2002; 193:302.
37. Gibbons AJ, Sugar AW. Evidence for continuing warfarin during dental extractions. Br Dent J 2003;194:65.
38. Balderston RH. Warfarin and extraction. Br Dent J 2003;194:408–9.
39. Brown AE. Warfarin and extractions. Br Dent J 2002;193:668.
40. Gibbons AJ, Sugar AW. Can warfarin be continued during dental extraction? Results of a randomized controlled trial. Br J Oral Maxillofac Surg 2003;41:280.
41. Ansell J. Issues in thrombosis management and anticoagulation: warfarin versus new agents: interpreting the data. Hematology 2010;2010:221–8.

42. Johnson-Leong C, Rada RE. The use of low-molecular-weight heparins in outpatient oral surgery for patients receiving anticoagulation therapy. J Am Dent Assoc 2002;133:1083–7.

43. Morimoto Y, Niwa H, Minematsu K. Risk factors affecting postoperative hemorrhage after tooth extraction in patients receiving oral antithrombotic therapy. J Oral Maxillofac Surg 2011;69:1550–6.

44. Roser SM, Rosenbloom B. Continued anticoagulation in oral surgery procedures. Oral Surg Oral Med Oral Pathol 1975;40:448–57.

45. Aldridge E, Cunningham LL Jr. Current thoughts on treatment of patients receiving anticoagulation therapy. J Oral Maxillofac Surg 2010;68:2879–87.

46. Al-Belasy FA, Amer MZ. Hemostatic effect of n-butyl-2-cyanoacrylate (histoacryl) glue in warfarin treated patients undergoing oral surgery. J Oral Maxillofac Surg 2003;61:1405–9.

47. Kim JC, Choi SS, Wang SJ, et al. Minor complications after mandibular third molar surgery: type, incidence, and possible prevention. Oral Surg Oral Med Oral Pathol Oral Radiol Endod 2006;102:4–11.

48. Borea G, Montebugnoli L, Capuzzi P, et al. Tranexamic acid as a mouthwash in anticoagulant-treated patients undergoing oral surgery. An alternative method to discontinuing anticoagulant therapy. Oral Surg Oral Med Oral Pathol 1993;75:29–31.

49. Carter G, Goss A. Tranexamic acid mouthwash—a prospective randomized study of a 2-day regimen vs 5-day regimen to prevent postoperative bleeding in anticoagulated patients requiring dental extractions. Int J Oral Maxillofac Surg 2003;32:504–7.

50. Sindet-Pedersen S, Ramstrom G, Bernvil S, et al. Hemostatic effect of tranexamic acid mouthwash in anticoagulant-treated patients undergoing oral surgery. N Engl J Med 1989;320:840–3.

51. Carter G, Goss A, Lloyd J, et al. Tranexamic acid mouthwash versus autologous fibrin glue in patients taking warfarin undergoing dental extraction: a randomized prospective clinical study. J Oral Maxillofac Surg 2003;62:1432–5.

52. Kaewpradub P, Apipan B, Rummasak D. Does tranexamic acid in an irrigating fluid reduce intraoperative blood loss in orthognathic surgery: a double blind randomized clinical trial. J Oral Maxillofac Surg 2011;69:186–9.

53. Brewer AK. Advances in minor oral surgery in patients with congenital bleeding disorders. Haemophilia 2008;14:119–21.

54. Kaddour Brahim A, Stieltjes N, Roussel-Robert V, et al. Dental extractions in children with congenital coagulation disorders: therapeutic protocol and results. Rev Stomatol Chir Maxillofac 2006;107:331–7.

55. Mokhtari H, Roosendaal G, Koole R, et al. Oral surgery in hemophilia patients. Ned Tijdschr Tandheelkd 2003;110:74–7.

56. Zanon E, Martinelli F, Bacci C, et al. Proposal of a standard approach to dental extraction in haemophilia patients. A case-control study with good results. Haemophilia 2000;6:533–6.

57. Campbell JH, Alvarado F, Murray RA. Anticoagulation and minor oral surgery: should the anticoagulation regimen be altered? J Oral Maxillofac Surg 2000;58:131–5.

58. Ward B, Smith M. Dentoalveolar procedures for the anticoagulated patient: literature recommendations versus current practice. J Oral Maxillofac Surg 2007;65:1454–60.

59. Carter G, Goss AN, Lloyd J, et al. Current concepts of the management of dental extractions for patients taking warfarin. Aust Dent J 2003;48:89–96.

60. Thomas S, Jeske AH, Suchko GD. Lack of scientific basis for routine discontinuation of oral anticoagulation therapy before dental treatment. J Am Dent Assoc 2003;134:1492–7.
61. Lloyd RE. Dental surgery in the anticoagulated patient. Br Dent J 2003;194:530.
62. Della Valle A, Sammartino G, Marenzi G, et al. Prevention of postoperative bleeding in anticoagulated patients undergoing oral surgery: use of platelet-rich plasma gel. J Oral Maxillofac Surg 2003;61:1275–8.
63. Muthukrishnan A, Bishop K. An assessment of the management of patients on warfarin by general dental practitioners in South West Wales. Br Dent J 2003; 195:567–70.
64. Webster K, Wilde J. Management of anticoagulation in patients with prosthetic heart valves undergoing oral and maxillofacial operations. Br J Oral Maxillofac Surg 2000;38:124–6.
65. Muthukrishnan A. Re: Webster K, Wilde J. Management of anticoagulation in patients with prosthetic heart valves undergoing oral and maxillofacial operations. Br J Oral Maxillofac Surg 2002;40:226.

Biopsy Techniques and Diagnoses & Treatment of Mucocutaneous Lesions

Michael H. Chan, DDS[a,b,*], Joshua C. Wolf, DDS[b]

KEYWORDS

- Biopsy • Mucocutaneous • Vesiculobullous
- Immune-based lesions • Treatment

Oral mucosal lesions are commonly encountered in clinical practice. A study conducted in the United States reported that they occurred in approximately 27.9% of patients aged 17 years and older[1] and in 10.3% of children aged 2 to 17 years.[2] The diagnosis and treatment of mucosal diseases should be an integral part of the general practitioner's practice. According to an American Dental (ADA) survey conducted in 2007, of 315,210 biopsies, 138,810 (44%) were performed by a general practitioner.[3] Understanding of the fundamentals of diagnosing mucocutaneous lesions requires a sound knowledge of its origin and clinical course, and of biopsy methods using contemporary diagnostic tools and techniques.

APPROACH TO LESIONS

A through systematic approach should be sought for every oral lesion, with the chief complaint as the starting point of the investigation.

Health History

A complete medical history should be obtained for all patients before performing an examination. An existing systemic condition can contribute to the cause of the lesion.

The authors have nothing to disclose.

[a] Oral & Maxillofacial Surgery/Dental Service, Department of Veterans Affairs, New York Harbor Healthcare Systems (Brooklyn Campus), 800 Poly Place (Bk-160), Brooklyn, NY 11209, USA
[b] Department of Oral and Maxillofacial Surgery, The Brooklyn Hospital Center, 121 DeKalb Avenue, Box 187, Brooklyn, NY 11201, USA
* Corresponding author. Oral & Maxillofacial Surgery/Dental Service, Department of Veterans Affairs, New York Harbor Healthcare Systems (Brooklyn Campus), 800 Poly Place (Bk-160), Brooklyn, NY 11209.
E-mail address: Michael.chan2@va.gov

Dent Clin N Am 56 (2012) 43–73
doi:10.1016/j.cden.2011.09.004
0011-8532/12/$ – see front matter Published by Elsevier Inc.

dental.theclinics.com

For instance, does the patient have lupus erythematosus, a sexually transmitted disease, tuberculosis, or an immune-compromised condition [eg, HIV, AIDS, leukemia], is the patient currently undergoing chemotherapy treatment, or has the patient been prescribed any new medications by another provider that may be causing a lichenoid reaction. Social history is particularly important if the patient has a smoking, alcohol, or beetle quid habit, because these are well-known carcinogens.

Lesion History

The focus of the examination should then shift to the history of the lesion. The usual initial questions are how long has the lesion been present, was it noticed by the patient or during a routine oral screening, has the lesion changed in size, and is any associated paresthesia present. A benign lesion usually has a slower growth as opposed to one that is malignant, which is more aggressive and has associated paresthesia. Patients should be asked if any associated symptoms are present, such as pain, fever, headaches, chills, or lymphadenopathy, and whether the characteristics of the lesion changed (eg, did the ulcer start as crops of vesicles or was it always an ulcer). A change in its features would highly suggest vesiculobullous disease or a disease of viral origin. Furthermore, did any recent memorable events lead up to discovery of the lesion (eg, trauma, local irritant, exposure to allergens). For instance, if the lesion was caused by a sharp cup rubbing against the tongue, it would be best remedied by smoothing the offending origin, with an appropriate follow-up to determine if the lesion needs further investigation.

Clinical Examination

An understanding of the normal anatomy will help the general practitioner differentiate between normal mucosa and an oral lesion. The general practitioner should be able to describe the presentation of the lesion in terms of location, size, shape, growth pattern, the sharpness of lesion borders, mobility, and consistency of the lesion on palpation. The general practitioner must also be aware of the possibility of two or more different lesions or one lesion with different presentation. A head and neck examination with lymph node inspection is *mandatory* before any oral biopsy. Lymphadenopathy can result from the surgical biopsy itself and can be confusing if TMN cancer staging were deemed necessary in the future.

With the information gathered during the history and physical examination, the general practitioner can develop a working differential diagnosis. Developing a differential diagnosis helps the general practitioner in using certain biopsy techniques and diagnostic tools that can facilitate a correct diagnosis. This article addresses mucocutaneous lesions that will be encountered in the dental practice.

MUCOCUTANEOUS DISEASES
Primary Herpetic Gingivostomatitis and Recurrent Herpes Lesions (Labialis or Stomatitis)

Two strains of herpes simplex viruses (HSV) exist. HSV-1 is usually responsible for perioral/orofacial infections and HSV-2 for genital infections. Two clinical manifestations of HSV-1 can occur: primary herpetic gingivostomatitis and recurrent herpetic-lesion labialis (lips) or stomatitis (intraoral). The route of transmission is through infected saliva, active perioral lesions, and sores on skin. Transmission easily occurs through intimate contact, kissing, sharing eating utensils, and toothbrushes. Only 1% of the population that gets the primary infection develops full-blown symptoms. This condition is called *primary herpetic gingivostomatitis*. The other 60% to 90% of children and young adults seroconvert to HSV antibodies without any clinical symptoms.[4]

After a period of incubation (usually 7 days), patients can experience a variety of symptoms, including headaches, irritability, muscle soreness (myalgia), pain on swallowing, fever, and painful lymphadenopathy. Crops of vesicles appear and rupture within 24 hours and then coalesce to form ulcers in the oral mucosa involving the gingiva (keratinized and nonkeratinized), tongue, and lips (**Fig. 1**). New lesions can continue to develop up to 7 more days and usually heal without scarring within 3 weeks.

After the primary HSV infection, the virus lays dormant in a regional nerve ganglion (ie, trigeminal ganglion) until a stimulus triggers it to cause a secondary or recurrent infection. This stimulus may be sunlight (sun sores), physical or emotional stress, hormonal changes (menstrual cycle), preceding upper respiratory infection (fever blister or cold sores), or suppression of the immune system (caused by HIV, AIDS, or current chemotherapy). The two clinical manifestations include the labialis and stomatitis. Herpes labialis is the more common of the two recurrent HSV infections. The clinical course starts with a tingling or itching sensation (prodrome phase) after which these crops of vesicles will coalesce and rupture within 48 hours. It proceeds to ulcerate, leaving behind a crusted brownish lesion on the lip (**Fig. 2**). The intraoral component (stomatitis) appears on keratinized gingiva (ie, hard palate or attached gingiva) and the tongue. The commonest region is the posterior hard palate over the greater palatine foramen (**Fig. 3**).[5] Unlike herpes labialis, these intraoral herpes seldom form vesicles, and proceed to ulcerate, leaving behind an erythematous macular base. Both clinical forms heal without scarring within 7 to 10 days.

Recurrent Aphthous Stomatitis

Recurrent aphthous stomatitis (RAS) affects 20% of the population worldwide between ages 10 and 30 years, with 50% being college students.[4] It occurs more common in women than men. The clinical signs and symptoms can include a tingling

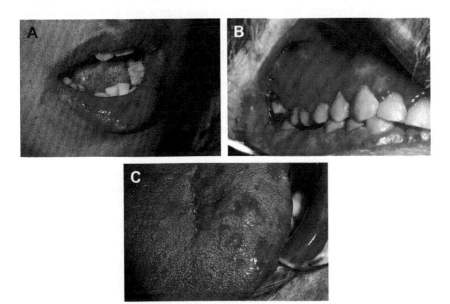

Fig. 1. Acute primary herpetic gingivostomatitis. Multiple shallow punctate lesions on both keratinizing and gland-bearing mucosa. (*A*) Lower lip, (*B*) gingiva, and (*C*) tongue. (*From* Sapp JP, Eversole LR, Wysocki GP. Contemporary oral and maxillofacial pathology. 2nd edition. Mosby; 2004. p. 210; with permission.)

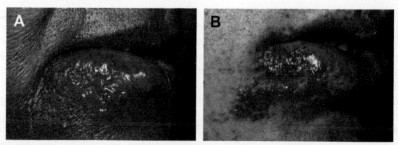

Fig. 2. Recurrent herpes labialis. (A) Early stages consisting of fluid-filled viral vesicles. (B) Late stage showing brownish crusted lesions. (From Sapp JP, Eversole LR, Wysocki GP. Contemporary oral and maxillofacial pathology. 2nd edition. Mosby; 2004. p. 211; with permission.)

or burning sensation, a well-delineated white ulcer with erythematous halo, and the absence of a vesicular stage. Although the cause of RAS is still unknown, local and systemic predisposing factors can contribute to its development. Local injuries to the oral mucosa, such as from trauma or tobacco smoke, can be offending agents. Systemic diseases, such as Behçet's disease, MAGIC (mouth and genital ulcers with inflamed cartilage) syndrome, PFAPA (periodic fever, aphthous-stomatitis, pharyngitis, adenitis) syndrome, cyclic neutropenia, HIV disease, and hematologic deficiencies (eg, iron, folic acid, vitamin B_{12}), could produce aphthous-like ulcerations in the oral cavity.[6]

Three forms of RAS exist: (1) minor (canker sore), (2) major (Sutton disease, periadenitis mucosa necrotica recurrens), and (3) herpetiform ulcerations.[6]

The minor form (canker sore) is the most common form of RASs, accounting for 80% of patients. Typically, these lesions are less than 5 mm in diameter, round, or oval-shaped with a grayish-white pseudomembrane and an erythematous halo. They appear on nonkeratinized surfaces on labial and buccal mucosa, the floor of the mouth, movable gingiva, the palate, and the dorsum of tongue (**Fig. 4**). The lesions heal in 10 to 14 days uneventfully.

The major form affects 10% of the patients with RAS. The lesions are greater than 1.0 cm in diameter. They tend to locate on the lips, soft palate, and fauces (**Fig. 5**). They last longer than the minor form and heal without scarring in 6 weeks. Major RAS has its onset after puberty and can persist for 20 years or more.[7]

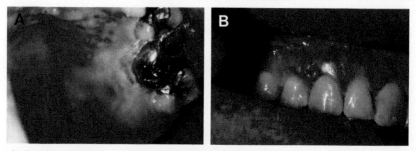

Fig. 3. Recurrent intraoral herpes. (A) Common intraoral site on posterior palate over greater palatine foramina. (B) Occasionally encountered gingival lesions. (From Sapp JP, Eversole LR, Wysocki GP. Contemporary oral and maxillofacial pathology. 2nd edition. Mosby; 2004. p. 211; with permission.)

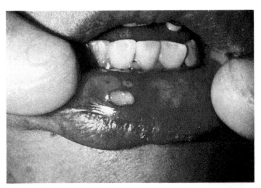

Fig. 4. Minor RAS. Lesions are shallow crateriform ulcers with a whitish-yellow base and an erythematous halo. (*From* Sapp JP, Eversole LR, Wysocki GP. Contemporary oral and maxillofacial pathology. 2nd edition. Mosby; 2004. p. 254; with permission.)

Herpetiform ulcerations present in 1% to 10% of patients with RAS. The lesions are usually 2 to 3 mm in diameter, with 100 ulcers appearing at a time. They can congregate into large lesions or diffuse throughout the oral cavity (**Fig. 6**).

Lichen Planus

Lichen planus (LP) is a chronic mucocutaneous disease of unknown origin. It generally develops in patients between 40 and 70 years old, with a predilection for women (2:1).[8] It affects the oral mucosa, tongue, and skin. The skin lesions occur on the flexor surface of the extremities with the four Ps (purple, pruritic, polygonal papules) (**Fig. 7**).[9] Although oral LP is prevalent in 2% of the population, skin lesions show along side with oral lesions in 12% to 14% of the time.[10] Oral LP can be classified into two types: reticular (reticular, plaque-like) and erosive (atrophic, bullous, ulcerative) (**Fig. 8**).[11] Reticular LP is much more common than the erosive form, with a higher predilection for buccal mucosa (bilateral 85% of the time), the dorsum surface of tongue, and attached gingiva. The reticular form is asymptomatic. It gets its name because of the interlacing white lines patterns known as Wickham striae (**Fig. 9**). These lesions wax and wane over weeks and months. However, the erosive type can have a long painful clinical course. Clinically, atrophic and erythematous areas are present, with central ulceration of

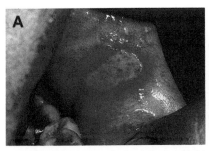
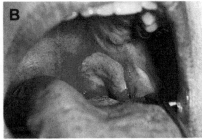

Fig. 5. Major RAS. Large shallow ulcers of labial mucosa (*A*) and lateral soft palate (*B*). Lesions are painful and exhibit characteristic erythematous halo. (*From* Sapp JP, Eversole LR, Wysocki GP. Contemporary oral and maxillofacial pathology. 2nd edition. Mosby; 2004. p. 255; with permission.)

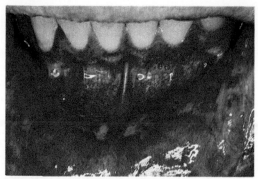

Fig. 6. Herpetiform (aphthous) ulcers. Clusters of small shallow aphthous ulcers of the labial mucosa that resemble lesions of a herpes simplex infection. (*From* Sapp JP, Eversole LR, Wysocki GP. Contemporary oral and maxillofacial pathology. 2nd edition. Mosby; 2004. p. 256; with permission.)

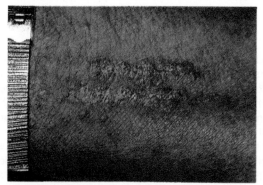

Fig. 7. LP. Papular skin lesions distributed in a linear pattern on the flexor surface of the wrist. (*From* Sapp JP, Eversole LR, Wysocki GP. Contemporary oral and maxillofacial pathology. 2nd edition. Mosby; 2004. p. 259; with permission.)

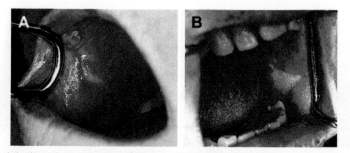

Fig. 8. LP. (*A*) Clinical appearance of the symptomatic erosive form of the disease on the buccal mucosa, exhibiting a large area of erosion against an erythematous background. (*B*) Plaque form of LP on the buccal mucosa. (*From* Sapp JP, Eversole LR, Wysocki GP. Contemporary oral and maxillofacial pathology. 2nd edition. Mosby; 2004. p. 258; with permission.)

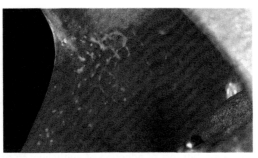

Fig. 9. LP. Clinical appearance of the lacework pattern of the reticular form of the disease. (*From* Sapp JP, Eversole LR, Wysocki GP. Contemporary oral and maxillofacial pathology. 2nd edition. Mosby; 2004. p. 258; with permission.)

varying degrees. The periphery is usually bordered by fine, white, radiating striae. Sometimes the atrophy and ulceration are confined to the gingival mucosa, called *desquamative gingivitis*. If the erosive component is severe, epithelial separation from the underlying connective tissue may occur, followed by minor trauma. This rare presentation is known as *bullous lichen planus*. Controversy exists over the actual malignant transformation of erosive LP to squamous cell carcinoma (1.5%–2.5%).[4]

Mucous Membrane Pemphigoid

Mucous membrane pemphigoid (MMP) is an autoimmune disease that affects many mucosal surfaces, including oral, ocular, nasal, esophageal, laryngeal, pharyngeal, genital, and skin. Oral and ocular surfaces remain the most common sites. The mean age of onset is older than 40 years, with predilection for women (2:1). Oral manifestations include vesiculobullous eruptions, desquamative gingivitis, and ulcerations (**Fig. 10**). With gingiva being the most common site, these lesions begin as painful fluid-filled blisters that then slough off, leaving behind a denuded ulcerative base (**Fig. 11**). Epithelial sloughing with digital pressure or perilesional manipulation indicates a positive Nikolsky sign, and resembles the skin falling off of a sour grape. Healing may take days to weeks, and scarring is usually not seen. The ocular component

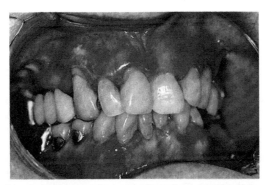

Fig. 10. MMP. Gingiva containing patchy areas of erythema and atrophy with loss of normal stippling. (*From* Sapp JP, Eversole LR, Wysocki GP. Contemporary oral and maxillofacial pathology. 2nd edition. Mosby; 2004. p. 16; with permission.)

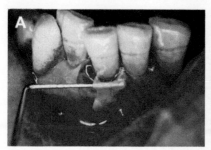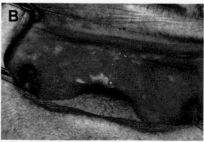

Fig. 11. MMP. (*A*) Gingiva exhibits loss of adhesion of epithelium to connective tissue. (*B*) Multiple diffuse areas of superficial erosions (*white*) against an erythematous background caused by mechanical forces of a denture on the fragile atrophic epithelium. (*From* Sapp JP, Eversole LR, Wysocki GP. Contemporary oral and maxillofacial pathology. 2nd edition. Mosby; 2004. p. 264; with permission.)

can progress to scarring, resulting in fusion of the eyelid and conjunctiva (symblepharon) (11%–61%). Poorly treated or untreated ocular lesions can ultimately lead to blindness.[12–14] Lesions on the laryngeal mucosa can also lead to severe scarring, resulting in stricture. Skin involvement is only a small component and is manifested in 0% to 11% of cases.[12–14] A proper referral to the ophthalmology; otolaryngology; urology; or dermatology department is necessary for proper care.

Pemphigus Vulgaris

Pemphigus vulgaris (PV) is an autoimmune disease involving the skin and mucous membrane that can be life-threatening. It affects a wide age range, from children to adults, with a predilection for people in their fourth to sixth decade. The condition is seen more often in individuals of Ashkenazi Jewish or Mediterranean descent. The overall incident is 0.1 to 0.5 patients per 100,000 population per year.[15]

The oral component of PV begins as a bulla formation, which will quickly rupture and leave behind a painful ulcerative base. The oral cavity is commonly the first site for PV development and can be found in the buccal mucosa, palatal mucosa, and lips (**Fig. 12**). Lesions confined in the oral cavity are not life-threatening, whereas cutaneous involvement is considerably more severe and fatal. Death is caused by septicemia or a fluid and electrolyte imbalance. Other mucous membranes may be affected, including the conjunctiva, nasal mucosa, pharynx, larynx, esophagus, and genital mucosa. Referral to a specialist is necessary for appropriate treatment. The clinical course has a rapid onset with a variable and unpredictable resolution.

Erythema Multiforme

Erythema multiforme (EM) is an acute immune-based inflammatory disease that affect both mucous membrane and skin (target lesion). The mucosal lesions include ocular, oral, and genital surfaces. EM seems to be a disease of children and young adults between 20 and 30 years of age. The origin is thought to be triggered by precipitating factors, such as infection, drugs, gastrointestinal conditions, malignancies, radiation therapy, or vaccination, with an explosive onset.

EM has two clinical forms, EM minor and EM major. EM minor more often affects the skin than the oral cavity (25%). The minor form can affect no more than one mucosal surface, with skin involvement. The minor form has a prodrome phase characterized by symptoms such as headache, fever, and malaise, followed by the formation of a papule or bulla that collapses to form "target lesions" (**Fig. 13**). The oral presentation

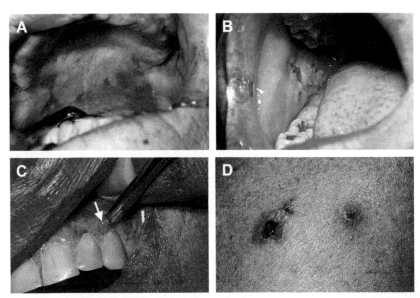

Fig. 12. PV. (A) Multiple erosive lesions of the soft palate. (*B*) Erosive lesions of the posterior buccal mucosa. (*C*) Blister formation (*arrow*) on normal-appearing gingiva after the movement of mirror handle under pressure, indicating positive Nikolsky sign. (*D*) Dry, crusted lesions on the skin. (*From* Sapp JP, Eversole LR, Wysocki GP. Contemporary oral and maxillofacial pathology. 2nd edition. Mosby; 2004. p. 267; with permission.)

of EM minor has the same characteristics, ranging from similar to aphthous-like ulcers to diffused erythematous erosion spots. The condition is self-limiting, with resolution in 2 to 3 weeks. A correlation of oral and cutaneous findings is needed to make the diagnosis. Tissue biopsy is not necessary to rule out this lesion; however, ruling out other vesiculobullous diseases may be helpful.

EM major is characterized by involvement of two or more mucosal surfaces and skin surfaces. The bulla develops and later pops, leaving a dark-red crusted lesion. EM major has two forms: (1) Stevens-Johnson syndrome and toxic epidermal necrolysis (TEN), or Lyell syndrome. The Stevens-Johnson syndrome is characterized by an

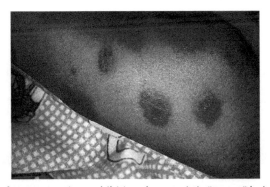

Fig. 13. EM. Skin of a young patient exhibiting characteristic "target" lesions. (*From* Sapp JP, Eversole LR, Wysocki GP. Contemporary oral and maxillofacial pathology. 2nd edition. Mosby; 2004. p. 271; with permission.)

extensive oral lesion commonly found in keratinized and nonkeratinized gingiva and bloody crusted lips (**Figs. 14** and **15**). Extraoral involvement includes ocular, esophageal, and genital surfaces. Scarring and partial blindness can result from ocular involvement. The mortality rate is 5% for Stevens-Johnsons syndrome. TEN is an even more extreme form of EM major, with a mortality rate as high as 30% to 35%.[5] The skin lesions are extensive and can resemble severe burns. Death occurs because of substantial loss of electrolytes and fluids, and widespread infection.

Lupus Erythematosus

Lupus erythematosus is a chronic inflammatory disease that targets the oral and cutaneous surfaces, and the end organs associated with circulating autoantibodies. Its origin is not fully understood, but it is thought to be caused by environmental, genetic, and hormonal factors. Three forms of lupus erythematosus exist: (1) discoid lupus erythematosus (DLE), (2) subacute cutaneous lupus erythematosus (SCLE), and (3) systemic lupus erythematosus (SLE). DLE is the mildest form and is confined to the cutaneous surface of the face; the scalp, with associated hair loss (alopecia); the ears, and occasionally the oral mucosa. The intermediate form is SCLE, which affects the head and neck and upper trunk, and extensor surfaces of the arm. Myalgia, arthralgia, fatigue, and malaise are common symptoms. The most severe and commonest form is SLE. These circulating autoantibodies target end organs, resulting in inflammation to the heart (pericarditis), lungs (pleurisy or pleural effusion), kidneys (lupus nephritis), and vasculature (vasculitis). Bone marrow with an anemia profile is present. The classic "butterfly rash" is found across the malar region (**Fig. 16**). The disease affects primarily women (9:1) during childbearing years, with an oral manifestation around 21%.[5]

The oral manifestation of lupus can have a variety of appearances, ranging from leukoplakia, to erythematous erosions, to chronic ulcerations. The leukoplakia lesions can be longstanding in the oral cavity without any symptoms. Patients will complain of burning mouth symptoms associated with the erythema and ulcerative conditions (**Fig. 17**).

BIOPSY/BIOPSY TECHNIQUES

Understanding the role of biopsy for oral mucocutaneous lesion will help general practitioners not only make a correct definitive diagnosis but also understand how to perform a biopsy that will be most beneficial for the pathologist (**Fig. 18**).

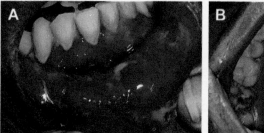
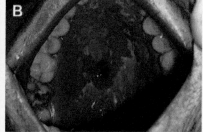

Fig. 14. Erythema multiforme. (*A*) Erosive lesions of the labial mucosa and gingiva. (*B*) Diffuse area of superficial sloughing and focal erosions of the palate. (*From* Sapp JP, Eversole LR, Wysocki GP. Contemporary oral and maxillofacial pathology. 2nd edition. Mosby; 2004. p. 272; with permission.)

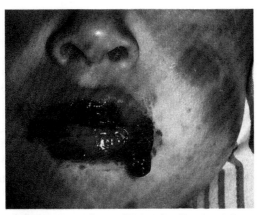

Fig. 15. Erythema multiforme. Acute form of EM major (Stevens-Johnson syndrome [SJS]) in 2-year-old male, exhibiting characteristic "target" lesions of the skin and hemorrhagic encrustations of the lips. (*From* Sapp JP, Eversole LR, Wysocki GP. Contemporary oral and maxillofacial pathology. 2nd edition. Mosby; 2004. p. 273; with permission.)

Indications

A biopsy involves obtaining tissue for histologic examination and definitive diagnosis. A biopsy is indicated for the following reasons:

> To rule out malignancy for any lip or oral lesion that persists for longer than 2 weeks after the exclusion of local irritants. If the lesion is a longstanding ulcer, some adjacent clinically normal epithelium should be included in the biopsy for comparison, and because the center of ulcers are usually necrotic tissue and have no diagnostic value.
> To evaluate any mucosa showing erythroplakia or leukoplakia, which may indicate a precancerous lesion. Lesions with erythroplakia or that are speckled with different appearances are now known to have a higher incidence of dysplasia

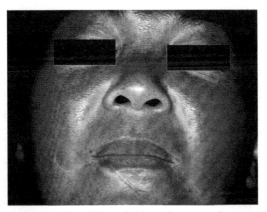

Fig. 16. Lupus erythematosus. Vasculitis and skin rash over malar areas of face ("butterfly rash") that intensify with exposure to sunlight are common in most forms of the disease. (*From* Sapp JP, Eversole LR, Wysocki GP. Contemporary oral and maxillofacial pathology. 2nd edition. Mosby; 2004. p. 275; with permission.)

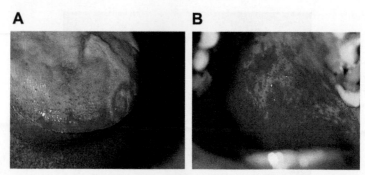

Fig. 17. Lupus erythematosus (LE). Patient with oral mucosal lesions of the tongue (*A*) and palate, consisting of diffuse and annular leukoplakic lesions, erythematous areas, and chronic ulcerations (*B*). Intraoral lesions are most frequently found in patients with the discoid form of LE but may be present to a lesser degree in all forms of the disease. (*From* Sapp JP, Eversole LR, Wysocki GP. Contemporary oral and maxillofacial pathology. 2nd edition. Mosby; 2004. p. 275; with permission.)

and should be the areas of biopsy. Multiple biopsies may be needed for large or multiple lesions.

To confirm a clinical diagnosis of LP or blistering lesions like pemphigus or pemphigoid. In a suspected LP lesion, sampling should be from a nonerosive area of the lesion, because the erosive areas will show nonspecific inflammatory changes and will not aid in the diagnosis. In the vesiculobullous lesions, the biopsy site should be adjacent to the bulla, where the epithelium is still intact. For these lesions, the laboratory should receive a fresh specimen in addition to a formalin one to allow for direct immunofluorescence.

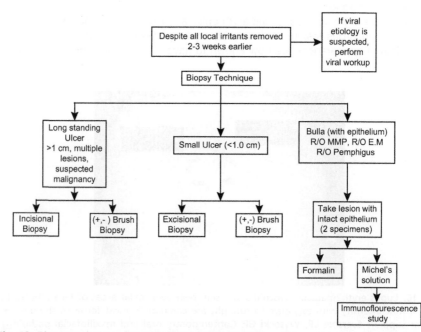

Fig. 18. Biopsy technique for oral mucocutaneous lesion.

Contraindications

Contraindications to biopsy exist in several instances:

- In seriously ill patients, in patients with systemic disorder that may worsen, or when secondary complications may develop postoperatively
- In areas that are difficult to access, where the surgery is difficult or hazardous because of the risk of injuring vital structures
- In cases of suspected vascular lesions or unstable coagulopathy, when an incisional biopsy should never be performed because of the risk of massive and persistent bleeding
- When the clinical diagnosis is a normal anatomic variant, such as physiologic gingival pigmentation, geographic tongue, linea alba, and fordyce granules.

Once the decision to biopsy is made, the general practitioner must decide which type to perform. This article describes the techniques of exfoliative cytology (brush biopsy), incisional biopsy, and excisional biopsy.

Oral transepithelial brush biopsy with computer-assisted analysis (TBBCA) was introduced in 1999 (patented by OralCDx, CDx Laboratories, Suffern, NY, USA) to allow clinicians to differentiate between precancerous and cancerous cells. This procedure is not designed to identify processes other than epithelial dysplasia and squamous cell carcinoma, and therefore if candidiasis or LP is suspected, other biopsy modalities should be used. The OralCDx kit contains a glass slide, slide holder, fixative package (95% ethanol alcohol and 5% carbowax), and a brush instrument. No topical anesthesia is needed because this may interfere with cell collection. The clinician must rotate the brush until mild bleeding is seen. The collected sample must be placed on the glass slide and the fixative material immediately poured on the specimen. The slide should dry for 15 to 20 minutes and then placed in the slide holder. The clinician should then place the slide in the prepaid Priority Mail package with the patient information sheet filled out and sent to Oral Scan Laboratory.[16] The current ADA Current Procedure Terminology (CPT) code for brush biopsy is D7288 and the procedure is compensated by the usual dental insurance plans.

Four results from the OralCDx biopsy are possible. Negative results indicate no epithelial disease and require no further treatment. Atypical results indicate abnormal epithelial structure of uncertain diagnosis, and positive results indicate definitive dysplasia. Both of these results warrant a scalpel biopsy to confirm a definitive tissue diagnosis. Inadequate results indicate an incomplete transepithelial biopsy, and rebiopsy of the lesion is required. The general practitioner may elect to either reperform the brush biopsy or perform a conventional scalpel biopsy.

Initial data from brush biopsies performed in 1999 showed promising results, with a sensitivity of 96% and specificity of 97%. The procedure has a false-negative rate of 4% and a false-positive rate of 10%.[17] An updated study conducted in Germany found the sensitivity and specificity of OralCDx to be 52% and 29%, respectively.[18] This is much lower than the initial report given by Sciubba.[17] The brush biopsy can also be used as a follow-up tool and for patients who are unable or refuse to undergo other traditional biopsy methods.

Incisional biopsy is reserved for lesions that are generally large (>1.0 cm), multiple, diffuse, or suspected malignancies. The biopsy sample is meant to serve as a representative portion of the lesion and part of healthy tissue. An incisional biopsy should be narrow and deep rather than broad and shallow. The depth of the incision should be three times the width.[19] As a general rule, the biopsy sample of an ulcerative lesion should include representative abnormal tissue with 2 to 3 mm of normal tissue (**Fig. 19**). This specimen will give the pathologist a representative lesion for microscopic examination. Lesions that contain areas of erythroplakia and leukoplakia should have multiple samples removed; if this is not possible, then areas with erythroplakia should be prioritized, because these have the most active cellular activity (**Fig. 20**).

Excisional biopsy is reserved for lesions that can be cured through complete removal, that are smaller than 1 cm, that are presumed clinically benign, and are surgically accessible. Removal of the lesion must include 2 to 3 mm of normal tissue (**Fig. 21**).

Ultimately, the differential diagnosis of a lesion dictates how a biopsy should be taken. For example, if an immune-based vesicle or ulcer is suspected, such as LP, pemphigoids, pemphigus, or SLE, then the biopsy should include clinically involved areas with some adjacent normal-appearing tissue and suspected lesion while avoiding ulcerated or ruptured vesicular areas, because this will yield a nonspecific inflammatory response.[20] Certain immune-based diseases will require a second biopsy so that an immunofluorescence study can performed to serve as a diagnostic adjunct.

TYPES OF INSTRUMENTS

The scalpel biopsy remains the gold standard for establishing a definitive diagnosis. The size, shape, and depth of the biopsy can be tailored based on the differential diagnosis. Punch and laser biopsies are an alternatives to the scalpel technique (**Box 1**).

Punch biopsy is a useful alternative to traditional scalpel biopsy. This technique can be used to diagnose multiple mucocutaneous lesions. The Keyes biopsy punches come in sizes ranging from 1.0 to 12.0 cm in 0.5-cm increments.[21] The advantages of this technique are its low surgical morbidity, that it generally requires no sutures, and that it can be used in any accessible oral mucosal region. The disadvantage is the limitation of depth that the punch can reach (the epithelial or superficial mesenchymal layer). The ideal surgical sites are the labial, buccal mucosa, and tongue surfaces. This technique requires the biopsy blade to be placed over the specimen and the handle rotated gently with the index and thumb until the external bevel of the blade is no longer visible. Counterpressure is needed to provide adequate pressure during the procedure. The blade should reach to the depth of connective tissue layer. If a base layer is still left, it can be released by a conventional No. 15 scalpel blade.

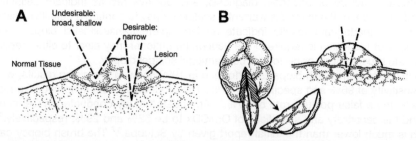

Fig. 19. (*A*) Illustration showing desirability of obtaining deep specimen rather than broad and shallow specimen when incisional biopsy is performed. If malignant cells are present only at base of lesion, broad and shallow biopsy might not obtain these diagnostic cells. (*B*) Illustration showing desirability of obtaining incisional biopsy at margin of soft tissue lesion. Junction of lesion with normal tissue frequently provides pathologist with more diagnostic information than if biopsy were taken only from center of lesion. This is particularly important when a biopsy of an ulcer is performed. (*From* Hupp JR, Ellis III E, Tucker MR. Contemporary oral and maxillofacial surgery. 5th edition. St Louis: CV Mosby; 2008. p. 436; with permission.)

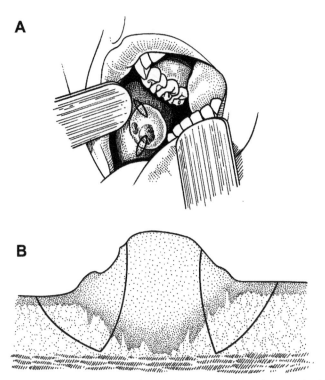

Fig. 20. Illustration demonstrating desirability of obtaining more than one incisional biopsy if characteristics of lesion differ from one area to another. (*A*) Frequently, one area of lesion appears histologically different from another. (*B*) When obtaining biopsy on buccal or labial mucosa, incision is usually carried to depth of musculature. (*From* Hupp JR, Ellis III E, Tucker MR. Contemporary oral and maxillofacial surgery. 5th edition. St Louis: CV Mosby; 2008. p. 436; with permission.)

Laser is an acronym for "Light Amplification by Stimulated Emission of Radiation." Any laser device can produce light energy through a power source and an active medium. The light energy produced by the laser emits and produces light at different wavelengths. It is the spectrum of wavelengths that determine the absorption into the various bodily tissues. Wavelength at the lower spectrum tends to attract soft tissue whereas mid and far infrared range attract water and hydroxyapatite crystals (eg, teeth and bones). For example, laser light is generated by an internal power source and then through an active mediums such as neodymium:yttrium-aluminium-garnet (Nd:YAG), carbon dioxide (CO_2) or diodes. This laser light travels through a fiber-optic cable which gets directed to the target tissue. This energy of light gets converted into heat upon direct tissue contact thus causing tissue vaporization.

Nd:Yag and CO_2 lasers can be useful for treating oral mucosal lesions. Since their initial use in the excision of malignant and premalignant lesions in the oral cavity, lasers have offered clinicians precise surgical management of oral soft tissue lesions, with minimal postoperative pain and successful postoperative healing. CO_2 laser produces light at 10,600 nm wavelength. It is highly absorbed by water, and hydroxyapatite. The CO_2 laser used in continuous wave, noncontact mode (coagulation) has a large beam diameter that is advantageous for removing large leukoplakia lesions,

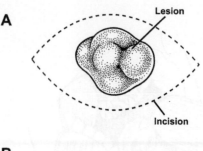

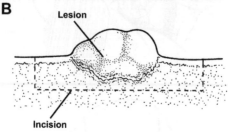

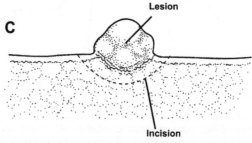

Fig. 21. Illustration of excisional biopsy of soft tissue lesion. (*A*) Surface view. Elliptical incision is made around lesion, at least 3 mm away from lesion. (*B*) Side view. Incision is made deep enough to remove lesion completely. (*C*) End view. Incisions are made convergent to depth of wound. Excision made in this way facilitates closure. (*From* Hupp JR, Ellis III E, Tucker MR. Contemporary oral and maxillofacial surgery. 5th edition. St Louis: CV Mosby; 2008. p. 436.)

Box 1
Instruments for biopsy
Gauze
Local anesthesia
Syringe
Scalpel with No. 15 blade
Tissue Pick-up (eg, Adson forceps with serrated teeth)
Suction
Needle holder
Scissors
Biopsy bottle with 10% formalin
Suture (3-0, 4-0 silk or chromic gut)
Michel's solution and container for immunofluorescence study

such as those on the cheek and tongue. Nd:Yag produces light at 1,064 nm wavelength and unlike the CO_2 laser, it does not get well absorbed by water or hydroxyapatite. The Nd:YAG laser can operate in either noncontact (coagulation) or contact mode (excision). It emits pulsed noncontinuous energy through a solid core silica fiber the width of three human hairs. This mechanism makes the Nd:YAG extremely precise and easy to use in areas around the dentition, where access is more difficult for the CO_2 laser or scalpel. The Nd:YAG is also less likely to cause collateral damage to adjacent hard and soft tissue because of its smaller beam size and short interaction times compared with continuous wave laser devices. Local anesthesia is not needed if the setting is kept at 2W, 20 Hz. When selecting the power setting for all laser devices, the minimum power required to produce the desired effect should be chosen.[22]

New innovations in laser technology include the Odyssey Diode Laser by Ivoclar Vivadent. It has both continuous and pulsed mode that produces light at 810+/20 nm wavelength. This wavelength is at the lower end of the infrared-spectrum making it ideal for soft tissue biopsy and other soft tissue applications. There are 2 models available Odyssey 2.4G and Odyssey Navigator. The Odyssey 2.4G is a table top version and the Odyssey Navigator is more portable weighing in at 2.5 lbs. Another Diode laser is the Picasso Laser by AMD Laser, LLC. There are 2 models available: Picasso at 7 watts and Picasso Lite at 2.5 watts. Both laser units can provide GP the power to treat most soft tissue procedures in office. The Picasso Lite 2.5 watts laser, starts at $2495 making it an affordable entry unit.

COMMUNICATION WITH PATHOLOGIST

In performing a biopsy, the surgeon is communicating to the pathologist that the specimen is a representation of the lesion itself. Surgeons can optimize that representation in several ways.

Handling of Tissue

When performing the biopsy, the surgeon must avoid damaging the specimen. Local anesthesia should be delivered as a field block or at least 1 cm away from the lesion to avoid distorting the specimen. An Adson forceps with serrated teeth is the preferred instrument to stabilize the lesion. Crushing the specimen is the commonest mistake made by general practitioners.[23]

Orientation of Specimen

The orientation of the representative sample to the larger lesion or lesion margins is often important to communicate to the pathologist. This information can be conveyed by placing a suture through the edge of the lesion and marking it by a direction (ie, anterior or superior). If the results indicate a malignancy, the general practitioner can relay this information to the referring head and neck surgeon.

Describe Lesion to the Pathologist

Describing the lesion and providing important patient and clinical background information (ie, size, shape, duration, growth pattern, color, mobility, lymph node involvement) could help the pathologist diagnose the lesion. Description of the site of each biopsy is especially important if more than one biopsy is being performed from one lesion or numerous lesions.

Transportation of the Specimen

To ensure the pathologist receives a correct representation, the specimen must not be distorted during transportation from the general practitioner to the pathologist. Soon after the specimen is removed, it should be placed in 10% formalin 10 the times the volume of the specimen. If the general practitioner has vesiculobullous disease as a differential diagnosis, the lesion should be placed in Michel's solution for an immunofluorescence study. CPT codes are D0482 and D0483 for direct and indirect immunofluorescence studies, respectively.

DIAGNOSIS AND TREATMENT
Primary and Recurrent HSV

History and clinical presentation are usually enough to deduce a clinical diagnosis of herpes virus infection. If uncertainty remains, laboratory tests are available to help confirm the diagnosis. Before using any of the tests discussed, the general practitioner should contact a local laboratory to determine the availability and turnaround time for each test (**Fig. 22**).

Viral culture is a collection of the virus at its most virulent stage. An excisional biopsy of the intact vesicle is the most ideal procedure to capture the virus. Alternatively, a needle aspiration from an intact vesicle would yield the best viral content. If a needle aspiration is not available or the general practitioner is uncomfortable with this technique, then the viral fluid can be collected through bursting a fresh vesicle and using a cotton swab for sampling. A skin sample must also be collected for viral culture because the virus hides in the skin cells; this is why the virus is very contagious in shedding stages during an active outbreak. Results of the culture will take 2 to 4 days depending on the laboratory's methods. The CPT code for reimbursement for viral culture is D0416.

A herpes virus antigen detection test requires fresh sores to be obtained. It detects marker antigens on the infected host's cell. A positive test indicates herpes virus. This test can be substituted for the viral culture.

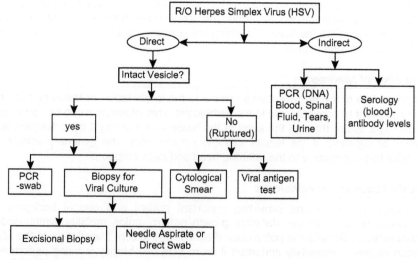

Fig. 22. HSV flow chart.

Unlike with viral culture, samples for cytology are collected from a ruptured vesicle. A cytology smear requires viral fluid from the vesicle to be placed on the glass slide so that it can viewed under a microscope. The CPT code for reimbursement for exfoliative cytology is D7287. This test, however, is not specific for HSV-1 because HSV-2 can have similar histologic features.

Although not as readily available as viral culture, polymerase chain reaction (PCR) test helps to detect the herpes virus's DNA. PCR is performed using the same collection method as the viral culture. Samples can also be collected from blood, spinal fluid, urine, or tears.

For an indirect test method, serology requires blood collection to detect HSV antibody level in the serum against specific viral antigens. The presence of the antibodies cannot be distinguished between an active or previous infection; this only reveals the host's immune response to the herpes virus. A false-positive can also occur for recent infection when the body has not mounted an immune response.

A common microscopic feature seen in a herpes virus infection is ballooning degeneration of the keratinocytes, multinucleated epithelial cells, and inclusion bodies (**Fig. 23**).

Treatment of primary herpetic gingivostomatitis is nonspecific and consists of palliative care during the acute phase (eg, increased fluid intake, antipyretics, topical or elixir analgesia). Topical benzocaine 20% (oral gel) applied to affected regions can

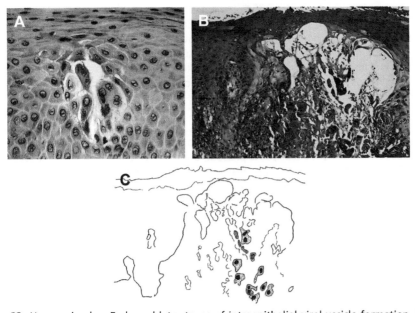

Fig. 23. Herpes simplex. Early and late stages of intraepithelial viral vesicle formation. (*A*) Incipient vesicle formation early in prodromal stage before presence of a clinically visible vesicle exhibiting ballooning degeneration, nuclear margination, and multinucleation of the spinous layer of keratinocytes (viral cytopathic changes) (Hematoxylin and eosin [H&E], high power magnification). (*B*) Fully developed but intact intraepithelial viral vesicle that contains fluid, virally altered keratinocytes, large numbers of viruses, and necrotic debris (H&E, medium power magnification). (*C*) Photomicrograph of cytologic smear of viral vesicle contents that reveals enlarged and ballooned keratinocytes and associated leukocytes. (*From* Sapp JP, Eversole LR, Wysocki GP. Contemporary oral and maxillofacial pathology. 2nd edition. Mosby; 2004. p. 214; with permission.)

provide temporary relief. If lesions are diffuse, then 1 to 2 teaspoons of Hurricane elixir in 500 mL can be swished and expectorated every 2 hours as needed for pain. Hurricane elixir has three active ingredients in equal quantity in the mixture: Mylanta, 2% Xylocaine, and 12.5 mg/5 mL diphenhydramine. Mylanta helps to coat the lining of the mouth thus giving the elixir a longer-lasting effect (**Box 2**). Acyclovir is not indicated for healthy patients and has little clinical effects on established lesions.

Although recurrent intraoral herpes (stomatitis) responds poorly to local antiviral agents, palliative remedies are usually prescribed for this condition until the virus runs its course. Over-the-counter (OTC), topical analgesia Lipactin gel and Zilactin can help control pain. However, treatment for recurrent herpes labialis using antiviral agents is effective only during the prodrome phase (**Box 3**). This treatment helps reduce healing time, viral shedding, and pain. The only available OTC medication is docosanol (Abreva) 10% cream, which helps to reduce healing time. Acyclovir (Zovirax) and penciclovir (Denavir) creams are antiviral agents approved by the U.S. Food and Drug Administration (FDA) for the treatment of herpes labialis. To be effective, acyclovir cream 0.5% must be applied five times per day for 4 days, and penciclovir (Denavir) topical cream 1% applied every 2 hours for 4 days. In 2009, the FDA approved a combination of 5% acyclovir and 1% hydrocortisone cream (Xerese) for the treatment of recurrent herpes labialis. The added corticosteroids help decrease local inflammation, which helps shorten the clinical course and vesicular outbreaks compared with acyclovir alone.[24] For patients who experience recurrent outbreaks (ie, two in 4 months), three antiviral oral medications are approved by the FDA to help shorten the clinical course. Acyclovir (Zovirax), 400 mg, taken orally five times per day for 4 days, valacyclovir (Valtrex), 2.0 g, taken orally every 12 hours for 1 day, and famciclovir (Famvir), 1500 mg, taken orally for 1 day. Acyclovir is used for immunocompetent patients, whereas famciclovir is reserved for those who are immunocompromised.

Recurrent Aphthous Stomatitis

Recurrent aphthous stomatitis is diagnosed based on clinical appearance alone. If any associated systemic disease is present, the patient should be referred to a physician. The mainstay of treatment of RAS is still corticosteroids, although topical analgesia can be used to alleviate pain. The topical form is used to treat mild to moderate conditions, whereas systemic is reserved for severe conditions (**Box 4**). Clobetasol propionate 0.05% and triamcinolone in Orabase 0.1%, with 15 g each equally mixed,

---

Box 2
Topical and elixir analgesia for primary herpetic gingivostomatitis

Local sites

Benzocaine (oral gel) 20%

Disp: 1 tube

Sig: apply to lesion every day as needed

Diffuse lesions

Hurricane elixir

Disp: 500 mL

Sig: 1–2 teaspoons every 2 hours as needed, swish and expectorate

---

Box 3
Antiviral medications[a]

Over-the-counter

Docosanol (Abreva)

    Disp: 2 g tube

    Sig: apply to lesion five times per day for 4 days

Topical prescription

Acyclovir 0.5% (Zovirax) cream

    Disp: 5 g tube

    Sig: apply five times per day

Penciclovir 1% (Denavir) cream

    Disp: 1.5 g

    Sig: apply to lesion every 2 hours for 4 days

Acyclovir 5% and Hydrocortisone 1% (Xerese)

    Disp: 1 tube

    Sig: apply five times per day

Oral prescription

Acyclovir (Zovirax), 400 mg

    Disp: 20 tablet

    Sig: 1 tablet by mouth five times per day

Valacyclovir (Valtrex), 2000 mg

    Disp: 2 tablets

    Sig: 1 tablet by mouth every 12 hours for 1 day

Famciclovir (Famvir), 1500 mg

    Disp: 1 tablet

    Sig: 1 tablet by mouth for 1 day

[a] Applied or used when symptoms first occur.

---

should be applied (but not rubbed) to affected areas three times daily.[4] For diffused lesions, one teaspoon of dexamethasone elixir, swished and expectorated 4 to 5 times per day, can be very effective. One study suggested that this local corticosteroid therapy does not produce any adrenal suppression despite long-term or repeated use.[6] Intralesional triamcinolone 0.1% in 1 mL can be used to treat large aphthae lesions.

Alternatives to topical corticosteroids are available for treating RAS. Amlexanox (Aphthasol) is an FDA-approved noncorticosteroid medication that has antiallergic and antiinflammatory properties. It comes in a 5% paste and should be applied two to four times daily. It helps reduce size and pain level, which speeds up recovery.[25–29] The only adverse effects of this drug is a stinging sensation at the site of application.[30] Hurricane elixir is good for diffused intraoral lesions. Chlorhexidine helps reduce the duration of RAS through its antimicrobial effects.[31–34]

Other agents on the market are notable for treating RAS. Tacrolimus ointment 0.1% is an immunosuppressant medication that should only be used in healthy patients. It

---

Box 4
Treatment for recurrent aphthous stomatitis

Clobetasol propionate 0.05% and triamcinolone in Orabase 0.1%

   Disp: 15 g each

   Sig: mix and apply to lesion (do not rub) three times daily

Hurricane elixir

   Disp: 500 mL

   Sig: 1 to 2 teaspoons every 2 hours as needed, swish and expectorate

Dexamethasone 0.5 mg/mL elixir

   Disp: 500 mL

   Sig: 1 teaspoon every 6 hours, swish and expectorate

Noncorticosteroid alternative

Amlexanox 5% oral paste (Aphthasol)

   Disp: 5 g tube

   Sig: apply to lesion every 6 hours as needed for pain

Chlorhexidine oral rinse

   Disp: 1 bottle (2-week supply)

   Sig: 20 mL for 30 seconds three times daily, swish and expectorate

---

inhibits T-lymphocyte activation, which can be detrimental in immunocompromised patients. Triclosan mouthrinse has antiinflammatory, analgesic, and antimicrobial properties, which help reduce the duration of ulcers in the oral cavity.[35] Tetracycline (eg, aureomycin, chlortetracycline, and tetracycline) helps reduce the healing time and pain. The British National Formulary included 100 mg of doxycycline mixed in 10 mL of water for 2 to 3 minutes every day for 3 days for the treatment of RAS.[36–39] Referral to a physician is prudent if systemic agents are needed. Prednisone or azathioprine should be reserved for patients with severe RAS otherwise refractory to local treatments. Thalidomide has been an effective alternative agent to steroids. It is a water-soluble macrolide that has antiinflammatory and anti-immunologic properties for suppressing T-cell function. Thalidomide used in 50- to 100 mg dosages every day has significant clinical effects against RAS. However, serious adverse reaction haven been reported with this drug, including teratogenicity, neuropathy, somnolence, constipation, rash, thromboembolic, and neutropenia.[40] Furthermore, one tablet at taken at day 20 of pregnancy can cause phocomelia.[41] Lastly, dapsone is an immunomodulatory agent that has shown to be effective in the treatment of RAS.[42]

Lichen Planus

Diagnosis of LP is based on clinical examination, histology, and direct immunofluorescence studies. Reticular LP can often be diagnosed through clinical findings alone. For erosive LP, a biopsy is often necessary to rule out other ulcerative diseases or premalignant changes. Histologic features of LP include epithelial acanthosis, hyperkeratosis, basal cell layer vacuolation, sawtooth rete, and dense band-like infiltrate of

T lymphocytes below the basement membrane (subbasilar) (**Fig. 24**). Direct immuno-fluorescence study will show a linear deposit of fibrinogen at the basement membrane (**Fig. 25**).

Reticular LP typically produces no symptoms and no treatment is required. Erosive LP, however, is often painful because of open sores. Because it is an immune-based disease, corticosteroids are recommended. The objective is to use the shortest course (1–2 weeks) of steroids without causing potential side effects (eg, immunosuppression, fungal over growth). Topical corticosteroids, such as clobetasol propionate 0.05% with triamcinolone in Orabase 0.1%, and dexamethasone elixir can be used as first-line therapy (**Box 5**). Intralesional injection of triamcinolone 0.1% in 1 mL has been used for resistant local steroid therapy. One study suggests *Portulaca oleracea L* or Purslane, 235 mg, orally every day is effective in treating oral lichen planus, with an 83% success rate after 2 weeks.[43] Purslane is a herbaceous weed found in the Tehran province in Iran that has anti-inflammatory, antiulcerogenic, antifungal, and antioxidant properties. Topical or systemic thalidomide has shown to be effective as an alternative for steroid therapy after 1 week of application,[40] with 54.5% and 66.7% of patients treated success-fully after 1 week and 1 month, respectively. Again, physicians should use this medication cautiously with the understanding that significant adverse reactions were reported in other studies.

Mucous Membrane Pemphigoid

A dominant histopathologic picture of MMP shows a separation of the epithelium from the connective tissue layer (**Fig. 26**). These autoantibodies (IgG, IgA, or both) are

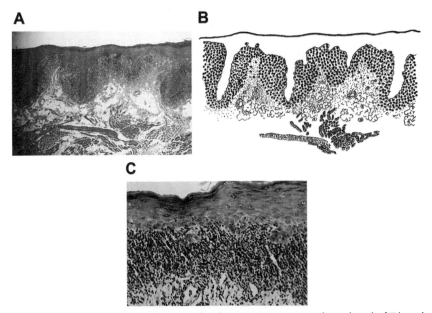

Fig. 24. LP. Microscopic features showing the characteristic narrow dense band of T lympho-cytes in the immediately adjacent connective tissue of reticular LP (*A*) and atrophic and erosive LP (*B*). (*C*) High power magnification of A. (*A, C,* H&E; *A,* low power; *B,* medium power and it's a diagram; *C,* high power.) (*From* Sapp JP, Eversole LR, Wysocki GP. Contem-porary oral and maxillofacial pathology. 2nd edition. Mosby; 2004. p. 260; with permission.)

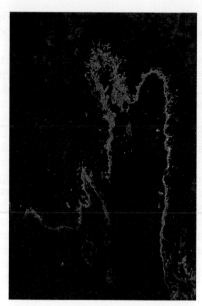

Fig. 25. LP. Photomicrograph of immunofluorescent pattern of linear deposit of fibrinogen at the basement membrane (low power magnification). (*From* Sapp JP, Eversole LR, Wysocki GP. Contemporary oral and maxillofacial pathology. 2nd edition. Mosby; 2004. p. 261; with permission.)

believed to attack the antigen sites between this layer, causing a separation. The antigen sites are BP180[44,45] and Laminin-5.[46,47] Direct immunofluorescence shows a linear deposition of complement (IgG, IgA, C3, or a combination) at the basement membrane zone. Indirect immunofluorescence has no value because circulating antibodies are not detectable at the basement membrane (**Fig. 27**).

Treatment of oral MMP depends on the severity and location of the lesion. If the lesion is mild to moderate and is confined to the gingiva and palate, then a custom tray with clobetasol propionate 0.05% and triamcinolone in Orabase 0.1% can be used.[9] Dexamethasone elixir is a good first choice for diffused intraoral lesions

---

Box 5
Treatment for oral erosive lichen planus

Clobetasol propionate 0.05% and triamcinolone in Orabase 0.1%

    Disp: 15 g each

    Sig: mix and apply to lesion (do not rub) three times daily

Dexamethasone 0.5 mg/mL elixir

    Disp: 500 mL (1-week supply with refills as needed)

    Sig: 1 teaspoon every 6 hours, swish and expectorate

Purslane, 235 mg

    Disp: 14 tablets

    Sig: 1 tablet by mouth every day

A   **B**

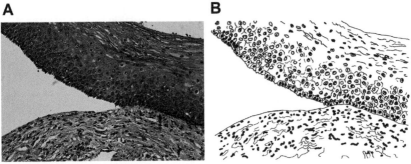

Fig. 26. MMP. Photomicrograph of mucosa showing lack of rete pegs and loss of adhesion of the epithelium with cleavage at the level of the basement membrane. (*A*) H&E, medium power magnification; (*B*) it is a diagram of *A*. (*From* Sapp JP, Eversole LR, Wysocki GP. Contemporary oral and maxillofacial pathology. 2nd edition. Mosby; 2004. p. 265; with permission.)

(**Box 6**). Large local lesions can be treated with intralesional injection of triamcinolone 0.1%. Systemic corticosteroids are reserved for patients who experience no response to local therapy. Burst therapy is described as a short course of 60–80 mg of systemic prednisone for several days, followed by 7 to 10 days of maintenance and tapered dosage. Alternative or "steroid sparing" medications are available. Dapsone (Avlosulfon) is an antimicrobial agent with immunosuppressive activity that has been shown to be somewhat effective.[48–50] Tacrolimus, retinoids, and cyclosporine have been used effectively against vesiculobullous disease.[51–53] Immunosuppressive agents, such as

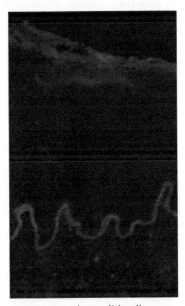

Fig. 27. MMP. Immunofluorescence reveals a solid yellow-green line, indicating the presence of IgG antibody complexed to the antigen at the basement membrane. (*From* Sapp JP, Eversole LR, Wysocki GP. Contemporary oral and maxillofacial pathology. 2nd edition. Mosby; 2004. p. 265; with permission.)

> **Box 6**
> **Treatment for oral mucous membrane pemphigoid**
>
> Clobetasol propionate 0.05% and triamcinolone in Orabase 0.1%
>
> Disp: 15 g each
>
> Sig: mix and apply to lesion (do not rub) three times daily
>
> Dexamethasone 0.5 mg/mL elixir
>
> Disp: 500 mL
>
> Sig: 1 teaspoon every 6 hours, swish and expectorate

azathioprine, methotrexate, and cyclophosphamide, in combination with systemic steroids is also effective in treating severe cases.

Pemphigus Vulgaris

PV is diagnosed based on clinical, histologic, and direct and indirect immunofluorescence studies. Histologically, PV has a typical blister formation showing edematous keratinocytes (Tzanck cells) detached from surrounding cells (acantholysis). An inflammatory infiltrate is dominated by mononuclear cells in the connective tissue (**Fig. 28**). Unlike MMP, which has a subepithelial separation, PV has intraepithelial separation caused by antibody (IgG) binding to antigen desmoglein 3. Direct immunofluorescence is used as an adjunct to confirm the diagnosis. This study shows binding of IgG and C3 in the intercellular epithelium resulting in a reticular pattern, which is classically known as the "chicken wire" appearance (**Fig. 29**). No staining occurs in the basement membrane zone; however, indirect immunofluorescence study shows a positive detection of autoantibodies at the basement.

Topical and elixir corticosteroids are used to treat oral PV (**Box 7**).[54] Intralesional triamcinolone may be used as second-line treatment. Systemic corticosteroids are reserved for severe cases (**Box 8**). In the first week, 60 to 80 mg of prednisone to be taken orally every day is prescribed. Follow-up after the first week will dictate how the remainder of the regimen is prescribed. If the blisters continue to appear,

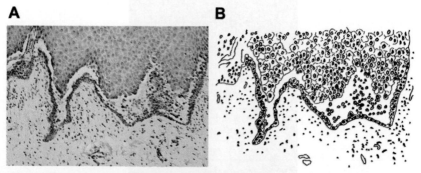

A   **B**

Fig. 28. PV. Photomicrograph of epithelium exhibiting rete pegs and a zone of acantholysis above the basal cell layer. Spinous cells (Tzanck cells) are present and floating freely in the fluid-filled intraepithelial space. (*A*) High power magnification, (*B*) it is a diagram of *A*. (*From* Sapp JP, Eversole LR, Wysocki GP. Contemporary oral & maxillofacial pathology. 2nd edition. Mosby; 2004. p. 268; with permission.)

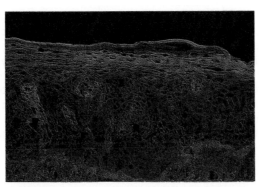

Fig. 29. PV. Immunofluorescent pattern of the IgG antibody adherence to the desmosomal protein (desmoglein) located on the periphery of epithelial intermediate cells, producing a "fishnet" pattern of binding sites (high power magnification). (*From* Sapp JP, Eversole LR, Wysocki GP. Contemporary oral and maxillofacial pathology. 2nd edition. Mosby; 2004. p. 268; with permission.)

Box 7
Treatment for oral pemphigus vulgaris

Clobestasol propionate 0.05% and triamcinolone in Orabase 0.1%

    Disp: 15 g each

    Sig: mix and apply to lesion (do not rub) three times daily

Dexamethasone 0.5 mg/mL elixir

    Disp: 500 mL

    Sig: 1 teaspoon every 6 hours, swish and expectorate

Box 8
Systemic steroids (Consult M.D.)

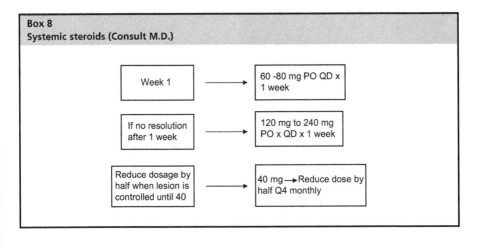

then the physician can increase the dose to 120 mg or up to 240 mg to be taken orally every day for the following week. If clinical evidence shows tight control of disease progression, the current dosage can be reduced by half weekly until 40 mg/d is reached. At that time, the 40 mg dosage is then decreased every 4 months.[55] For most patients, low maintenance doses, usually every other day, are needed for years. High-dose pulses of corticosteroids may be delivered for relapsing or resistant cases, either orally or intravenously. Adverse side effects of corticosteroids can overwhelm the patient's adrenal system, causing cushingoid symptoms. As an alternative to systemic corticosteroids, immunosuppressant and antimicrobial agents, similar to those used for MMP, can be applied to PV successfully.

Erythema Mulitforme

EM is diagnosed based on the exclusion of other vesiculobullous diseases. The histopathology is not pathognomonic. Intercellular and intracellular edema overlying the epithelium is seen, with focal microvesicle formation (**Fig. 30**). Direct and indirect immunofluorescence studies have no diagnostic value. Treatment is directed toward treating or removing the offending agent (eg, HSV, drug-induced). Mild symptoms can be controlled by administering analgesic and antipyretics or topical steroids. Patients with severe symptoms should be admitted in the hospital to control body fluid, electrolyte losses, and infection. Systemic steroid or immunosuppressant therapy may be needed to control lesion progression.

Lupus Erythematosus

Lupus erythematosus is diagnosed using the following tests. Direct immunofluorescence will be positive for IgA, IgM, and IgG immunoglobulins, fibrinogen, and C3. Indirect immunofluorescence will be negative. SLE is diagnosed based on analysis of antinuclear antibodies to doubled-stranded DNA, detection of and serum rheumatoid factors, and a lupus erythematosus cell test.

Treatment of DLE is with topical steroid antimalarials and sulfones. The more severe form requires steroids or combination of steroids and immunosuppressive drugs, such as cyclophosphamide and azathioprine. Systemic steroid are reserved for oral forms that are refractory to local treatment.

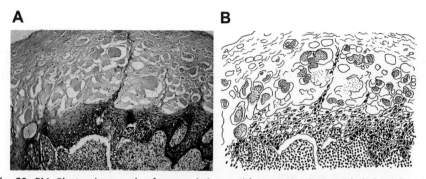

Fig. 30. EM. Photomicrograph of mucosal tissue with extensive intraepithelial pooling of eosinophilic coagulum, separation of the epithelium from connective tissue (bulla formation), and intense chronic inflammatory cell infiltrates. (*A*) High power magnification with H&E stain, (*B*) it is a diagram of *A*. (*From* Shklar G. Oral lesions of erythema multiforme: histologic and histochemical observations. Arch Dermatol 1965;92:495; and Sapp JP, Eversole LR, Wysocki GP. Contemporary oral and maxillofacial pathology. 2nd edition. Mosby; 2004. p. 273; with permission.)

SUMMARY

Oral mucocutaneous diseases are common encounters in the daily dental practices, the general practitioner should have a heightened ability to recognize abnormal tissues. A through and systemic approach to these lesions requires a working diagnosis through history, clinical examination, and biopsying of lesions. Proper referral to medical specialists can prevent certain comorbidities and mortalities.

ACKNOWLEDGMENTS

The authors want to extend a very special thanks to Fran Tidona (Chief, Library Service at Brooklyn Campus) for her tireless pursuit to help gather numerous articles for us.

REFERENCES

1. Shulman J, Beach M, Rivera-Hidalgo F. The prevalence of oral mucosal lesions in U.S. adults: data from the Third National Health and Nutrition Examination Survey, 1988-1994. J Am Dent Assoc 2004;135:1279.
2. Shulman J, Beach M, Rivera-Hidalgo F. Prevalence of oral mucosal lesions in children and youths in the USA. Int J Paediatr Dent 2005;15:89.
3. American Dental Association. The 2005-06 Survey of Dental Services Rendered. ADA; 2007.
4. Kerpel S, Freedman P, Reich R. A comprehensive review course in oral pathology [handout]. 2002.
5. Sapp JP, Eversole LR, Wysocki GP. Contempoary oral & maxillofacial pathology. 2nd edition. St. Louis (MO): Mosby; 2004. p. 210–3.
6. Scully C, Porter S. Oral mucosal disease: recurrent aphthous stomatitis. Br J Oral Maxillofac Surg 2008;46:198–206.
7. Scully C, Porter S. Recurrent aphthous stomatitis: current concepts of etiology, pathogenesis and management. J Oral Pathol Med 1989;18:21–7.
8. Thorn JJ, Holstrupp P, Rindum H, et al. Course of various clinical forms of oral lichen planus. A prospective follow-up study of all 611patients. J Oral Pathol Med 1988;17:213–318.
9. Toscano NJ, Holtzclaw DJ, Shumaker ND. Surgical considerations and management of patients with mucocutaneous disorders. Compend Contin Educ Dent 2010;31:346.
10. Rogers RS III, Eisen D. Erosive OLP with genital lesions. The vulvovaginal-gingival syndrome and peno-gingival syndrome. Dermatol Clin 2003;21(1): 79–89.
11. Anderson JO. OLP: a clinical evaluation of 115 cases. Oral Surg Med Oral Pathol 1968;23(1):31–41.
12. Lourenco SV, Boggio P, Agner Macado Martins LE, et al. childhood oral mucous membrane pemphigoid presenting as desquamative gingivitis in a 4-year-old girl. Acta Derm Venereol 2006;86(4):351–4.
13. Endo H, Rees TD, Kuyama K, et al. Clinical and diagnostic features of mucous membrane pemphigoid. Compend Contin Educ Dent 2006;27(9):512–8.
14. Suresh L, Kumar V. Significance of IgG4 in the diagnosis of mucous membrane pemphiogoid. Oral Surg Oral Med Oral Pathol Oral Radiol Endod 2007;104(3): 359–62.
15. Scully C, Challacombe SJ. Pemphigus: update on etiopathogenesis, oral manifestations, and management. Crit Rev Oral Boil Med 2002;13(5):397–408.

16. Zunt S. Transepithelial brush biopsy: an adjunctive diagnostic procedure. J Indiana Dent Assoc 2001;80(2):6–8.

17. Sciubba J. Improving detection of precancerous and cancerous oral lesions. Computer-assisted analysis of the oral brush biopsy. U.S. Collaborative OralCDx Study Grooup. J Am Dent Assoc 1999;(30):1445–57.

18. Hohlweg-Majert B, Deppe H, Metzger MC. Sensitivity and specificity of oral brush biopsy. Cancer Invest 2009;27:293–7.

19. Golden D, Hooley J. Oral mucosal biopsy procedures. Excisional and incisional. Dent Clin North Am 1994;38(2):279–300.

20. Marx RE, Stern D. Oral and maxillofacial pathology: a rationale for diagnosis and treatment. Carol Stream (IL): Quintessence books; 2003. p. 1–15.

21. Lynch D, Morris L. The oral mucosal punch biopsy: indications and technique. J Am Dent Assoc 1990;121:145–9.

22. White J, Chaudhry S. Nd:Yag and CO2 Laser Therapy of Oral mucosal Lesions. J Clin Laser Med Surg 1998;16(6):299–304.

23. Oliver R, Sloan P. Oral Biopsies: methods and applications. Br Dent J 2004; 196(6):329–33.

24. Hull C, Brunton S. The role of topical 5% acyclovir and 1% hydrocortisone cream (xerses) in the treatment of recurrent herpes simplex labialis. Postgrad Med 2010; 122(5):1–6.

25. Kwandala A. 5% amlexanox oral paste, a new treatment for recurrent minor aphthous ulcers: I. Clinical demonstration of acceleration of healing and resolution of pain. Oral Surg Oral Med Oral Pathol Oral Radiol Endod 1997;83(2):222–30.

26. Greer RO Jr, Lindenmuth JE. A double-blind study of topically applied 5% amlexanox in the treatment of aphthous ulcers. J Oral Maxillofac Surg 1993;51(3):243–8 [discussion: 248–9].

27. Binnie WH, Curro FA. Amlexanox oral paste: a novel treatment that accelerates the healing of aphthous ulcers. Compend Contin Educ Dent 1997;18(11): 1116–8, 1120–2, 1124 passim.

28. Murray B, McGuinness N, Biagioni P, et al. A comparative study of the efficacy of Aphtheal in the management of recurrent minor aphthous ulceration. J Oral Pathol Med 2005;34(7):413–9.

29. Murray B, Biagioni PA, Lamey PJ. The efficacy of amlexanox OraDisc on the prevention of recurrent minor aphthous ulceration. J Oral Pathol Med 2006; 35(2):117–22.

30. Khandwala A, Van Inwegen RG, Charney MR, et al. 5% amlexanox oral paste, a new treatment for recurrent minor aphthous ulcers: II. Pharmacokinetics and demonstration of clinical safety. Oral Surg Oral Med Oral Pathol Oral Radiol Endod 1997;83(2):231–8.

31. Addy M, Tapper-Jones L, Seal M. Trial of astringent and antibacterial mouthwashes in the management of recurrent aphthous ulceration. Br Dent J 1974; 136(11):452–5.

32. Addy M, Carpenter R, Roberts WR. Management of recurrent aphthous ulceration. A trial of chlorhexidine gluconate gel. Br Dent J 1976;141(4):118–20.

33. Addy M. Hibitane in the treatment of aphthous ulceration. J Clin Periodontol 1977; 4(5):108–16.

34. Hunter L, Addy M. Chlorhexidine gluconate mouthwash in the management of minor aphthous ulceration.A double-blind, placebo-controlled cross-over trial. Br Dent J 1987;162(3):106–10.

35. Greenspan JS, Gadol N, Olson JA, et al. Antibody-dependent cellular cytotoxicity in recurrent aphthous ulceration. Clin Exp Immunol 1981;44(3):603–10.

36. Guggenheimer J, Brightman VJ, Ship II. Effect of chlortetracycline mouthrinses on the healing of recurrent aphthous ulcers: a double-blind controlled trial. J Oral Ther Pharmacol 1968;4(5):406–8.
37. Graykowski EA, Kingman A. Double-blind trial of tetracycline in recurrent aphthous ulceration. J Oral Pathol 1978;7(6):376–82.
38. Denman AM, Schiff AA. Recurrent oral ulceration treated with Mysteclin: a controlled study. Br Med J 1979;1(6173):1248–9.
39. Häyrinen-Immonen R, Sorsa T, Pettilä J, et al. Effect of tetracyclines on collagenase activity in patients with recurrent aphthous ulcers. J Oral Pathol Med 1994;23(6):269–72.
40. Wu Y, Zhou G, Zeng H. A Randomized double-blind, positive-control trail of topical thalidomide in erosive oral lichen planus. Oral Surg Oral Med Oral Pathol Oral Radiol Endod 2010;10:188–95.
41. Porter SR, Jorge J Jr. Thalidomide: a role in oral oncology? Oral Oncol 2002;38: 527–31.
42. Handfield-Jones S, Allen BR, Littlewood SM. Dapsone use with oral-genital ulcers. Br J Dermatol 1985;113:501.
43. Agha-Hosseini F, Borhan-Mojabi K, Monsef-Esfahani HR. Efficacy of purslane in the treatment of oral lichen planus. Phytother Res 2010;24:240–4.
44. Kromminga A, Sitaru C, Meyer J, et al. Cicatricial pemphigoid differs from bullous pemphigoid and pemphigoid gestationis regarding the fine specificity of autoantibodies to the BP180 NC16A domain. J Dermatol Sci 2002;28(1):68–75.
45. Roh JY, Yee C, Lazarova Z, et al. The 120-kDa soluble ectodomain of type XVII collagen is recognized by autoantibodies in patients with pemphigoid and linear IgA dermatosis. Br J Dermatol 2000;143(1):104–11.
46. Sakamoto K, Mori K, Hashimoto T, et al. Antiepiligrin cicatricial pemphigoid of the larynx successfully treated with a combination of tetracycline and niacinamide. Arch Otolaryngol Head Neck Surg 2002;128(12):1420–3.
47. Parisi E, Raghavendra S, Werth VP, et al. Modification to the approach of the diagnosis of mucous membrane pemphigoid: A case report and literature review. Oral Surg Oral Med Oral Pathol Oral Radiol Endod 2003;95(2):182–6.
48. Ciarrocca KN, Greenberg MS. A retrospective study of the management of oral mucous membrane pemphigoid with dapsone. Oral Surg Oral Med Oral Pathol Oral Radiol Endod 1999;88(2):159–63.
49. Ahmed AR, Colón JE. Comparison between intravenous immunoglobulin and conventional immunosuppressive therapy regimens in patients with severe oral pemphigoid: effects on disease progression in patients nonresponsive to dapsone therapy. Arch Dermatol 2001;137(9):1181–9.
50. Kirtschig G, Murrell D, Wojnarowska F, et al. Interventions for mucous membrane pemphigoid/cicatricial pemphigoid and epidermolysis bullosa acquisita: a systematic literature review. Arch Dermatol 2002;138(3):380–4.
51. Chainani-Wu N, Silverman S Jr, Lozada-Nur F, et al. Oral lichen planus: patient profile, disease progression and treatment responses. J Am Dent Assoc 2001; 132(7):901–9.
52. Stanley JR. Therapy of pemphigus vulgaris. Arch Dermatol 1999;135(1):76–8.
53. Fine JD. Management of acquired bullous skin diseases. N Engl J Med 1995; 333(22):1475–84.
54. Darling M, Daley T. Blistering mucocutaneous disease of the oral mucosa—a review: part 1. Mucous membrane pemphigoid. J Can Dent Assoc 2005;71:851–4.
55. Darling MR, Daley T. Blistering mucocutaneous diseases of the oral mucosa— a review: part 2. Pemphigus vulgaris. J Can Dent Assoc 2006;72(1):63–6.

Diagnosis and Management of Common Postextraction Complications

Joseph E. Pierse, DMD, MA, Harry Dym, DDS*, Earl Clarkson, DDS

KEYWORDS

- Diagnosis • Management • Postextraction complications
- Impacted teeth

Extraction of impacted teeth is one of the most common surgical procedures performed by oral and maxillofacial surgeons. Extensive training, skill, and experience are necessary to perform this procedure with minimal trauma to the surrounding soft and hard tissue. When the clinician is untrained or inexperienced, the incidence of complications rises exponentially.[1–3] Treatment planning for the removal of asymptomatic teeth is no less problematic. In many situations the course of treatment depends on the clinician's experience, professional judgment, and knowledge of current evidence-based literature.

Every surgical procedure results in some degree of postoperative bleeding and inflammation, typically manifesting as pain and edema. Through the inflammatory response and the natural progression of the body to heal itself, wound repair and tissue regeneration are activated, and physiologic mediators are concentrated in the wound area, resulting in the induction of nociceptive pathways and a change in vascular permeability. Although the complex physiology of the human body is beyond the scope of this article, the educated clinician should have an understanding of the time line associated with these processes so as to determine whether a patient's complaint of postoperative bleeding, pain, or swelling represents a normal response to surgical trauma or an aberrant reaction.[4]

SURGICAL DAMAGE TO ADJACENT STRUCTURES

Occasionally an impacted tooth is located such that its removal may seriously compromise adjacent vital structures, making it prudent to leave the impacted tooth in situ. The potential risks, benefits, and alternatives must be discussed thoroughly

Department of Dentistry/Oral & Maxillofacial Surgery, The Brooklyn Hospital Center, 121 DeKalb Avenue, Box 187, Brooklyn, NY 11201, USA
* Corresponding author.
E-mail address: Hdymdds@yahoo.com

Dent Clin N Am 56 (2012) 75–93
doi:10.1016/j.cden.2011.09.008
0011-8532/12/$ – see front matter © 2012 Elsevier Inc. All rights reserved.

dental.theclinics.com

with the patient before consent. At the completion of development, full bony impacted third molars may be positioned in close proximity or through the inferior alveolar nerve canal. It may be prudent to leave the impacted tooth (if asymptomatic) in place and not risk paresthesia or anesthesia of the inferior alveolar nerve. Surgical extraction of impacted third molars can result in significant bony defects that may not heal adequately in elderly or medically compromised patients and may result in the loss of adjacent teeth rather than the improvement or preservation of periodontal health.

EVALUATION AND DETERMINATION OF SURGICAL DIFFICULTY

Preoperative assessment of the third molar, both clinically and radiographically, is paramount during the surgical procedure for the removal of impacted teeth. Classification is based on the angulation of the impacted tooth, the relationship of the impacted tooth to the anterior border of the ramus and the second molar, the depth of the impaction, and the type of tissue overlying the impacted tooth. According to the literature, the mesioangular impaction, which accounts for 45% of all impacted mandibular third molars, is the least difficult to remove. The vertical impaction (40% of all impactions) and the horizontal impaction (10%) are intermediate in difficulty, whereas the distoangular impaction (5%) is the most difficult.[5–11]

The relationship of the impacted tooth to the anterior border of the ramus indicates the space available for tooth eruption as well as the planned extraction. If the length of the alveolar process anterior to the anterior border of the ramus is adequate enough to allow tooth eruption, the tooth is generally easier to deliver. The depth of the impaction under the hard and soft tissues is also an important consideration in determining the degree of difficulty. Root morphology also plays a significant role. Root anatomy can be either conical and fused, or separate and divergent, with the latter being more difficult to manage.[5–11]

Another important determinant of difficulty of extraction is the age of the patient. When impacted teeth are removed before the age of 20 years, there are fewer complications. The roots are usually two-thirds formed, and often separated from the inferior alveolar nerve, therefore allowing minimal bone removal and fewer complications during tooth extraction. There is usually a broader pericoronal space formed by the follicle of the tooth, which provides additional access for tooth extraction without large quantities of bone removal. However, extraction of impacted teeth in patients of older age groups (>40 years) proves to be more challenging, with increased risk of complications. The longer roots are often completely formed, which requires more bone removal, and their apical location is closer to the inferior alveolar canal, which increases the risk of postsurgical anesthesia or paresthesia. Furthermore, there is an increased density and decreased elasticity in the bone with age.[12]

EXPECTED POSTOPERATIVE COURSE

Surgical removal of impacted third molars is associated with a moderate incidence of complications. These complications range from the expected and predictable outcomes, such as edema, pain, trismus, and minor bleeding, to more severe and permanent complications, including inferior alveolar nerve anesthesia and fracture of the alveolus. The overall incidence of complication and the severity of these complications are proportional to the depth of the impaction. Extraction of impacted teeth in the elderly or medically compromised patient is associated with a higher incidence of postoperative complications, especially alveolar osteitis, infections, mandible fracture, tooth fracture, sinus communication, and inferior alveolar nerve paresthesia.[13–17]

Another determinant of the incidence of complications of third molar surgery is the relative experience and training of the clinician. After the surgical removal of an impacted third molar, certain normal physiologic responses occur. These responses include such sequelae as mild bleeding, edema, trismus, and pain. With experience, the oral and maxillofacial surgeon develops an understanding as to how this surgical procedure affects the patient's quality of life.[18,19] As expected, third molar removal has a profoundly negative impact for the first 4 to 7 days after surgery, but longer follow-up reveals improved quality of life, mostly resulting from the elimination of chronic pain and inflammation.[20]

BLEEDING

Bleeding can be minimized by using an ideal surgical technique and by avoiding untoward force, the tearing of flaps, or excessive trauma to the overlying soft tissue. When a vessel is cut or severed, the bleeding should be stopped by some measure to prevent secondary hemorrhage after surgery. The most efficient approach to obtaining hemostasis after surgery is to apply a moist gauze pack and have the patient bite down directly over the site with adequate application of pressure.

The clinician can prevent excessive postoperative bleeding by meticulous tissue management intraoperatively. However, in some patients, immediate postoperative hemostasis is difficult. In such situations a variety of measures can be used to promote local hemostasis, which include additional sutures, the application of topical thrombin, oxidized cellulose, chitosin bandage, absorbable gelatin sponge, and the use of a local anesthetic with epinephrine. Patients who have known acquired or congenital coagulopathies require extensive preparation and preoperative planning.

Postoperative bleeding is a common sequela of any dentoalveolar procedure. In healthy patients, postoperative bleeding is typically minimal and self-limited by the clotting cascade of the body. The timeline for clot formation is typically 6 to 12 hours postoperatively. Continuous active bleeding after the twelfth hour is considered excessive and should warrant concern. The patient should be taken to the emergency room for immediate attention.

It is important to distinguish and discuss the difference between active bleeding from surgical site and oozing. Patients are often concerned with excessive bleeding because they observed traces of blood in their saliva. Oozing should resolve within 36 to 72 hours postoperatively, and should respond positively to pressure. However, patients with a hemorrhagic bleed present with their mouth actively filling with blood immediately after removing the hemostatic dressing.

Among the most important measures in the management of excessive postoperative bleeding is recognition of the compromised patient. During the preoperative assessment, a detailed medical history should be obtained, including disorders associated with coagulopathies, use of anticoagulants because of comorbidities, and an individual or family history of bleeding affiliated with surgical procedures, excessive bleeding during exfoliation of deciduous teeth, and, in women, a history of menorrhagia. Appropriate adjunct therapy, such as discontinuation of anticoagulant medications, factor infusions, or use of clot-stabilizing pharmacotherapy, should be considered in patients with risk factors or known bleeding diatheses.[21,22]

Patients on warfarin, for instance, pose a common problem for the clinician performing surgical procedures. The underlying medical problem, like long-standing atrial fibrillation, deep vein thrombosis, prosthetic heart valve, or myocardial infarction, often prohibits discontinuing the anticoagulant. An acceptable management strategy is to hospitalize the patient, discontinue the medication, and maintain the patient on a step-down heparin regimen until the prothrombin time (PT)-international normalized ratio (INR) are at therapeutic levels.

Caution should be taken during treatment planning when considering the type of dentoalveolar surgery being performed. Many minor oral surgical procedures can be performed while the patient is anticoagulated.[2] In general, for patients on warfarin, a PT-INR less than 2.5 is acceptable if multiple extractions are required. For extraction of 1 to 3 teeth, without posterior teeth or surgical extractions, an INR of less than 3.0 is acceptable. Therefore, for patients requiring multiple extractions, staged visits are appropriate to prevent discontinuation of the anticoagulants.

It is common to identify an incompletely formed clot, or liver clot. This clot is often mobile and continues to aggravate the surgical site. Careful removal of the clot is critical to successfully promote hemostasis. As mentioned earlier, the use of vasoconstrictor anesthetics is appropriate once the source of bleeding has been identified. If the vasoconstrictor is applied to the area before the identification of the bleed, determining the site of origin is complicated. The wound may need to be repacked with a local hemostatic agent and sutured. Arterial bleeds that cannot be controlled with local measures should be treated with ligation or electrocautery. If bleeding persists, embolization, proximal vessel ligation, or other endovascular procedures should be considered in conjunction with interventional radiology.[23,24]

EDEMA

Postsurgical edema or swelling is an expected side effect of third molar surgery. The onset of swelling is typically between 12 and 24 hours, with a peak incidence noted 48 to 72 hours postoperatively. Edema typically begins to subside at 4 days postoperatively, with most patients experiencing complete resolution within 5 to 7 days. A cold compress may be used to minimize the onset of edema and aid in the reduction of chronic throbbing pain.[23,25–27]

It is important to educate patients of this time course and that edema is often anticipated. In addition, patients should be informed to sleep with their head elevated and not to sleep on their side, to avoid any dependent swelling. Furthermore, perioperative steroids may be used to prevent swelling in patients undergoing invasive procedures (ie, complete bony impacted third molar extraction). Perioperative steroids produce moderate to marked decreases in edema, but are short-acting in their effects **(Table 1)**.[28–35]

INFECTION

Another postsurgical complication related to the removal of impacted third molars is infection. The incidence of infection after the removal of third molars is low, at only 1.7% to 2.7%.[36] About 50% are localized subperiosteal abscess infections, which occur 2 to 4 weeks after an uneventful postoperative course. These infections are often attributed to debris remaining under the mucoperiosteal flap. Treatment is simply surgical debridement and drainage. Of the remaining 50%, few postoperative infections are significant enough to warrant surgery, antibiotics, or hospitalization. Infections occur only within the first 7 days 0.5% to 1% of the time.[8] According to the literature, this situation is considered an acceptable infection rate, which would not warrant administration of prophylactic antibiotics.[37] The oral cavity harbors a broad spectrum of bacterial flora. Therefore, any intraoral wound is exposed to certain aerobic, anaerobic, and facultative organisms with pathogenic potential. The routine use of antibiotics is used for the prevention of postoperative infections **(Table 2)**.[38]

Table 1
Steroid medications

Medication	Preoperative Evening	Day of Surgery	Postoperative Day 1	Postoperative Day 2
Methylprednisolone sodium succinate (Solu-Medrol)	16 mg by mouth at bedtime for a morning case Nothing for an afternoon case	Morning case: 125 mg intravenously at start of case Afternoon case: give 16 mg by mouth 4 h before start of case; 125 mg intravenously at start of case Night of surgery: 16 mg by mouth at bedtime	8 mg by mouth every 6 h	8 mg by mouth every 6 h
Methylprednisolone acetate (Depo-Medrol) long-acting	16 mg by mouth at bedtime for a morning case Nothing for an afternoon case	Morning case: 40 mg intramuscularly after local anesthesia administration Afternoon case: 16 mg by mouth 4 h before start of case; 40 mg intramuscularly after local anesthesia administration	Nothing	Nothing
Dexamethasone (Decadron)	8 mg by mouth at bedtime for morning case Nothing for an afternoon case	Morning case: 16 mg by mouth 4 h before start of case or 8–12 mg intravenously at start of case Afternoon case: give 16 mg by mouth 4 h before start of case; 16 mg by mouth 4 h before or 8–12 mg intravenously at start of case 8 mg by mouth night of surgery	16 mg by mouth in the morning	Nothing

Table 2
Antibiotics

Medication	Indication	Coverage	Adult Dose/Route of Administration	Pediatric Dose/Route of Administration
Penicillin VK	First line for odontogenic infections	Streptococci, oral anaerobes	250–500 mg by mouth every 6 h for 7 d	25–50 mg/kg/d every 6–12 h for 7 d (suspension 125, 250 mg/5 mL)
Cephalexin, cephadroxil	Need for bacteriocidal broader coverage	Gram-positive cocci, some gram-negative rods, oral anaerobes	250–500 mg by mouth every 6 h for 7 d	25–50 mg/kg/d divided every 12 h for 7 d. Severe infections 100 mg/kg/d (suspension 100, 125, 250 mg/5 mL)
Amoxicillin	Need for broad-spectrum infections >3 d	Gram-positive cocci, *Escherichia coli, Haemophilus influenzae,* oral anaerobes	250–500 mg by mouth every 8 h or 500–875 by mouth every 12 h for 7 d	40 mg/kg/d by mouth divided every 8 h or 45 mg/kg/d every 12 h for 7 d (suspension 125, 250 mg/5 mL)
Clindamycin	Need for broad-spectrum, oral anaerobes, penicillin-allergic patient	Gram-positive cocci, anaerobes	150–450 mg by mouth every 6 h for 7 d	8–25 mg/kg/d suspension by mouth divided every 8 h or every 6 h for 7 d (suspension 75 mg/5 mL)

Prevention of postoperative infection starts with the identification of the medically compromised patient. Furthermore, the incidence of postoperative inflammatory complications increases with age, smoking, preexisting infection/disease in the surgical area, oral contraceptive pharmacotherapy in women, and ultimately the clinician's lack of surgical experience.

When dealing with impacted teeth, mandibular third molars have been shown to have a higher rate of postoperative infections than maxillary teeth. As with other common complications, careful tissue management, debridement/curettage of necrotic/infected tissue, and thorough irrigation of the wound site with normal saline or chlorhexidine reduces the amount of detrimental bacteria within the wound site, thus decreasing the possibility of infection.[2,39]

Patients presenting with infections often complain of persistent pain and swelling that is not improving with time, a foul taste, drainage from the wound, and trismus. The patient may be febrile, but this is variable and dependent on the magnitude of the infection. Early recognition of an infectious process, like a cellulitis, requires prompt treatment with an initial course of antibiotics with broad-spectrum coverage for gram-positive and anaerobic organisms (see **Table 2**). If the symptoms persist for more than 48 to 72 hours after the procedure, with possible abscess formation, incision and drainage of the abscess may be indicated, with collection of the purulent exudate for culture and sensitivity testing to provide adequate antibiotic therapy. Prompt recognition and treatment are necessary to prevent the spread of infection into the spaces of the head and neck through the facial planes, which can result in airway embarrassment, severe infection, and morbidity.[36,40–51]

ALVEOLAR FRACTURE

Fractures of the alveolus should be considered in the differential diagnosis of persistent pain or swelling after dentoalveolar procedures. Fractures are the result of using excessive force during tooth extraction. If left unrecognized and untreated, such fractures can progress into malocclusion, malunion, infection, and paresthesia.

During the initial assessment, a primary risk factor should include the patient's age because loss of bone density, elasticity, and strength are often correlated with elderly patients. Furthermore, atrophic mandibles, or mandibles with large intrabony defects, are also at an increased risk for fracture.[52–54]

Recognition of the fracture is the most important management. It can manifest as a mobile alveolar segment or malocclusion. Postoperatively, any patient complaining of malocclusion, pain and edema disproportionate to the procedure, tooth displacement or mobility, or persistent paresthesia should be evaluated for a possible alveolar fracture.

Once a fracture is identified using panoramic radiographs or computed tomography (CT), treatment is guided by the nature of the fracture and functional limitation. Treatment ranges from modifications in the patient's diet and early immobilization to internal reduction and fixation of the fracture.

ROOT FRACTURE

One of the most frequent problems encountered in removing third molars is the fracture of the root, which may be difficult to retrieve. In these situations the root fragment may be displaced into the submandibular space, the inferior alveolar canal, or the maxillary sinus. Uninfected roots left within the alveolar bone have been shown to remain in place without postoperative complications.[55] The pulpal tissue undergoes fibrosis, and the root becomes completely incorporated within the alveolar bone. Aggressive attempts to remove portions of roots that are in precarious positions cause more damage than benefit, when radiographic follow-up may be all that is required. When such excessive forces are applied to the tooth, the torque generated causes a fracture at the junction between that portion of the root still attached to the alveolar bone and that portion already released from the socket wall.

The prevention of root fractures is primarily based on meticulous surgical technique, minimizing excessive force, and ensuring that the dentition is adequately luxated, providing an atraumatic delivery. Recognition of teeth at risk for root fracture is also an important preventative measure. Multirooted posterior teeth, curved roots, anterior dentition with root dilacerations, or teeth with widely spaced, thin roots all pose an increased risk for fracture. Thus, inadvertent root fractures can be avoided by prudent treatment planning and sectioning of a tooth before elevation and removal. Once the tooth has been delivered, it should be examined carefully to confirm that the roots were completely removed. Furthermore, it is important to reconstitute the fragments of a sectioned tooth to confirm that no remnants remain in the socket.

If a root fracture is noted, the socket should be irrigated copiously with normal saline, and an attempt should be made to directly visualize the retained root or root tip. For teeth without preoperative evidence of periapical disease or infection, small root tips, less than 3 mm, can be retained without adverse effects. For posterior teeth, the risk of causing damage to the maxillary sinus or inferior alveolar nerve may often outweigh the risk of leaving the fragment in place. However, if there is associated disease with the tooth preoperatively, it is imperative that the root fragment be removed. Once the fragment is directly visualized, root tip picks or elevators should be used to separate the fragment from the alveolar socket without apical pressure. Gentle manipulation should be used until the root is mobilized, at which point it can be delivered.

ALVEOLAR OSTEITIS

The incidence of alveolar osteitis or dry socket after the removal of impacted mandibular third molars is 3% to 30%. When dry socket is defined in terms of pain that requires the patient to seek follow-up, the incidence is between 20% and 25%. The pathogenesis of alveolar osteitis has not been clearly defined, but the condition is most likely the result of lysis of a fully formed blood clot before the clot is replaced with granulation tissue, thus leaving the alveolar bone exposed. The process of fibrinolysis occurs 3 to 4 days after extraction. Patients present with a severe throbbing, radiating pain, often associated with a malodor from the surgical site, and trismus. The source of the fibrinolytic agents may come from tissue, saliva, or bacteria.[2,23,56–64]

The incidence of dry socket is higher in patients with a social history of smoking. Female patients who take oral contraceptives are also at risk of alveolar osteitis. Its occurrence can be reduced by diminishing the bacterial contamination of the surgical site. This objective can be accomplished initially by presurgical rinsing with chlorohexidine, which reduces the incidence of dry socket by up to 50%. Copious irrigation of the surgical site with normal saline throughout the procedure is also effective. The solution to pollution is dilution. The use of topical medicaments, antibiotics like tetracycline, clot stabilizers (Gelfoam [Pfizer, Distributed by Pharmacia & UpJohn Company, Division of Pfizer INC., New York, NY, USA]), platelet-rich plasma, and medicated mouth rinses have also been suggested for prevention of alveolar osteitis.[2,37,57–62,65–68]

The treatment of the dry socket is palliative in nature during the delayed healing process. This treatment is usually accomplished by irrigation of the involved socket, gentle mechanical debridement, and placement of an obtundent dressing. The dressing is changed daily for approximately 7 days. The pain usually resolves within 3 to 5 days, although it may take as long as 10 to 14 days in some patients.

The lack of fever, edema, or purulent discharge may help to distinguish alveolar osteitis from an infection. This distinction is important, because antibiotic treatment does not resolve dry socket. Clinical findings may include a cryptlike socket with exposed bone and erythematous soft tissue margins, food debris or other detritus in the socket, and extreme tenderness to palpation. Radiographic examination should also be obtained to rule out the presence of any retained tooth structure or other surgical site complication, like alveolar fracture. Once a diagnosis of a dry socket has been made, treatment should commence immediately. Because the condition is self-limiting, pain control (**Table 3**) and increased oral hygiene are the primary goals.

PARESTHESIA/ANESTHESIA

Surgical removal of mandibular third molars places both the lingual and inferior alveolar branches at risk for possible injury. The lingual nerve is most often injured during soft tissue flap reflection, whereas the inferior alveolar nerve is injured during the extraction process itself. According to the literature, the accepted incidence of injury to the inferior alveolar and lingual nerves after third molar surgery is about 3%. Episodes of paresthesia should only be transient after routine surgical extractions. However, as many as 45% of nerve compression injuries, which are typical in third molar surgery, result in a permanent neurosensory abnormality.[13–16,69–72]

The most common predisposing factor is complete bony impaction of mandibular third molar, involving mesioangular and vertical impaction predominantly. In some cases, nerve proximity to the root is indicated by an apparent narrowing of the inferior alveolar canal as it crosses the root or root dilaceration adjacent to the canal. Other radiographic findings include diversion of the path of the canal by the tooth, darkening of the apical end of the root (indicating that it is included within the canal), and discontinuity of the white line of the canal.[73]

During the preoperative radiographic evaluation, the clinician should take extraordinary precautions to avoid injury to the nerve, such as additional bone removal or sectioning of the tooth. The patient should be thoroughly informed regarding the increased risk of nerve injury. When an injury to the lingual or inferior alveolar nerve is diagnosed in the postoperative period, the clinician should begin planning for its management, including referral to a neurologist or a microneurosurgeon.[74]

SINUS COMMUNICATION

After extraction of maxillary posterior teeth, sinus communications are common, often unrecognized, and do not require treatment. Persistent, symptomatic sinus communications are rare, with a frequency of less than 1%.[23] Oral-antral communications may result from excessive manipulation of the operative site or poor technique. Communications typically result from intimate anatomic associations between the roots of the teeth and the floor of the maxillary sinus, especially when the antrum is pneumatized.

As with displacement of teeth into the maxillary sinus, prevention of such communications starts with identification of the at-risk patient. Meticulous evaluation of preoperative radiographs for evidence of encroachment of the roots on the floor of the sinus should alert the clinician to the likelihood of this complication. On extraction, the socket should be curetted delicately if necessary. If the tooth is not removed completely, judicious exploration should be undertaken, so as not to displace the remnant into the sinus, or perforate the sinus floor while attempting to remove the fragment. A self-limiting communication may be an unavoidable side effect of tooth removal because of the anatomic relationship between the roots and the sinus, especially in patients of increasing age, because of the increased size of the antrum.

Table 3
Pain medication

Medication	Mode of Action	Indication	Adult Dose	Pediatric Dose	Common Side Effects
Acetaminophen (APAP)	Central prostaglandin synthesis inhibition	Mild to moderate pain	325–650 mg every 4–6 h not to exceed 4 g daily, 2 g daily in liver-compromised patients	<12 years of age, 10–15 mg/kg every 4–6 h, not to exceed 2500 mg daily	Hepatotoxic in high doses or when given in the presence of ethanol
Ibuprofen/ aspirin	Peripheral prostaglandin synthesis inhibition	Mild to moderate pain	Aspirin: 325–650 mg every 4–6 h not to exceed 3500 mg daily. Ibuprofen: 200, 400, 600 every 4–6 h or 800 mg every 8 h not to exceed 3200 mg daily	Ibuprofen: >6 months of age 5–10 mg/kg by mouth every 6–8 h (suspension 50 mg/1.25 mL, 100 mg/ 5 mL)	Gastrointestinal upset, platelet suppression, renal hypoperfusion: consider coadministration of antacid or proton pump inhibitor
Opioids: codeine hydrocodone oxycodone	Opioid receptor antagonist	Moderate to severe pain	In combination with APAP: 30 mg codeine, 300 mg APAP 5 mg hydrocodone, 500 mg APAP (Vicodin) 5 mg oxycodone 325 mg APAP (Percocet)	Codeine, 0.5–1 mg/kg, combined with APAP (see above dosing) every 4–6 h	Addictive constipation: consider coadministration of stool softener or laxative; may cause drowsiness or sedation

Diagnosis of a sinus communication is often made by having the patient force air through the nasal cavity while the nares are deliberately closed. If a large communication exists, air bubbles are visible in the socket, although this method may prove ineffective for small communications. If a communication is discovered, either by tactile sensation or forced air maneuver, the size of the defect and patient complaint guide the treatment.[75] As a general principle, any patient with a communication should be placed on sinus precautions, including broad spectrum antibiotics (see **Table 2**) and nasal decongestants (pseudoephedrine). Most oroantral communications heal spontaneously with little intervention.

The clinician should monitor the patient closely over the postoperative period to confirm closure of the oroantral communication. If an oroantral fistula develops, standard procedures to produce a layered closure of the wound and management of the sinus are indicated. The size of the clinical fistula is smaller than the bony defect.

TEMPOROMANDIBULAR DISORDER

Can a dentist cause a temporomandibular disorder (TMD)? The short answer is yes. In a survey of 230 patients with a TMD, 30% related the onset of their symptoms to some form of dental treatment.[75] Patients who undergo difficult mandibular exodontia procedures can develop temporomandibular joint (TMJ) symptoms immediately after the procedure. This situation often results from trauma to the TMJ that occurs during mandibular extractions if no support is given to counteract the lateral forces during difficult and prolonged exodontia procedures.

These lateral forces can be counteracted by providing support to the mandible with the other hand or the use of a bite block.[76,77] If you have failed to use a bite block, patients often tell you that they are experiencing joint pain while undergoing a difficult lower extraction. The risk of developing a postextraction TMJ problem is highest in those patients who have a previous history of TMJ problems, and those patients should be advised before any extensive procedure that they may develop a recurrence or exacerbation of their preexisting disease; be aware that this complication can also occur in someone with no preexisting TMD condition. It is also prudent to ask a question directly to the patient about any preexisting history of TMD disorders before beginning any complicated exodontias, to perform a brief TMJ examination on all patients before beginning any dental or oral surgical procedures, and to document these findings in your patient records (before rendering any patient treatment). The best way to limit or eliminate TMJ problems as a potential postsurgical complication is to attempt to do one or all (if needed) of the following.

A. Limit the amount of forces used during exodontia
B. Always use a bite block for mandibular extraction
C. Allow the patient to rest their joint during the procedure if the procedure is taking considerable time
D. Surgically remove some buccal or palatal bone or section the tooth involved to allow you to decrease the forces needed to complete the extraction.

If a patient returns to your office after a difficult exodontia procedure showing TMJ symptoms, such as TM joint pain or, limitation of opening, they should be placed on the usual TMJ/TMD treatment regimen. The usual TMJ regimen should include:

1. Recommend the patient be placed on a soft nonchew diet for 1 to 2 weeks
2. Apply moist heat to the affected side several times a day

3. Prescription for nonsteroidal antiinflammatories for 2 weeks or more
4. Prescription for muscle relaxant.

The patient should be followed up until symptoms are significantly improved, and all patient encounters and responses should be documented in the patient records.

TRISMUS

The inability to fully open one's mouth (40 mm is considered the norm) after difficult surgical exodontia is not unusual, especially in the immediate postoperative period. This situation is caused directly by swelling that occurs and most likely often peaks at 24 to 48 hours.

The severity of the facial swelling is caused by multiple factors, including length of surgical procedures, amount of soft tissue resection, and the complexity of the procedure. One week after most surgical extractions or surgical procedures, most patients should return to their presurgical level of mouth opening. If this situation does not occur and the patient presents with limited jaw opening (<20 mm), the treating dentist should be concerned enough to perform a thorough clinical examination and attempt to determine the most likely cause.

Prolonged trismus after oral surgical procedures can have multiple causes:
1. TMD/TMJ disorder
2. Patient has pain and is guarding or splinting; this is a reflexive protective measure
3. Masticator space infection
4. Fibrotic reaction secondary to inferior alveolar nerve block
5. Fractured jaw.

Diagnostic radiographs may be indicated to help establish a diagnosis but if the dentist is not certain as to the underlying cause, timely referral to an oral and maxillofacial surgeon may be of value.

TISSUE EMPHYSEMA

Tissue emphysema is an uncommon condition that follows a surgical extraction in which a regular dental handpiece was used to section a tooth or remove bone. The condition can present itself while the patient is in the dental chair or at a later time (24–48 hours). The condition can present dramatically with soft tissue facial or neck swelling that spreads and when palpitated has a popping or grafting sensation referred to as crepitus. The patient may also experience acute chest pain and shortness of breath. The cause of this soft tissue swelling is air forced under pressure below the periosteum and into, for example, the submandibular space, lateral pharyngeal space, and ultimately the mediastinum and pericardial space by the back air ejected from a dental handpiece while a surgical extraction is performed. This complication can be best avoided by using a special surgical handpiece that is either electric powered or blows the compressed air out the back.

Treatment consists of ice application to the affected site, antibiotics, and frequent monitoring. The condition is usually resolved in several days; however, severe cases require hospitalization because this condition can sometimes be life-threatening and lead to mediastinitis or meningitis.[78]

DISPLACEMENT OF TEETH AND ROOTS

Teeth and roots can be displaced into various anatomic sites depending on the location of the tooth involved (**Box 1**).

> **Box 1**
> **Various anatomic areas into which teeth have been displaced**
>
> - Maxillary sinus
> - Sublingual space
> - Submandibular space
> - Intratemporal space
> - Lateral pharyngeal space
> - Floor of nose

Multiple factors and reasons have been explained as possible causes, including:

- Surgeon's experience level
- Anatomic variants, such as thin lingual plate of mandible or sinus that is close to molar roots
- Excessive forces
- Poor visualization because of inadequate surgical exposure.

In all cases, when the tooth or root disappears, good suction and light should be used to search the extraction socket before assuming the tooth has been displaced. Often, simply by gently irrigating the socket and using a fine suction tip and good light, the missing tooth/root can be seen and retrieved. If the tooth has been displaced into the infratemporal space, it would be best to abort the procedure and close the site and refer the patient to an oral and maxillofacial surgeon. Most often, the tooth is allowed to fibrose, and then a CT scan is taken to determine the exact location of the tooth and a decision is made on whether retrieval is necessary. If a decision is made to search and retrieve the displaced tooth, this most often requires a hemicoronal flap,; although occasionally it can be accessed through an intraoral approach.

Teeth or roots can often be pushed out through a thin lingual mandibular plate into the sublingual space. If this situation occurs, this displaced tooth or root can often be palpated in the floor of the mouth and gently guided back into the socket. If this strategy is not possible, timely referral to an oral and maxillofacial surgeon is again advised.

FOREIGN BODIES

Within the past few years, because of the advent of implant placement, we have seen an increased incidence of foreign bodies displaced into the maxillary sinus, such as paralleling pins, implants, and roots. Our discussion is limited to the retrieval of such items. The key to prevention of such complications is proper preoperative planning. This planning begins with thorough clinical examination, study models, pictures, and most importantly adequate and current radiographic imaging. Periapical, occlusal, and panorex images may not be adequate. The information required to plan a complex or even a simple case of placement of multiple maxillary posterior implants may include CT scans or cone beam studies. These studies allow the dentist to view the surgical site in a three-dimensional (3D) format. The information gathered from these studies not only gives information about implant selection, placement, and need for sinus augmentation but also reveals disease that otherwise may be missed. Chronic sinusitis, infected sinus, cyst, polyps, bony defects, and quality and quantity of bone can be evaluated with these studies.

Selection of the proper implant, based on available bone, is key to prevention of mishaps (**Box 2**). Once the dimensions of the implant site are known, the proper depth to drill prevents the dentist from entering the maxillary sinus. It is advisable to have a 0-mm to 2-mm distance between implant and sinus floor. Even when properly planned an implant may still escape into the maxillary sinus. If this situation occurs, abort the procedure and reposition the patient with the occlusal plan parallel to the floor. Suction can be tried to pull the implant into the oral cavity, but the suction has to be powerful. If this strategy fails, take a radiograph. It may be periapical, occlusal, or panorex, depending on what is available in the office. If the implant was partially displaced, you should be able to locate it with these radiographic techniques.

However, if you cannot locate the implant, it may have displaced to the posterior of the maxillary sinus. Ask the patient to bend their head forward between their knees and repeat the radiographs. This maneuver should move the implant into the anterior sinus. If the implant is located close to the surgical site, reflecting a buccal flap and creating a buccal window may be used to retrieve the implant. If the implant cannot be located, check the oral cavity, gauze drapes, and suction canister for the implant. If the implant still cannot be located, the authors suggest suturing the surgical fold, placing the patient on antibiotics, pain medication, and sinus medication, and referring them to a radiologist or oral and maxillofacial surgeon for sinus radiographs. Based on your surgical training, a decision has to be made on referring the patient for treatment or doing it yourself.

On locating the implant radiographically, a surgical procedure, like a Caldwell-Luc procedure, may be required to remove the implant. If the implant was displaced because of insufficient bone height, sinus augmentation can be performed at the time and the implant placed later. If bone is adequate, then the proper implant can be selected and placed at this time.

NEEDLE BREAKAGE

Needle breakage is an uncommon occurrence in dentistry. Anesthetic techniques used in dentistry, especially the interior alveolar and lingual nerve blocks, suggest contacting the bone, then withdrawing the needle 1 mm before injecting the solution. Also, with a bite block in the mouth, when administering inferior alveolar nerve block, the needle may have to be bent to deliver the anesthetic into the pterygomandibular depression. In the pediatric population the patient may not sit still, and you should wait until movement has stopped before delivering an anesthetic.

Box 2
Steps to follow: foreign body displaced into maxillary sinus

1. Adequately evaluate posterior maxilla
2. Select proper implant
3. Suction, oral cavity
4. Radiographic studies
5. Retrieve implant, close surgical site
6. Antibiotics, pain medication, sinus medication
7. Referral to oral and maxillofacial surgeon

Avoid inserting small-diameter needles up to the hub, because this increases the chance of breakage. Once the needle has been inserted in the tissue, try to reduce redirecting the needle. This action can tear muscle, vessels, or nerves and may contribute to hematoma formation. If the needle has to be removed and the anesthetic agent delivered in the new position, try not to bend the needle, but if it must be bent, do not bend it at the hub.[79]

If breakage occurs, try to remove the needle immediately if part of it is visible. In the office avoid lengthy procedures, which may complicate the situation. Close the surgical site and refer the patient to your hospital or to a surgeon. However, the patient should be informed of the occurrence and made aware of your plan for removal of the needle. Having admitting privileges at a local hospital can be advantageous, because one can participate in the patient care. To retrieve the needle, a CT scan with 1.5-mm slices that can be reconstructed three-dimensionally is necessary. If the patient is not symptomatic a delayed removal can be planned. This strategy helps the tissue stabilize and encapsulate the needle. When immediate removal is necessary, the patient should be admitted to the hospital for management. The removal of a needle should be performed by someone who has experience in the procedure because otherwise undesirable trismus and even infection may result and prevent an early successful operation. Radiology services, including the use of a C arm and localizing needles, are needed.

Needle Breakage
- Avoid movement of patient
- Avoid insertion to close the hub
- Avoid bending the needle.

Management
- Removal of hemostat
- Notify patient
- Document event
- Referral to experienced surgeon
- Radiographic films: 3D CT
- Delayed removal.

REFERENCES

1. Sisk AL, Hammer WB, Shelton DW, et al. Complications following removal of impacted third molars: the role of the experience of the surgeon. J Oral Maxillofac Surg 1986;44:855–9.
2. Larsen PE. The effect of chlorhexidine rinse on the incidence of alveolar osteitis following the surgical removal of impacted mandibular third molars. J Oral Maxillofac Surg 1991;49:932–7.
3. Capuzzi P, Montebugnoli L, Vaccaro MA. Extraction of impacted 3rd molars– a longitudinal prospective study on factors that affect postoperative recovery. Oral Surg Oral Med Oral Pathol 1994;77:341–3.
4. Nordenram A, Hultin M, Kjellman O, et al. Indications for surgical removal of the mandibular third molar. Swed Dent J 1987;2:23–9.
5. Ng F, Bums M, Ken WJ. The impacted lower third molar and its relationship to tooth size and arch form. Eur J Orthod 1986;8:254–8.
6. Forsberg CM. Tooth size, spacing, and crowding in relation to eruption or impaction of third molars. Am J Orthod Dentofacial Orthop 1988;94:57–62.
7. Venta I, Turtola L, Ylipaavalniemi P. Radiographic follow-up of impacted third molars from age 20 to 32 years. Int J Oral Maxillofac Surg 2001;30:54–7.

8. Lysell L, Rohlin M. A study of indications used for removal of the mandibular third molar. Int J Oral Maxillofac Surg 1988;17:161–4.
9. Hattab FN, Abu Alhaija ES. Radiographic evaluation of third molar eruption space. Oral Surg Oral Med Oral Pathol Oral Radiol Endod 1999;88:285–91.
10. Ades AG, Joondeph DR, Little RM, et al. A long-term study of the relationship of third molars to changes in the mandibular dental arch. Am J Orthod Dentofacial Orthop 1990;97:323–35.
11. Larsen PE, Mesieha ZS, Peterson LJ, et al. Impacted third molars: radiographic features used to predict extraction difficulty. J Dent Res 1991;70:551–7.
12. Amler MH. The age factor in human extraction wound healing. J Oral Surg 1977; 35:193–7.
13. Nordenram A. Postoperative complications in oral surgery. Swed Dent J 1983;7: 109–14.
14. Goldberg MH, Nemarich AN, Marco WP. Complications after mandibular third molar surgery: a statistical analysis of 500 consecutive procedures in private practice. J Am Dent Assoc 1985;111:277–9.
15. Bruce RA, Frederickson GC, Small CS. Age of patients and morbidity associated with mandibular third molar surgery. J Am Dent Assoc 1980;101:240–5.
16. Osborn TP, Frederickson C, Small IA, et al. A prospective study of complications related to mandibular third molar surgery. J Oral Maxillofac Surg 1985;43:767–9.
17. Hinds EC, Frey KF. Hazards of retained third molars in older persons: report of 15 cases. J Am Dent Assoc 1980;101:246–50.
18. McGrath C, Comfort MB, Lo EC, et al. Changes in life quality following third molar surgery–the immediate postoperative period. Br Dent J 2003;194:265–8.
19. Shafer DM, Frank ME, Gent JF, et al. Gustatory function after third molar extraction. Oral Surg Oral Med Oral Pathol Oral Radiol Endod 1999;87:419–28.
20. White RP, Shugars DA, Shafer DM, et al. Recovery after third molar surgery: clinical and health-related quality of life outcomes. J Oral Maxillofac Surg 2003;61:535–44.
21. Partridge CG, Campbell JH, Alvarado F. The effect of platelet-altering medications on bleeding from minor oral surgery procedures. J Oral Maxillofac Surg 2008;66:93–7.
22. Dodson TB. Strategies for managing anticoagulated patients requiring dental extractions: an exercise in evidence-based clinical practice. J Mass Dent Soc 2002;50:44–50.
23. Susarla SM, Blaeser BF, Magalnick D. Third molar surgery and associated complications. Oral Maxillofac Surg Clin N Am 2003;15:177–86.
24. Rodesch G, Soupre V, Vazquez MP, et al. Arteriovenous malformations of the dental arcades. The place of endovascular therapy: results in 12 cases are presented. J Craniomaxillofac Surg 1998;26:306–13.
25. Forsgren H, Heimdahl AN, Johansson B, et al. Effect of application of cold dressings on the postoperative course in oral surgery. Int J Oral Surg 1985;14:223–8.
26. Peterson LJ. Post-operative patient management. In: Peterson LJ, Ellis E III, Hupp JR, et al, editors. Contemporary oral and maxillofacial surgery. 3rd edition. New York: Mosby; 1998. p. 249–56.
27. Haug RH, Perrott DH, Gonzalez ML, et al. The American Association of Oral and Maxillofacial Surgeons Age-Related Third Molar Study. J Oral Maxillofac Surg 2005;63:1106–14.
28. Hooley JR, Francis FH. Betamethasone in traumatic oral surgery. J Oral Surg 1969;27:398–403.
29. Huffman GG. Use of methylprednisolone sodium succinate to reduce postoperative edema after removal of impacted third molars. J Oral Surg 1977;35:198–9.

30. Pedersen A. Decadron phosphate in the relief of complaints after third molar surgery. Int J Oral Surg 1985;14:235–40.
31. Beirne OH, Hollander B. The effect of methylprednisolone on pain, trismus, and swelling after removal of third molars. Oral Surg Oral Med Oral Pathol 1986;61:134–8.
32. Bustedt H, Nordenram A. Effect of methylprednisolone on complications after removal of impacted mandibular third molars. Swed Dent J 1985;9:65–9.
33. Alexander RE, Throndson RR. A review of perioperative corticosteroid use in dentoalveolar surgery. Oral Surg Oral Med Oral Pathol 2000;90:406–15.
34. Green SM, editor. Tarascon pocket pharmacopoeia. Redlands (CA): Tarascon Publishing; 2007.
35. Salerno A, Hermann R. Efficacy and safety of steroid use for postoperative pain relief. Update and review of the medical literature. J Bone Joint Surg Am 2006;88:1361–72.
36. Nordenram A, Grave S. Alveolitis sicca dolorosa after removal of impacted mandibular third molars. Int J Oral Surg 1983;12:226–31.
37. Heimdahl A, Nord CE. Treatment of orofacial infections of odontogenic origin. Scand J Infect Dis 1985;46(Suppl):101–5.
38. Ren YF, Malmstrom HS. Effectiveness of antibiotic prophylaxis in third molar surgery: a meta-analysis of randomized controlled clinical trials. J Oral Maxillofac Surg 2007;65:1909–21.
39. Sweet JB, Butler DP, Drager JL. Effects of lavage techniques with third molar surgery. Oral Surg Oral Med Oral Pathol 1976;42:152–68.
40. Loukota RA. The incidence of infection after third molar removal. Br J Oral Maxillofac Surg 1991;29:336–7.
41. Happonen RP, Backstrom AC, Ylipaavalniemi P. Prophylactic use of phenoxymethyl penicillin and tinidazole in mandibular third molar surgery, a comparative placebo controlled clinical trial. Br J Oral Maxillofac Surg 1990;28:12–5.
42. Bystedt H, Nord CE. Effect of antibiotic treatment on postoperative infections after surgical removal of mandibular third molars. Swed Dent J 1980;4:27–38.
43. Bystedt H, yon Konow L, Nord CE. Effect of tinidazole on postoperative complications after surgical removal of impacted mandibular third molars. Scand J Infect Dis 1981;26(Suppl):135–9.
44. Hellem S, Nordenra A. Prevention of postoperative symptoms by general antibiotic treatment and local bandage in removal of mandibular third molars. Int J Oral Surg 1973;2:273–8.
45. Kariro GS. Metronidazole (Flagyl) and *Arnica montana* in the prevention of postsurgical complications; a comparative placebo controlled clinical trial. Br J Oral Maxillofac Surg 1984;22:42–9.
46. Krekmanov L, Nordenram A. Postoperative complications after surgical removal of mandibular third molars. Int J Oral Maxillofac Surg 1986;15:25–9.
47. Krekmanov L, Hallander HO. Relationship between bacterial contamination and alveolitis after third molar surgery. Int J Oral Surg 1950;9:274–80.
48. Krekmanov L. Alveolitis after operative removal of third molars in the mandible. Int J Oral Surg 1981;10:173–9.
49. Macgregor AJ, Addy A. Value of penicillin in the prevention of pain, swelling and trismus following the removal of ectopic mandibular third molars. Int J Oral Surg 1980;9(3):166–72.
50. Rood JP, Murgatroyd JM. Metronidazole in the prevention of "dry socket." Br J Oral Surg 1979;17:62–70.
51. Flynn T. Principles of management of odontogenic infections. In: Miloro M, Ghali GE, Larsen P, et al, editors. Peterson's principles of oral and maxillofacial surgery. 2nd edition. Ontario (Canada): BC Decker; 2004. p. 277–93.

52. Safdar N, Meechan JG. Relationship between fractures of the mandibular angle and the presence and state of eruption of the lower 3rd molar. Oral Surg Oral Med Oral Pathol Oral Radiol Endod 1995;79:680–4.
53. Tevepaugh DB, Dodson TB. Are mandibular third molars a risk factor for angle fractures? A retrospective cohort study. J Oral Maxillofac Surg 1995;53:646–9.
54. Peterson LJ. Principles of management of impacted teeth. In: Peterson LJ, Ellis E III, Hupp JR, et al, editors. Contemporary oral and maxillofacial surgery. 4th edition. St Louis (MO): CV Mosby; 2003. p. 184–213.
55. Knutsson K, Lysell L, Rohlin M. Postoperative status after partial removal of the mandibular third molar. Swed Dent J 1989;13:15–22.
56. Nitzan DN. On the genesis of "dry socket." J Oral Maxillofac Surg 1983;41: 706–10.
57. Sweet JB, Butler DP. The relationship of smoking to localized osteitis. J Oral Surg 1979;37:732–5.
58. Meechan JG, MacGregor ID, Rogers SN, et al. The effect of smoking on immediate postextraction socket filling with blood and the incidence of painful socket. Br J Oral Maxillofac Surg 1988;26:402–9.
59. Swanson AE. A double-blind study on the effectiveness of tetracycline in reducing the incidence of fibrinolytic alveolitis. J Oral Maxillofac Surg 1989;47:165–7.
60. Goldman DR, Kilgore DS, Panzer JD, et al. Prevention of dry socket by local application of lincomycin in Gelfoam. Oral Surg Oral Med Oral Pathol 1973;35: 472–4.
61. Hall HD, Bildman BS, Hand CD. Prevention of dry socket with local application of tetracycline. J Oral Surg 1971;29:35–7.
62. Mitchell L. Topical metronidazole in the treatment of "dry socket." Br Dent J 1984; 156:132–4.
63. Larsen PE. Alveolar osteitis after surgical removal of impacted mandibular third molars. Identification of the patient at risk. Oral Surg Oral Med Oral Pathol 1992;73:393–7.
64. Berwick JE, Lessin ME. Effects of a chlorhexidine gluconate oral rinse on the incidence of alveolar osteitis in mandibular third molar surgery. J Oral Maxillofac Surg 1990;48:444–8.
65. Hita-Iglesias P, Torres-Lagares D, Flores-Ruiz R, et al. Effectiveness of chlorhexidine gel versus chlorhexidine rinse in reducing alveolar osteitis in mandibular third molar surgery. J Oral Maxillofac Surg 2008;66:441–5.
66. Shepherd J. Pre-operative chlorhexidine mouth rinses reduce the incidence of alveolar osteitis. Evid Based Dent 2007;8:43.
67. Halpern LR, Dodson TB. Does prophylactic administration of systemic antibiotics prevent postoperative inflammatory complications after third molar surgery? J Oral Maxillofac Surg 2007;65:177–85.
68. Rutkowski JL, Fennell JW, Kern JC, et al. Inhibition of alveolar osteitis in mandibular tooth extraction sites using platelet-rich plasma. J Oral Implantol 2007;33:116–21.
69. Kipp DP, Goldstein BH, Weiss WW Jr. Dysesthesia after mandibular third molar surgery: a retrospective study and analysis of 1,377 surgical procedures. J Am Dent Assoc 1980;100:185–92.
70. Wofford DT, Miller RI. Prospective study of dysesthesia following odontectomy of impacted mandibular third molars. J Oral Maxillofac Surg 1987;45:15–9.
71. Mason DA. Lingual nerve damage following lower third molar surgery. Int J Oral Maxillofac Surg 1988;17:290–4.
72. Robinson PP. Observations on the recovery of sensation following inferior alveolar nerve injuries. Br J Oral Maxillofac Surg 1988;26:177–89.

73. Rood JP. The radiological prediction of inferior alveolar nerve injury during third molar surgery. Br J Oral Maxillofac Surg 1990;28:20–5.
74. Blaeser BF, August MA, Donoff RB, et al. Panoramic radiographic risk factors for inferior alveolar nerve injury after third molar extraction. J Oral Maxillofac Surg 2003;61:417–21.
75. Peterson LJ. Prevention and management of surgical complications. In: Peterson LJ, Ellis E III, Hupp JR, et al, editors. Contemporary oral and maxillofacial surgery. 3rd edition. New York: Mosby; 1998. p. 257–75.
76. Wright E. Manual of temporomandibular disorders. Ames (IA): Blackwell; 2005.
77. Spinnato G, Alberto PL. Complications of dentoalveolar surgery in Fonseca. 2nd edition, vol. 1. Oral and maxillofacial surgery. St. Louis (MO): Elsevier; 2009.
78. Henderson SJ. Risk management in clinical practice. Part II. Oral surgery. Br Dent J 2011;210(1).
79. Thoma KH. Local anesthesia. Oral surgery, vol. 1. Boston (MA): Mosby; 1969.

Management of Acute Postoperative Pain after Oral Surgery

Mark C. Fletcher, DMD, MD[a,b,c,d,*], Joseph F. Spera, DMD[e,f,g]

KEYWORDS

- Oral surgery • Pain management • Postoperative pain
- Acute pain

Pain after oral surgical procedures is one of the most studied models in pharmacology and pain research. Sensory nociception in the head and oral cavity is disproportionately greater than in most other areas of the body. Because of this phenomenon, appropriate preemptive and postoperative pain management is critical to achieve a successful outcome. This article provides the practitioner with a brief review of the acute pain mechanism as it relates to the effects of a surgical insult. An understanding of the physiologic modulation of acute pain establishes a rational framework for the concept of preemptive and postoperative analgesia. A brief review of commonly used analgesic agents is presented. Research in pain management and new drug development is ongoing as new concepts in neurophysiology and pharmacology are being elucidated.

ACUTE PAIN MECHANISMS

When examining how to manage acute postoperative pain in the oral and maxillofacial surgery patient, it is important to review the physiologic mechanisms involved in acute

A version of this article originally appeared in the May 2002 issue of *Oral and Maxillofacial Surgery Clinics of North America*.

[a] Private Practice, Oral and Maxillofacial Surgery, 34 Dale Road, Suite 105, Avon, CT 06001, USA
[b] Division of Oral and Maxillofacial Surgery, University of Connecticut School of Dental Medicine, 263 Farmington Avenue, Farmington, CT 06030, USA
[c] Hartford Hospital, 80 Seymour Street, Hartford, CT 06102, USA
[d] Connecticut Children's Medical Center, 282 Washington Street Hartford, CT 06106, USA
[e] Private Practice, 2101 Foulk Road, Wilmington, DE 19810, USA
[f] Department of Oral and Maxillofacial Surgery and Hospital Dentistry, Christiana Care Health System, Wilmington, DE, USA
[g] Department of Oral and Maxillofacial Surgery, Thomas Jefferson University Hospital, Philadelphia, PA, USA
* Corresponding author. Private Practice, Oral and Maxillofacial Surgery, 34 Dale Road, Suite 105, Avon, CT 06001.
E-mail address: markcfletcher@att.net

postsurgical pain. Webster's dictionary describes pain as a basic bodily sensation induced by a harmful stimulus characterized by physical discomfort.[1] When tissue homeostasis is disrupted by a surgical insult, autonomic, hormonal, and chemical changes that play a role in the subjective perception of pain are observed physiologically.

This article does not address every detail involved in the acute pain mechanism. Nonetheless, a simplified understanding of the neurophysiology of acute pain is important when reviewing pharmacotherapy **Tables 1** and **2**.

Peripheral pain stimuli are initially encountered at the nociceptor level on skin, joint, or end-organ surfaces where they are processed and transmitted via first-order neurons to the dorsal horn neurons of the spinal cord. These first-order neurons vary in width and composition. These nerve fibers are classified into 2 general subtypes: A and C. A fibers tend to be myelinated and fast conducting, whereas C fibers tend to be unmyelinated, slower-conducting fibers. A fibers produce a more localized sharp pain, whereas C fibers produce a dull, poorly localized ache. These primary afferent fibers, through the release of specific neurotransmitters, transmit sensory information to the dorsal horn neurons of the spinal cord.

The spinal cord is comprised of various laminae, numbered 1 through 10. These laminar tracts are comprised of specific types of second-order neurons, each varying in function. Examples of dorsal horn neurons include nociceptive specific cells (NS), wide dynamic range cells (WDR), complex cells, viscerosomatic cells, and others. NS cells are specific for a small receptive field and respond to high-threshold noxious stimuli. Conversely, WDR cells respond to a wide spectrum of stimuli, receiving mainly multisynaptic input from both A and C fibers. WDR cells have a wider receptive field than NS cells. Complex, viscerosomatic, and other types of dorsal horn neurons may play excitatory and inhibitory roles on pain stimulus transmission while having various receptive field sizes and pain characteristics.[2]

Depending on the afferent fiber type and the neurotransmitters involved, primary afferent stimuli are directed to specific laminae within the spinal cord where they are processed and transmitted, via the spinothalamic tract, to the brain. Information is transmitted to third-order neurons in the thalamus for further processing. Afferent information is then relayed to the somatotopic areas of the cerebral cortex, where conscious pain perception arises. It is at this sophisticated supraspinal level that

Table 1
Commonly used oral narcotic analgesics

Drug	Trade Names	Usual Dose	Combination Drug
Codeine	Empirin with codeine Tylenol with codeine	30–60 mg	Aspirin (325 mg) Acetaminophen (300–650 mg)
Hydrocodone	Lortab, Norco, Vicodin, Maxidone	5.0, 7.5, 10.0 mg	Acetaminophen (500–750 mg)
Hydromorphone	Dilaudid	1–4 mg	
Oxycodone	Percocet, Percodan, Roxicet, Roxiprin, Tylox	2.25–5.0 mg, 7.5 mg	Acetaminophen (300–500 mg) Aspirin (325 mg)
Pentazocine	Talacen, Talwin	12.5–25.0 mg	Acetaminophen (650 mg) Aspirin (325 mg)
Meperidine	Demerol	50–150 mg	None

From Fletcher MC, Spera JF. Pre-emptive and postoperative analgesia for dentoalveolar surgery. Oral Maxillofacial Sur Clin N Am 2002;14:137–51; with permission.

Table 2 Properties of oral narcotic analgesics						
Drug	Analgesia	Sedation	Nausea or Vomiting	Constipation	Euphoria	Comment
Codeine	+	+++	++	++	+	Low potency
Hydrocodone	++	+	+	+	++	
Hydromorphone	++	++	+	+	+++	
Oxycodone	+++	++	+	+	+++	
Pentazocine	++	+	+	+	+	CNS side effects
Meperidine	++	++	++	+	+++	Rarely indicated

Plus and minus symbols indicate estimations of degree of negative or positive effect.
Abbreviation: CNS, central nervous system.
From Fletcher MC, Spera JF. Pre-emptive and postoperative analgesia for dentoalveolar surgery. Oral Maxillofacial Surg Clin N Am 2002;14:137–51; with permission.

such factors as anxiety, depression, fear, and learned behavior exert their influences on the phenomenon of perceived pain (**Figs. 1** and **2**).

Although pain transmission in the head is quite similar to transmission in the spinal system, some distinct differences exist. Sensory nociception is disproportionately greater in the head and oral cavity when compared with other parts of the body. This amplification probably results from speech, taste, and masticatory functions. Cranial nerves V, VII, IX, and X relay sensory information to the trigeminal ganglion. The spinal nucleus of the ganglion transmits afferent sensory information through the medullary dorsal horn of the spinal cord to the thalamus.[3] This amplification in sensory distribution is what makes postsurgical dental pain one of the most studied models in pharmacology and pain research.

MODULATION OF THE ACUTE PAIN MECHANISM
Peripheral Sensitization

With the basic neuroanatomic architecture previously described, the modulatory processes involved at the various levels of impulse transmission can be better understood. Free nerve endings, or nociceptors, are peripherally activated in response to tissue damage. Afferent conduction of information is transmitted through myelinated A fibers or unmyelinated C fibers to the dorsal horn neurons. At the level of the free nerve ending, there is interplay between the various surrounding structures, including blood vessels and mast cells. This interplay contributes to the release of pain mediators, such as substance P, glutamate, and metabolites of arachidonic acid, among others. The release of histamine and cytokine activity in the face of mast cell degranulation can sensitize other free nerve endings in the area of insult. Plasma components, platelets, and the products of surgically damaged cells themselves all contribute to the release of neuroactive substances involved in peripheral sensitization and hyperalgesia.[2,3]

Central Sensitization

Recent studies have demonstrated central sensitization of the dorsal horn neurons in the spinal cord. This concept was examined by using a surgical incision in the rat model. Three types of dorsal horn neurons, low-threshold, WDR, and high-threshold cells, were studied after surgical incision in the root foot. Decreased withdrawal thresholds to punctate mechanical stimuli after incision was observed. The activation

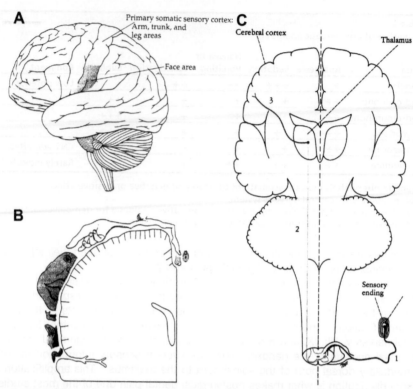

Fig. 1. (*A*) Primary somatic sensory cortex located in the postcentral gyrus. Note the large proportional area dedicated to the facial region. (*B*) Penfield and Rasmussen's homunculus[37] depicting disproportionately large areas dedicated to the face and jaw regions. (*C*) A simplified view of the ascending sensory pathway depicting first-, second-, and third-order neurons leading to the primary somatic sensory cortex. ([*B*] *From* Martin JH. Neuroanatomy text and atlas. 2nd edition. Old Tappan (NJ): Appleton and Lange; 1996. p. 379; with permission; and [*C*] Snell RS. Clinical neuroanatomy for medical students. 5th edition. Philadelphia: Lippincott Williams and Wilkins; 2001. p. 146. Copyright 2001; with permission.)

of various neuropeptides and excitatory amino acids upregulate centrally mediated impulse transmission. These findings suggest central sensitization and hyperalgesia in the face of surgical insult.[4] Additional studies on the concept of central sensitization are currently underway and may have significant implications in the concept of preemptive and preventive analgesia.

Neuropeptide and Amino Acid Modulators

Research in the area of neurophysiology has elucidated the existence of specific neuropeptides and excitatory amino acids released at central and peripheral nerve terminals.[2,5–7] Examples of such neuropeptides are substance P, calcitonin, gene-related peptide, cholecystokinin, and somatostatin. These neuropeptides play a role in the modulation of transmitted afferent pain stimuli. The principle excitatory amino acid is *N*-methyl-Daspartate (NMDA). Specific excitatory amino acid receptors also exist on postsynaptic dorsal horn neurons in the spinal cord. NMDA receptors are specific to A-and C-fiber stimulation.[8] These receptors, among others, have been the target of various experimental analgesic drugs.

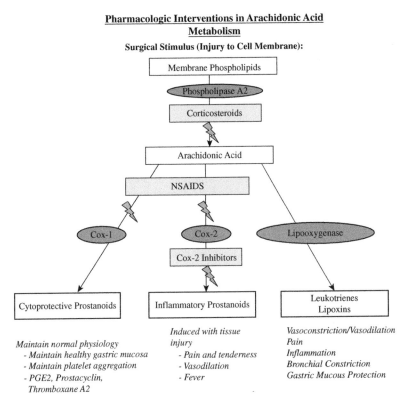

Pharmacologic Interventions in Arachidonic Acid Metabolism

Surgical Stimulus (Injury to Cell Membrane):

Membrane Phospholipids

Phospholipase A2

Corticosteroids

Arachidonic Acid

NSAIDS

Cox-1   Cox-2   Lipooxygenase

Cox-2 Inhibitors

| Cytoprotective Prostanoids | Inflammatory Prostanoids | Leukotrienes Lipoxins |

Maintain normal physiology
- *Maintain healthy gastric mucosa*
- *Maintain platelet aggregation*
- *PGE2, Prostacyclin, Thromboxane A2*

Induced with tissue injury
- *Pain and tenderness*
- *Vasodilation*
- *Fever*

Vasoconstriction/Vasodilation
Pain
Inflammation
Bronchial Constriction
Gastric Mucous Protection

Fig. 2. Pharmacologic interventions in arachidonic acid metabolism. COX, cyclooxygenase; NSAIDS, nonsteroidal antiinflammatory drugs. (*From* Fletcher MC, Spera JF. Pre-emptive and postoperative analgesia for dentoalveolar surgery. Oral Maxillofacial Surg Clin N Am 2002;14:137–51; with permission.)

Excitatory and inhibitory modulation was further studied at the spinal level. Wind-up pain hyperalgesia, whereby repeated stimulus frequency beyond a critical threshold leads to the enhancement of cellular responses, both in magnitude and duration, is thought to be a result of neurokinin excitatory modulation. Repeated stimulation of C fibers converging on WDR cells in dorsal horn neurons is thought to elicit the release of substance P and the excitatory amino acid NMDA, leading to this clinical phenomenon.[9,10] Pharmacologic agents, such as ketamine, have been found to antagonize at the NMDA receptor, thus, exhibiting some intrinsic analgesic properties.[11] Conversely, the release of inhibitory neuropeptides, such as γ-amino-butyric acid (GABA), from the dorsal horn neurons is associated with the inhibition of primary afferent pathways by primary afferent depolarization. It is this phenomenon that has provided the basis for dorsal spinal cord stimulation in the treatment of patients with chronic pain.[12] Enhancing the activity of inhibitory GABA provides another pharmacotherapeutic approach to analgesia. Pharmacologic agents, such as barbiturates and benzodiazepines, achieve their biologic effect as GABA receptor agonists.

Supraspinal Modulation

Supraspinal modulation of impulse transmission in the thalamus and cerebral cortex is also observed. Monoamines, such as serotonin and norepinephrine, and the release of endogenous enkephalins have been observed to downregulate the afferent pain stimulus in the spinal cord directly or through second-messenger activation and provide excellent avenues for pharmacotherapy. Similarly, anxiolysis and patient education can modify cortical processing of pain perception.[9,10] This factor is extremely relevant in ambulatory oral and maxillofacial surgery patients. Many new selective serotonin reuptake inhibitors and centrally acting analgesics, such as clonidine, achieve their biologic effect at this level.

PREEMPTIVE ANALGESIA

An understanding of the cascade of neurophysiologic events that stem from a surgical insult provides an excellent rationale for attempts at preemptive analgesia. Oral and maxillofacial surgery patients undergoing modern ambulatory dentoalveolar surgery require a rapid return to the activities of daily living. Unlike other surgical disciplines, inpatient hospital stays and prolonged recovery are not a tolerated outcome in most cases. It has been suggested that lessening pain during the surgical procedure itself will reduce overall postoperative analgesia requirements.[13] Preemptive analgesic intervention is aimed at attenuating or entirely blocking central pain sensitization, leading to reduced pain in the postoperative period. Preemptive goals are to attain reductions in analgesic rescue medication requirements and to hasten overall recovery.

Analgesia for postoperative dentoalveolar surgery has traditionally been approached by prescribing a particular analgesic drug of choice with instructions to take as needed for pain. Experience with this approach dictates that many patients will wait until the onset of significant pain before starting the medication. Recent studies have demonstrated efficacy in using adjunctive analgesic measures, such as the administration of long-acting local anesthesia, corticosteroids, and intraoperative nitrous oxide analgesia, with regard to reducing postoperative pain.[3] Also, the concept of using analgesic pain medication postoperatively, before the onset of significant pain (as preventive analgesia), is being used.[13] Each of these modalities have lead to decreased total pain after surgery and decreased pain intensity at fixed postoperative time intervals when measured by a visual analog scale.[8,13]

Investigators have retrospectively explored the concept of the preemptive blockade of central sensitization resulting from surgery.[14] In this analysis, the amount of time was measured between surgery and the first request of postoperative analgesia medication in patients who underwent a variety of surgical procedures under general anesthesia. Preoperative administration of local anesthesia delayed the postoperative request for analgesic medication by 6 hours when compared with control subjects. Preoperative opioid administration caused a 3-hour delay, and the contribution of both local anesthesia and an opioid showed additive effects on delaying the request of postoperative analgesic medications. This finding provided sound rationale for prospective investigational studies on preemptive analgesia.

Subsequent prospective studies on preemptive analgesia were initiated in the oral and maxillofacial ambulatory surgery model.[15,16] The preoperative use of 0.5% bupivacaine, when compared with lidocaine and saline placebo injections in patients undergoing third molar surgery under general anesthesia, lead to statistically significant decreased pain perception at 4 and 48 hours after surgery. Additional studies have suggested that the use of nonsteroidal antiinflammatory drugs (NSAIDs) before surgery, with the preincisional administration of long-acting local anesthesia, significantly reduced the amount of postoperative pain, as measured by a visual analog scale.[11] These results support the theory that blockade of factors leading to central sensitization will have a positive effect by decreasing postoperative pain perception.

It should be pointed out that these studies support the supposition that blocking central sensitization reduces overall pain perception and pain duration. Nevertheless, the question remains: At which point is preemptive intervention most important, blocking the nociceptive input at surgery or blocking the postoperative pain resulting from surgery in the immediate postoperative period? A recent study indicates that whether or not the nociceptive input of surgery was blocked through the administration of long-acting local anesthesia, overall postoperative pain perception was the same.[16] This finding suggests the important contribution of immediate postoperative pain toward the initiation of central sensitization in ambulatory oral and maxillofacial surgical patients. Additional studies are necessary to clarify this distinction.

When looking at the data available for patients undergoing complex dentoalveolar surgery, it would seem prudent for the practitioner to administer a long-acting local anesthetic, such as etidocaine or bupivacaine, at the time of surgery or, at the latest, in the immediate postoperative period. This practice would preemptively block the initiation of central sensitization and the resulting hyperalgesia. The use of nitrous oxide analgesia during surgery and corticosteroids for the reduction of postoperative inflammation and local tissue injury should also lead to the diminution of postoperative pain. Most recently, it has been demonstrated that pretreatment with NSAIDs also leads to decreased postoperative pain and edema in oral and maxillofacial surgery patients.[11,17] This treatment may prove to be another effective preemptive analgesic approach. Further studies regarding preemptive analgesia in surgical patients will undoubtedly change the standard approach to ambulatory surgical pain management.

POSTOPERATIVE ANALGESIC AGENTS
The Opioid Drug Class

Mechanism of action

Opioids in oral and maxillofacial surgery have long been the mainstay drug class for the management of moderate to severe postsurgical pain. References to the opium poppy can be found dating back to 300 BC in Sumerian and Egyptian culture. The opium poppy, *Papaver somniferum*, gives rise to more than 20 different alkaloids. Morphine was isolated in 1806, followed by codeine in 1832.[18] Opioid receptors are found throughout the body, providing sites for activation of endogenously released opioid substances. Beta-endorphins, enkephalins, and dynorphin compounds have been identified as agents for endogenous central analgesia.[19] These endogenous opioid receptors provide natural targets for centrally mediated pharmacotherapy.

Opioid receptors are subdivided into delta, kappa, and mu subtypes. They are located centrally in C-fiber terminals within the dorsal horn of the spinal cord. They are also found supraspinally in nociceptive processing areas of the brain. A peripheral component of opioid analgesia has also been described at the afferent C-fiber terminals on skin and joint surfaces.[9] Current terminology has now classified delta, kappa, and mu opioid receptors as OP1, OP2, and OP3, respectively. It is primarily the central analgesic action of opioids that makes them so effective in managing acute postsurgical pain.

Opioid receptors, neuronal pools, exogenous and endogenous ligands, routes of delivery, and dosage of various compounds have contributed immensely to our ability to effectively manage postoperative pain in oral and maxillofacial surgery patients.[19] All opioids act on stereo-specific, saturable membrane receptors. As previously mentioned, these receptors are widely but unevenly distributed throughout the central nervous system (CNS). In addition to the 3 opioid receptors, delta, kappa, and mu, 2 additional receptors, epsilon and sigma, also exist. Studies have indicated that only mu, kappa, and delta receptors (OP3, OP2, and OP1, respectively) have analgesic properties. Mu/OP3 receptors are located widely throughout the CNS and have been identified in the limbic system, thalamus, striatum, hypothalamus, and midbrain.[18] Kappa receptors are located primarily in the spinal cord and cerebral cortex. Opiate receptors are coupled with G-protein receptors, which function as positive and negative modulators of synaptic transmission via second-messenger activation. These G proteins provide amplification of physiologic activity at the receptor level. Opioid receptors differ with respect to distribution, ligand affinity, and proposed behavioral action. Research has confirmed that the mu/OP3 receptor is not only associated with analgesic properties but is also responsible for respiratory depression. Two mu receptor subtypes have been discovered. Although a certain degree of cross-reactivity exists, mu1 is mainly responsible for analgesia and mu2 for respiratory depression. This finding has opened the door to research aimed at developing mu1-specific analgesic agents.[19] Pure agonists, such as morphine sulfate, codeine, oxycodone, and meperidine, act on the mu/OP3 receptor.

The nomenclature for opioid classification is based on the type and degree of receptor activation. Drugs or neurotransmitters that act on receptors and cause a biologic effect are known as agonists. Opiate agonists produce analgesia by inhibiting excitatory neurotransmission of substance P, acetylcholine, noradrenaline, and dopamine. Opiate agonists also modulate the endocrine system and immune system. They inhibit the release of vasopressin, somatostatin, insulin, and glucagon.[18]

Opiate antagonists will act on receptors to reverse a biologic effect. They will occupy a receptor without eliciting a physiologic response. This factor has clinical significance with the use of certain narcotic-reversal agents and mixed agonist-antagonist agents. Mixed agonist-antagonist drugs can be considered for use in postoperative analgesia. These drugs have potent analgesic effects without the high potential for tolerance or dependency inherent in pure mu/OP3 agonists. The opioid agonist-antagonists have high affinity and low potency at the mu receptor while activating kappa, delta, and sigma receptors. Drugs in the agonist-antagonist class include such agents as butorphanol, pentazocine, and nalbuphine. The opioid agonist-antagonist agents have been proven effective for use in the control of moderate pain but have not proven to be potent enough analgesics for severe postoperative pain.

The most significant adverse reaction to the opioid agonists is respiratory depression. For this reason, most opioid agents used in outpatient postsurgical pain management are formulated in combination with non-narcotic analgesics. This formulation potentiates the analgesic effects of the individual agents within the formulation while minimizing the potentially life-threatening side effects of pure opioid administration. When these drugs are properly titrated and the recommended doses are not exceeded, the risk of respiratory depression is small because the tolerance to this effect develops rapidly. Allergic reactions to opiate agonists are uncommon. Opiates can cause histamine release, resulting in pruritus. The most common gastrointestinal (GI) effects include nausea, vomiting, and constipation.

Codeine

Codeine remains one of the most frequently prescribed narcotics to treat postoperative pain in the ambulatory surgical setting. It is also widely used for its antitussive properties. It is most commonly used in combination with acetaminophen. Codeine is closely related in structure to morphine, possessing a methyl group that protects it from rapid degradation in the liver. It is one-third as potent as morphine.[20] Doses of 120 mg will produce respiratory depression similar to that resulting from 10 mg of morphine sulfate. Because of its low degradation on the first pass, codeine's oral efficacy is two-thirds that of its parenteral activity. Studies assessing codeine's ability to relieve postoperative oral surgical pain have been equivocal and have indicated that 60 mg of codeine is required to achieve therapeutic benefit in dental pain. The usual adult dosage is 30 to 60 mg orally every 4 to 6 hours as needed, with a maximum dose of 360 mg in 24 hours. This dosage has led to formulations that combine codeine with other analgesics, such as acetaminophen. In doing so, analgesic synergism will reduce the total dose requirements for codeine. The maximum dosage of acetaminophen should not exceed 4 g in a 24-hour period. The most common side effects are constipation, nausea, vomiting, and sedation.

A small percentage of patients have been found to be nonresponders to codeine and codeine-based derivative analgesic agents, such as hydrocodone and oxycodone. These patients do not derive adequate analgesic efficacy from these types of analgesic agents. Manifestations of this phenomenon may be difficult to differentiate from drug-seeking behavior. It has been discovered that approximately 5% to 10% of Caucasians lack functional cytochrome P450 2D6, a liver enzyme involved in the metabolism of many drugs, including codeine.[21] Assays of codeine and its metabolites have been compared with CYP2D6 phenotypic activity in human patients, demonstrating a direct correlation between the two.[22] Although this phenomenon is still being investigated, there is a likely genetic contribution to poor codeine metabolism. Oral and maxillofacial surgery patients who do not respond to codeine-based analgesia in the immediate postoperative period may respond to alternative agents, such as meperidine or propoxyphene.

Hydrocodone

Hydrocodone was first synthesized in 1920. It is derived from the opioid alkaloid thebaine. It has antitussive and analgesic properties.[23] Hydrocodone is approximately 6 times more potent than codeine on a weight-per-weight basis.[24] Hydrocodone is an oral semisynthetic mu opiate receptor agonist. Structurally, hydrocodone is a ketone derivative of codeine. Equipotent doses of codeine and hydrocodone have similar efficacy and severity of adverse side effects.[17] The combination of acetaminophen and hydrocodone are used together to treat moderate to severe pain. Combination formulations of hydrocodone are available in doses of 5.0, 7.5, and 10.0 mg (such formulations include Vicodin, Vicodin ES, Norco, and Maxidone). Hydrocodone and ibuprofen have also been combined (Vicoprofen) for the treatment of moderate to severe pain. The usual dose of 5 to 10 mg is effective for approximately 3 hours. A 5-mg dose of hydrocodone is equipotent to 30 mg of codeine. Also, a 4-g/d ceiling dose of acetaminophen within the combination agents establishes daily dose limitations. Side effects of hydrocodone include constipation, nausea, vomiting, and sedation.

Oxycodone

Oxycodone is an oral semisynthetic opiate agonist derived from the opioid alkaloid thebaine. It has been in clinical use since the early 1900s. Its pharmacologic action is similar to that of morphine. Oxycodone, similar to hydrocodone, is a cogener to codeine. It is approximately 10 to 12 times more potent than codeine on a weight-per-weight basis.[24] Because of resistance to extensive first-pass metabolism, oxycodone is an excellent orally administered narcotic analgesic agent. Similar to other narcotic combination medications, acetaminophen-oxycodone formulations (Percocet, Roxicet, Tylox) work through a synergistic effect. Combinations produce additive analgesic effects compared with the same doses of either agent alone. Similar to the hydrocodone combination agents, increased dosage of oxycodone combination agents is limited by the maximum dose and ceiling effect of acetaminophen at 4 g/d. The typical dose of oxycodone is 5 to 10 mg. Oral administration of acetaminophen-oxycodone has an onset of analgesia in 30 minutes and a peak analgesic effect in 90 minutes. The duration of analgesia is 3 to 4 hours. The metabolism of both drugs is mediated through cytochrome P450. The administration of other drugs, which affect these isoenzymes, may affect the efficacy and incidence of adverse reactions from this formulation. As in the case of codeine, a small percentage of nonresponders may be related to decreased CYP2D6 expression. A 5-mg dose of oxycodone is equivalent to 50 to 60 mg of codeine.

Oxycodone is indicated for the treatment of moderate to severe postoperative pain. As a solo agent, 5.0 to 7.5 mg of oxycodone is administered orally every 6 hours, as needed for pain. Side effects to oxycodone are similar to all centrally acting narcotic agonists and include constipation, nausea, vomiting, and sedation. It is worthy to note that oxycodone can elicit a significant euphoric effect and carries an increased potential for abuse in both solo and combination formulations. Recent reports have shown this problem to be increasing in severity in the United States.[25] Sustained-release oxycodone compounds (eg, OxyContin) are not indicated in the management of acute pain after dentoalveolar surgery.

Meperidine (Demerol)

Meperidine hydrochloride is a synthetic opiate agonist belonging to the phenylpiperidine class. Other members of this group include alfentanil, fentanyl, loperamide, and sufentanil. Meperidine is recommended for moderate to severe acute pain and has the unique ability to interrupt postoperative shivers and chills. According to the Agency for Health Care Policy and Research Clinical Practice Guideline, for acute pain management in operative procedures, meperidine is recommended only for use in brief courses. Meperidine should be considered as a second-line agent to treat acute pain. Meperidine is metabolized to normeperidine, a compound capable of inducing seizures at high concentrations. Meperidine is available in oral and parenteral formulations and was approved for use by the Food and Drug Administration (FDA) in 1942.

Meperidine is primarily a kappa-opiate receptor agonist and has local anesthetic effects. Its affinity for the kappa receptor is greater than that of morphine. The oral form of meperidine undergoes extensive first-pass metabolism. To treat moderate to severe pain in adults, the dosage is 50 to 150 mg by mouth or intramuscularly (IM) every 3 to 4 hours. The drug has a short analgesic effect and a significant euphoric effect.[24] The recommended intravenous (IV) dose is 50 to 100 mg. After oral administration, the onset of analgesia is within 15 minutes and peak effects occur in 60 to 90 minutes. Protein binding is 65%, primarily to albumin and α-1-acid glycoprotein. In patients with normal hepatic and renal function, the half-life is 3 to 5 hours. As previously mentioned, meperidine is a reasonable alternative for the rare patients who have been determined to be nonresponders to codeine-derived analgesics or those with a true allergy to the codeine class. Its use needs to be limited to 10 to 14 days, however, because of the potential buildup of toxic normeperidine byproducts. Also, meperidine is strictly contraindicated in patients taking monoamine oxidase inhibitor–type antidepressants.

Pentazocine (Talwin Nx)

Pentazocine is a synthetic opiate agonist-antagonist analgesic used to treat moderate to severe pain. This drug is considered the prototype of the agonist-antagonist class of analgesics, with a potency of approximately one-sixth to one-third that of morphine. It was approved for use by the FDA in 1967 and reformulated to include naloxone and approved for use in 1982. At therapeutic doses, pentazocine has less respiratory depression than morphine. It does have a tendency to produce dysphoric reactions. Pentazocine is an agonist at the kappa receptor and weak antagonist at the mu receptor. Its antagonism at the mu receptor is weaker than both butorphanol and nalbuphine. It is given orally, parenterally, or IM. It is well absorbed in the GI tract, and the onset of action is 15 to 30 minutes after administration. The analgesic effect of 50 mg of pentazocine is equipotent to 60 mg of codeine. The recommended oral dosage is 50 mg every 3 to 4 hours.

Butorphanol (Stadol)

Butorphanol tartrate is a synthetic parenteral and intranasal opiate agonist-antagonist. There is good GI absorption of oral butorphanol but it undergoes extensive first-pass metabolism, making its bioavailability low. Transnasal administration of butorphanol has an absolute bioavailability of 60% to 70%.[26] Although it is structurally related to morphine, it is more similar in action to nalbuphine. Butorphanol is used to treat moderate to severe acute pain. Butorphanol injection was approved in 1978; the nasal spray was approved in 1991. Although butorphanol was not a controlled substance in the United States when it was introduced, the Drug Enforcement Administration recommended in June 1997 that both the injection and the nasal spray be classified as a controlled substance.

Butorphanol is an agonist at the kappa receptors but is a weak antagonist at the mu receptor. A recent study indicates that butorphanol delivered transnasally is an effective analgesic for postoperative pain. Butorphanol is administered transnasally by spraying once in 1 nostril. Each spray is equivalent to 1 mg. In this study, the threshold dose for adequate analgesia was 1 mg. A 2-mg dose produced better analgesia, with an increased incidence in adverse events, namely dizziness and drowsiness. Butorphanol is reportedly being considered as an option for preoperative and intraoperative analgesia. Additional studies will be needed to establish the exact role of butorphanol in perioperative pain management.[27]

Tramadol (Ultram, Ultram ER, Ryzolt)

Tramadol is a centrally acting opioid analgesic, it was introduced to the US market in 1994 and is utilized for treatment of moderate to severe pain. It is a synthetic analog of codeine and is converted to the active metabolite O-desmethyltramadol, a more potent mu opioid agonist causing inhibition of ascending pain pathways in the central nervous system. Tramadol also acts as a serotonin releasing agent and a norepineph-rine re-uptake inhibitor making it unique when compared to other opiate formula-tions.[28] For these reasons, it is considered to have atypical opiate properties. When initially introduced to the US market, tramadol was thought to have a low dependence potential. Further experience with this medication has demonstrated more significant dependency and withdrawal properties than originally thought. This has resulted in its classification as a controlled substance regulated in similar fashion to other opioid analgesics. Immediate release tablets of tramadol are used for acute pain manage-ment and extended release formulations have been developed for around-the-clock pain management. Tramadol is available in 50 mg (scored) immediate release tablets and 100, 200, and 300 mg extended release tablets. Recommended adult dosing for oral surgical pain is 50 to 100 mg of the immediate release formulation every 4 to 6 hours, not to exceed 400 mg/day. Extended release formulations should not exceed 300 mg/day. Clinical studies have demonstrated tramadol and tramadol-acetaminophen combinations to be similar in efficacy, and with less adverse events when compared to hydrocodone/acetaminophen combinations, codeine, aspirin with codeine, and placebo for the management of post-operative oral surgical pain.[29,30]

The Nonsteroidal Antiinflammatory Drug Class

Mechanism of action

NSAIDS have been used since the discovery of sodium salicylate in 1875 and acetylsalicylic acid (aspirin) in 1899 for the treatment of pain, fever, and inflammation. Most recently, these drugs have become quite diverse and more specific in their mechanisms of action. The antiinflammatory and analgesic properties of these drugs without the narcotic-related side effects of drowsiness, constipation, respiratory depression, and addiction potential make NSAIDs very popular in ambulatory dentoalveolar surgical patients. With regard to analgesia, NSAIDs primarily act peripherally at the site of tissue injury. As previously discussed in this article, a cascade of events occurs at the tissue level immediately after making a surgical incision. Inflammatory mediators, such as histamine, serotonin, bradykinin, platelet-activating factor, interleukin-1, and derivatives of arachidonic acid metabolism, such as prostaglandins, thromboxanes, and leukotrienes, are released. These mediators have been found to sensitize peripheral nociceptors, leading to inflammatory pain and hyperalgesia. NSAIDs block this cascade of events, thus, leading to a reduction in inflammation and pain perception.

NSAIDs exert their effect by inhibiting the synthesis of prostaglandins within the endoperoxide pathway. Inflammation will prompt the enzyme phospholipase A2 to break down cell membrane components and yield arachidonic acid. The endoperoxide biosynthetic pathway leads to the metabolism of arachidonic acid and the synthesis of prostaglandins. The initial step of the endoperoxide pathway is driven by the enzyme cyclooxygenase (COX). Prostaglandins have varied physiologic effects that are both beneficial and detrimental to normal physiologic homeostasis. The beneficial effects of prostaglandins include the maintenance of renal blood flow through the activity of prostacyclin, gastric mucin production, and mucosal protection and the maintenance of platelet function. Conversely, pain, inflammation, fever, bronchial constriction, and decreased blood flow can also be attributed to the release of prostaglandins.

COX has been identified as a major actor in the endoperoxide pathway. COX is subdivided into 2 isoenzymes, COX-1 and COX-2. Physiologically, it has been determined that COX-1 is constitutively released and contributes to normal physiologic homeostasis. It provides the previously mentioned beneficial aspects of prostaglandin function. Alternatively, the isoenzyme, COX-2, is released primarily after tissue injury and plays an instrumental role in tissue inflammation and pain mediation. Interleukin-1, tumor necrosis factor, lipopolysaccharide, mitogens, and reactive oxygen intermediates are all mediators released after tissue injury, which have been found to induce COX-2 enzyme activity.[31]

NSAIDs have been designed over the years to inhibit enzymatic reactions in the endoperoxide cascade. Historically, most of the drugs were nonselective COX inhibitors. Sodium salicylate, aspirin, ibuprofen, and others are included in this group. During the past 10 years, COX-2 selective inhibitors have been developed. These drugs are aimed at blocking the inductive, detrimental effects of the COX-2–mediated prostaglandins while maintaining the physiologically beneficial effects of the COX-1 isoenzyme. The drug formulation known as celecoxib (Celebrex) is a COX-2 selective inhibitor. COX-2 inhibiting medications play a role in the management of mild to moderate pain, with reported diminished side-effect profiles when compared to the non-specific COX inhibitors.[32]

Adverse responses to NSAIDs are directly related to their mechanism of action. The most common are GI disturbances, gastric irritation, increased bleeding time, and renal impairment. Less common effects are allergic reactions and asthma. These effects are all related to prostaglandin inhibition. GI adverse effects are the most common adverse reaction to NSAIDs and constitute the greatest risk of death.[33] Patients with peptic ulcer disease and other disturbances in GI mucosal integrity should avoid the usage of NSAIDs altogether. Increased risk of postoperative hemorrhage has been reported with the usage of NSAIDs, mainly because of the drugs' antiplatelet effects. Spontaneous hemorrhage in the postoperative period is rarely the cause of NSAID use alone but may be significant in patients with thrombocytopenia, underlying bleeding dyscrasias, or concomitant use of anticoagulant drugs.[31] It is also worthy to note that patients who are taking aspirin daily for its antithrombotic effects should discontinue use of the drug for at least 5 days before the scheduled date of surgery. Also, NSAIDs' effect on renal function is related to the inhibition of renal prostacyclin, resulting in decreased renal blood flow and decreased glomerular filtration rate. This issue is important in patients with underlying renal compromise and the elderly who may be dependent on the vasodilatory effect of prostaglandins for baseline renal function.[33] Less commonly, aspirin and other NSAIDs can precipitate acute bronchospasm in patients with asthma. Approximately 5% to 10% of adult patients with asthma may be sensitive to NSAID administration.[33] When selecting NSAIDs for postoperative analgesia, the practitioner must evaluate not only which drug is most appropriate for patients but also the overall risk profile with regard to the above-mentioned issues.

Acetylsalicylic acid (aspirin)
Aspirin is the salicylic ester of acetic acid. Its uses are for analgesia, antiinflammatory action, antipyretic action, and antithrombosis. Aspirin is the classic NSAID. It was first introduced to medicine in 1899. It nonselectively inhibits COX (COX-1 and COX-2). For a long time, aspirin has been beneficial in oral and maxillofacial surgery for its antiinflammatory action by inhibiting the formation of prostaglandin E and F subtypes. This inhibition results in decreased vasodilation, tissue permeability, edema, and leukocytic infiltration. Its analgesic activity is likely the result of prostaglandin inhibition in the periphery at the site of tissue injury. There may also be a centrally mediated analgesic component to aspirin, although this mechanism has not been clearly elucidated.

The aspirin dosage for postoperative oral surgical pain is 325 to 650 mg by mouth every 4 hours or 1000 mg by mouth every 6 hours, as needed for pain in adult patients. Aspirin therapy is effective for mild to moderate pain. Aspirin has fallen out of favor as a primary drug of choice in postoperative analgesia, mainly because of its significant and permanent effect of platelet inhibition. The administration of aspirin before third molar surgery has actually been shown to increase postoperative edema. This effect is likely caused by decreased platelet aggregation. It is also associated with the classic adverse effects of the NSAID drug class, such as gastroenteric irritation and ulceration, renal impairment, and the potential for hemorrhage occurrence. Besides observing standard precautions with the usage of all NSAID drugs, absolute contraindications for aspirin usage include the incidence of aspirin-induced nasal polyps, salicylate hypersensitivity, and urticaria. It should also be used with extreme caution in patietns with asthma.[18]

Ibuprofen
Ibuprofen is an oral NSAID with antiinflammatory and antipyretic actions. It was initially approved for usage in 1974. It is most effective as an analgesic agent for mild to

moderate postoperative pain. Similar to the other NSAIDs, its analgesic properties result from the peripheral inhibition of prostaglandins. Ibuprofen is a nonselective COX inhibitor and is associated with the classic adverse effects of the NSAID drug class, including gastroenteric irritation and ulceration, renal impairment, and alterations in platelet function.

The dosage of ibuprofen in adults and adolescents is 400 mg by mouth every 4 to 6 hours as needed for pain. This dosage can be increased to 600 mg for severe pain. The half-life of ibuprofen is 2 to 5 hours. Absolute contraindications to ibuprofen are similar to other NSAIDs. They are to be avoided in patients with asthma, aspirin-induced nasal polyps, salicylate hypersensitivity, and urticaria.

Ibuprofen provides excellent pain relief in postsurgical oral and maxillofacial surgery patients. It can be used as a transition drug after the need for pure or combination narcotic-based pain control is obviated. Ibuprofen is available in combination form with hydrocodone (Vicoprofen) and provides significant relief of moderate to severe pain after third molar impaction surgery. This relief is accomplished by combining the centrally mediated analgesia of a narcotic with the peripherally mediated activity of an NSAID. Ibuprofen does not have the permanent effect on platelet activation that aspirin does but, nonetheless, is associated with the potential for postoperative hemorrhage. This potential was demonstrated in a pediatric population after tonsillectomy.[34] This factor should be a consideration when selecting any NSAID.

Naproxen (Naprosyn)

Naproxen is an NSAID with analgesic and antipyretic activity. It is a propionic acid derivative related structurally to ibuprofen. It was approved for use by the FDA in 1976 and became available over the counter in 1994 (Aleve). Like ibuprofen, naproxen is better tolerated than aspirin with regard to NSAID-related side effects. Naproxen is a nonselective inhibitor to the enzyme COX, providing peripheral analgesic properties by inhibiting the in vivo synthesis of prostaglandins. Nonspecific inhibition of the COX-1 isoenzyme contributes to this agent's adverse side effects, including decreased gastric mucosal cytoprotection, impaired renal function, and alteration in platelet function.

Naproxen is administered by mouth and has a half-life of 10 to 20 hours. It is an excellent drug of choice for mild to moderate pain, and compared with aspirin and ibuprofen, its extended half-life increases patient compliance through less-frequent dosing requirements. The oral dosage of naproxen sodium is initially 550 mg by mouth, followed by 275 mg by mouth every 6 to 8 hours, as needed. The maximum initial daily dose of naproxen sodium is 1375 mg and, therefore, should not exceed 1100 mg. Naproxen is available in enteric-coated and sustained-release tablets.

Ketorolac (Toradol)

Ketorolac is a NSAID that provides analgesic and antipyretic activity. It is similar in chemical structure to indomethacin. It was approved for parenteral usage in 1989 and oral usage in 1993. Like other NSAIDs, ketorolac is a peripheral analgesic agent. It inhibits prostaglandin synthesis through nonselective inhibition of COX. Ketorolac is an excellent drug for short-term postoperative pain control. Parenteral administration in the immediate postoperative period has been compared with morphine for adequacy of pain relief without the classic narcotic-related side effects.[35]

Ketorolac is administered in parenteral and oral forms. Doses are 30 mg IV or 60 mg IM in healthy adults who are greater than 50 kg in total body weight. It can be given as a single dose in the immediate postoperative period. If multiple parenteral dosing is desired, the drug can be repeated every 6 hours, with the maximum dose not to exceed 120 mg. Oral ketorolac can be administered for a maximum of 5 days postoperatively. In patients who have received IV or IM doses of ketorolac in the immediate postoperative period, 20 mg of ketorolac should be followed by 10 mg of the drug every 4 to 6 hours. The maximum oral daily dose should not exceed 40 mg.

Ketorolac has been found to be an excellent alternative to narcotics in ambulatory surgical patients. It is best administered after the completion of the surgical procedure. Similar to the other NSAIDs, contraindications and side effects are related to the drug's nonspecific inhibition of the enzyme COX. Ketorolac has been found to elicit more profound adverse side effects than other classic NSAIDs, probably because of its increased potency. Absolute contraindications include asthma, breast-feeding, cerebrovascular disease, dehydration or renal impairment, GI bleeding or peptic ulcer disease, aspirin-induced nasal polyps, urticaria, or salicylate hypersensitivity.

COX-2 inhibitors

The FDA has approved COX-2 inhibitors for the management of osteoarthritis, rheumatoid arthritis, primary dysmenorrhea, and acute pain management in adults. COX-2 inhibitors minimize the inflammatory response by inhibiting the release of the enzyme COX-2. COX-2 is released after tissue injury in macrophages, monocytes, synovial cells, leukocytes, and fibroblasts.[32] These COX-2 selective therapeutic agents alternatively leave the cytoprotective COX-1 enzymes intact. This process provides protection against such side effects as GI tract irritation and decreased platelet aggregation, which are commonly observed with the nonselective COX-inhibiting agents.

Advantages of COX-2–inhibiting agents include extended half-lives, decreased frequency of dosing, and little to no affect on bleeding parameters (because of their minimal effect on platelet aggregation). COX-2 inhibitors are rapidly becoming excellent therapeutic alternatives to standard nonspecific COX inhibitors, such as ibuprofen, in the postsurgical and acute dental pain model. Disadvantages of the COX-2 inhibitors include the relatively high price of these drugs.[32] Continued research and drug development is being done with COX-2–inhibiting agents and they seem to have a very promising role in the future of postoperative and preemptive analgesia.

Celecoxib (Celebrex)

Celecoxib (Celebrex) is a COX-2 inhibitor and has been found to be most beneficial in the management of chronic pain. It offers the advantage of having an extended half-life, allowing limitation of the dose frequency to once or twice a day. A recent study evaluating the use of celecoxib after orthopedic surgery demonstrated that 400 to 600 mg of celecoxib administered orally for 2 to 5 days after surgery was as effective as 10 mg of hydrocodone and 1 g of acetaminophen given orally 2 to 3 times daily.[36] Alternatively, other studies have shown celecoxib to be limited in efficacy when used for the management of acute pain after third molar extraction. It is evident that additional studies will be needed to clarify this issue.

Celecoxib is administered in 200-mg daily dosages or 100 mg twice daily in adults. It is used mainly in the management of chronic joint pain. As described previously, higher doses have been described for the management of severe postoperative orthopedic pain; 200 mg of celecoxib has been found to be equivalent to 400 mg of ibuprofen.[32] Absolute contraindications to celecoxib include aspirin-induced nasal polyps, asthma, salicylate and sulfonamide hypersensitivity, and urticaria.

SUMMARY

Oral surgical procedures provide a unique model for the study of pharmacology and pain. The role of central and peripheral sensitization and other modulating factors affecting the acute pain mechanism provide various opportunities for pharmacologic intervention in pain management. The concept of preemptive analgesia is rapidly being incorporated into the management of ambulatory surgical patients and has lead to hastened recovery and less pain medication requirements. The modern practitioner has access to a variety of pharmacologic agents for the treatment of acute pain. Opioids, NSAIDs, combination formulations, and new analgesic agents are constantly being put to the test in light of the many new discoveries in neurophysiology and pharmacology research. Basic knowledge of how these agents exert their effects should lead to the most appropriate selection of pharmacotherapy for each patient.

REFERENCES

1. Webster's new encyclopedic dictionary. New York: Black Dog and Leventhal Publishers Inc; 1993.
2. Klein CM, Coggeshall RE, Carlton SM, et al. The effects of A-and C-fiber stimulation on patterns of neuropeptide immunostaining in the rat superficial dorsal horn. Brain Res 1992;580:121–8.
3. Desjardins P. Patient pain and anxiety: the medical and psychologic challenges facing oral and maxillofacial surgery. J Oral Maxillofac Surg 2000; 58(Suppl 2):1–3.
4. Vandermeulen EP, Brennan T. Alterations in ascending dorsal horn neurons by a surgical incision in the rat foot. Anesthesiology 2000;93:1294–302.
5. Duggan AW, Hendry IA, Morton CR, et al. Cutaneous stimuli releasing immunoreactive substance P in the dorsal horn of the cat. Brain Res 1988;451:261–73.
6. Duggan AW, Morton ZR, Zhao ZQ, et al. Noxious heating of the skin releases immunoreactive substance P in the substantia gelatinosa of the cat: a study with antibody microprobes. Brain Res 1987;403:345–9.
7. Yaksh TL. Substance P release from knee joint afferent terminals: modulation by opioids. Brain Res 1988;458:319–24.
8. Dickenson AH, Sullivan AF. Differential effects of excitatory amino acid antagonists on dorsal horn nociceptive neurons in the rat. Brain Res 1990;506:31–9.
9. Crane M, Green P, Gordon N. Pharmacology of opioid and non-opioid analgesics. Oral Maxillofacial Surg Clin N Am 2001;13:1–13.
10. Sorkin L, Wallace M. Acute pain mechanisms. Surg Clin North Am 1999;79: 213–29.
11. Dionne RA. Suppression of dental pain by preoperative administration of flurbiprofen. Am J Med 1986;80:41–9.
12. Barolat G. Spinal cord stimulation for chronic pain management. Arch Med Res 2000;31:258–62.
13. Dionne R. Pharmacotherapy update: preemptive versus preventive analgesia: which approach improves clinical outcomes? Compendium 2000;21:48–56.
14. McQuay H. Do preemptive treatments provide better pain control? In: Gebhardt GF, Hammond DL, Jensen TS, editors. Proceedings of the Seventh World Pain Congress. Seattle (WA): IASP Press; 1994. p. 709–23.
15. Gordon SM, Dionne RA, Brahim J, et al. Blockade of peripheral neuronal barrage reduces postoperative pain. Pain 1997;70:209–15.
16. Gordon SM, Dionne RA, Brahim JS, et al. Differential effects of local anesthesia on central hyperalgesia [special issue]. J Dent Res 1997;76:153.
17. Troullos ES, Freeman RD, Dionne RA. The scientific basis for analgesic use in dentistry. Anesth Prog 1986;33(3):123–38.

18. Reents S, Vieson K. Opiate agonist overview. Clinical Pharmacology 2000, Copyright 2001, Gold Standard Multimedia. Available at: http://cponline.hitchcock.org.
19. Zuniga J. Current advances in anesthesia and pain control research, clinical relevance of neurotransmitter-receptor interactions. Oral Maxillofacial Surg Clin N Am 1992;4:875–85.
20. Houde RW, Wallensteine SL, Beaver WT. Clinical management of pain. In: deStevens G, editor. Analgesic. New York: Academic Press; 1965. p. 75–122.
21. Roberts R, Joyce P, Kennedy MA. Rapid and comprehensive determination of cytochrome P450 CYP2D6 poor metabolizer genotypes by multiplex polymerase chain reaction. Hum Mutat 2000;16:77–85.
22. Haffen E, Paintaud G, Berard M, et al. On the assessment of drug metabolism by assays of codeine and its main metabolites. Ther Drug Monit 2000;22:258–65.
23. Eddy NB, Halbeck H, Braenden OJ. Synthetic substances with morphine-like effect. Bull World Health Organ 1957;17:595–600, 705–9.
24. Turturro M, Paris P. Oral narcotic analgesics: choosing the most appropriate agent for acute pain. Postgrad Med 1991;90:89–90, 93–5.
25. Kalb C. Playing with painkillers. Newsweek 2001;137(15):44–8.
26. Bristol Myers Squibb Co. Stadol (butorphanol tartrate) injectable and Stadol NS nasal spray [package insert]. New York: Bristol Myers Squibb Co; 2001.
27. Desjardins PJ, Norris LA, Cooper SA, et al. Analgesic efficacy of intranasal butorphanol (Stadol NS) in the treatment of pain after dental impaction surgery. J Oral Maxillofac Surg 2000;58(Suppl 2):19–26.
28. Lexicomp On-Line for Oral Surgery, 2011 Lexi-Comp Inc. All rights Reserved.
29. Fricke JR Jr, Karim R, Jordan D, et al. A double-blind, single-dose comparison of the analgesic efficacy of tramadol/acetaminophen combination tablets, hydrocodone/acetaminophen combination tablets, and placebo after oral surgery. Clin Ther 2002;24(6):953–68.
30. Moore PA, Crout RJ, Jackson DL, et al. Tramadol hydrochloride: analgesic efficacy compared with codeine, aspirin with codeine, and placebo after dental extraction. J Clin Pharmacol 1998;38(6):554–60.
31. Power I, Barratt S. Analgesic agents for the postoperative period: nonopioids. Surg Clin North Am 1999;79:275–95.
32. Moore P, Hersh E. Celecoxib and rofecoxib, the role of COX-2 inhibitors in dental practice. J Am Dent Assoc 2001;132:451–6.
33. Cashman J, McAnulty G. Nonsteroidal anti-inflammatory drugs in perisurgical pain management. Drugs 1995;49:51–70.
34. Harley EH, Dattolo RA. Ibuprofen for tonsillectomy pain in children: efficacy and complications. Otolaryngol Head Neck Surg 1998;119:492–6.
35. Jelinek GA. Ketorolac versus morphine for severe pain. Ketorolac is more effective, cheaper, and has fewer side effects. BMJ 2000;321:1236–7.
36. Brugger AW, Richardson ET, Drupka DT, et al. Comparison of celecoxib, hydrocodone/acetaminophen, and placebo for relief of post-surgical pain (abstract/poster 880). Presented at the 1999 Annual Meeting of the American Pain Society. Available at: www.ampainsoc.org/abstract99/data/44/index.html. Accessed November 11, 1999.
37. Penfield W, Rasmussen T. The cerebral cortex of man: a classical study of the localization of function. New York: Macmillan; 1950.

Risk Management in the Dental Office

Harry Dym, DDS

KEYWORDS

- Oral surgical procedures • Lawsuits • Risk management
- Clinical negligence

This article is devoted to risk-management strategies and is most appropriate for this issue of *Dental Clinics*, whose main focus is on oral surgical procedures in the general dental office.

Lawsuits are more likely to be filed following poor outcomes related to oral surgical procedures rather than after operative or prosthetic dental procedures; in addition, the total dollar amount of the lawsuit awards are almost always significantly higher in cases involving poor oral surgical outcomes than in the case of general dental procedures most often performed.

This opening discourse is not meant to discourage or dissuade general practitioners from performing oral surgical procedures if they have the experience, training, and appropriate skill set to complete the planned procedure; rather, it is intended to advise practitioners as to the steps one can take to limit the chances of any litigation from ever occurring, and thus avoid the almost always emotionally and painful time-consuming process associated with a malpractice lawsuit (**Box 1**).

REASONS FOR LAWSUITS

Many factors contribute to the current climate that supports the ongoing litigious nature of clinical practice:

- Physicians and dentists are no longer looked on as community leaders
- Physicians and dentists are now viewed as business people rather than dedicated healers of the sick
- Due to decreased insurance payments related to managed care contracts, dentists/physicians can no longer afford the luxury to spend significant time periods with patients to help develop any meaningful rapport
- As the economy continues to weaken with high unemployment rates and significant underemployment, and patients are burdened with high levels of personal debts, they often see litigation as a possible solution to their money problems

Department of Dentistry/Oral and Maxillofacial Surgery, The Brooklyn Hospital Center, 121 DeKalb Avenue, Brooklyn, NY 11201, USA
E-mail address: hdymdds@yahoo.com

Dent Clin N Am 56 (2012) 113–120
doi:10.1016/j.cden.2011.07.001
0011-8532/12/$ – see front matter © 2012 Elsevier Inc. All rights reserved.

dental.theclinics.com

Box 1
Basic definitions

1. Malpractice: Failure to meet the duty of care and/or breach of accepted standards of care as defined by the profession

2. Standards of Care: The duty of a physician to use the care and skill ordinarily used by reputable members of the profession practicing under similar circumstances

3. Summons and Complaint: A document "served" to the dentist, which begins the actual lawsuit process listing a "Bill of particulars" (outlining the claimed negligence and injuries sustained)

4. Statute of Limitations: Each state has a specific law that specifies how long a patient has to file a lawsuit after an incident occurs

---

- *It's easy to sue*; the patient assumes no financial personal costs (other than their time), even if they lose
- There are plenty of lawyers willing to take almost all comers.

CLINICAL NEGLIGENCE

For a patient to succeed in any claim of negligence in a malpractice lawsuit, 4 essential features must be present and proved in a court of law.[1]

1. That a duty of care is owed by the dentist to the patient
2. That there was a breach of duty of care in failure to reach the standard of care expected
3. That the patient suffered harm/losses
4. That the patient's damages must have been directly caused by the dentist's breach of the standard of care.

All general dentists who perform oral surgical procedures in the office will at one time experience a poor outcome; whether it be acute or chronic bone infection, a post-surgical bleeding episode, numbness of the lip, and so forth. Of course all patients who experience poor results certainly do not begin malpractice suits, so what other related factors are involved that may trigger a patient or their family to initiate a lawsuit against their dentist?

Patients who perceive that their doctor and their office staff possess the following qualities are less likely to sue than those patients who have become frustrated with the doctors and his or her staff.

- Competence
- Commitment
- Compassion
- Caring
- Honesty
- Collaboration—with patient, family, and other
- Thoroughness
- Qualifications
- Humanity
- Did the best they could
- Did what they promised.

A patient who experiences a disappointing outcome is more likely to give a doctor who has these qualities the benefit of the doubt. When the patient perceives that the doctor has not shown these qualities or done these things, the "benefit of the doubt" factor lessens greatly.

DOCUMENTATION

Complete patient records are not only vital to good patient care but are considered a legal requirement by most state dental boards. Failure to maintain such records could lead to a loss of license to practice. A complete dental record

- Complies with licensure and accreditation standards
- Facilitates diagnosis and treatment of the patient
- Serves as basis for defense of a potential malpractice claim
- Provides basis for communication with different health care members
- Provides quality assurance data
- Serves as the means to obtain proper reimbursement and helps substantiate billing codes.

The ideal chart size is 8.5 × 11 in, thus not the small card system that offers little room for information and is always difficult to read. Each patient should have a separate record with all supplementary documents (radiographs, path records, and so forth) contained in one file. Entries must be made in a timely manner and must never be altered in response to a subpoena.

Entries are best made by the doctor, because staff entries expose the doctor to a weakened defense if the case should lead to litigation.

Each patient visit should be recorded with the date and a clear, comprehensive note using the subjective, objective, assessment, plan (SOAP) method, although some advocate the subjective, objective, opinion, options, assessment, agreed, plan (SOOOAAP) technique. Remember that lawsuits often occur years after patient treatment, and the doctor may not even recall seeing the patient. In such cases, patient records will often be the best witness for the defense.

The essentials of good documentation should also include all the elements listed in **Box 2** but should never include the following elements:

- Personal (other than medical/dental) opinions
- Speculation on causes of poor outcomes
- Derogatory statements about the patient or his/her family professional disputes
- Financial payments or plans (keep in separate part of record)
- Reference to legal actions, attorneys, or risk-management activities.

HANDWRITING

Malpractice cases have been lost purely because of the poor appearance of a patient's chart; as some people say, "a sloppy chart means a sloppy doctor." Therefore, attention to handwriting and legibility are vital to good care and a positive judgment. If a doctor has difficulty in this area, dictation and transcription services and computerized recording systems are available.

RADIOGRAPHIC STUDIES

All radiographic studies taken in the dental office must be dated, read, and noted in the patient's record. The general dentist will be held responsible if he or she fails to

---

Box 2
Essentials of good documentation

Required Patient Information

- Completed and signed patient medical and dental history form
- Radiographs (labeled and dated)
- Patient name, address, telephone number, date of birth, and age
- Physician's name and telephone number
- Emergency contact information
- Patient visit note
- Date and time at each entry
- Note of review of medical and allergic history (initial encounter)
- SOAP note
- Drugs administered to patient
- Prescription given to patient
- Instructions given to patient
- Referrals made and referrals or instructions not followed
- Telephone conversation with patient and physician
- Cancellation/new appointment
- Laboratory tests ordered
- Results of laboratory tests or consultants' reports

---

adequately interpret any of the films taken in his or her office whether they be periapicals, occlusal, panoramic, or computerized tomographic scans. If the dentist is not comfortable reading the radiographs taken in the office, an outside service should contracted to review the radiographic studies and issue a written report.

ALTERATION OF RECORDS

Medical records should never be altered. If a record is altered, its writer will lose all credibility. Aside from the dishonesty factor, an altered record will not stand up in court. There are numerous ways to determine that a record has been altered. Ink manufacturers add a new element to their ink each year, so the ink can be dated. In addition, written records can be carbon dated. In short, an altered record will be found.

Once a record has been determined to be altered, a case is no longer defensible. If the practitioner feels that the chart does not accordingly reflect all the events that have transpired regarding this particular patient, he or she can take steps to appropriately note any information that comes in after the fact, or any information that was overlooked at the time the patient was treated. There are several ways this can be addressed, but an altered record is not one of them.

TIME-OUT PROCEDURE

Before beginning any complicated oral surgical procedure, it would be good office policy for the practitioner to take a few seconds to perform a mental or actual checklist.

Time out should include the following:

- Do I have clear diagnostic radiographs?
- All necessary equipment readily available?
- Am I certain as to which tooth is being extracted?
- Have I explained the nature of the surgery and possible complications to the patient?

WHEN TO REFER

As stated earlier, a general dentist's decision to treat or refer patients for oral/implant or periodontal surgical services should be based on the clinician's ability as determined by his or her training and experience.

However, it would unethical to somehow transmit the perception to patients that the treating general practitioner is an educationally trained specialist, if that were not the case. Patients often prefer to not see a specialist, which requires leaving the office, and are more receptive to having their own dentists, with whom they have a close relationship, perform all required surgical procedures.

If the general dentist feels that he or she is not comfortable performing the necessary surgical procedures, he or she has an obligation to refer the patient to a specialist. The general dentist must document in the chart that a referral is made and also record in the chart whether the patient followed through with the appointment, as well as documenting whether the patient failed to visit the specialist.

INFORMED CONSENT

Obtaining informed consent from a patient before beginning any invasive dental procedure is a well-established necessity, but is particularly vital prior to performing any oral surgical procedure. A well-informed patient is more likely to have more reasonable expectations as to outcome and possible complications.

In fact, the courts have ruled (Schloendorff v Society of New York Hospitals 1914)[2] that doctors who fail to obtain consent before performing an operation can be held liable to criminal charges such as assault and battery. There is no state or national guideline recommended regarding exactly what elements should be contained in the informed consent process, but most risk-management consultants recommend that it be thorough and contain key multiple elements (**Box 3**).

It is highly advisable that the treating dentist be the person who engages the patient in the informed consent process and also takes the time to document in the patient's chart that such a discussion was held. Although oral consent is commonly taken by dentists and is acceptable; the best way to obtain and document a patient's informed consent after providing a diagnosis and treatment options, and discussing common risks is to use a printed standard form. It is often useful to use educational materials such as brochures, pamphlets, books, DVDs, or Internet-based patient interactive educational tools before proceeding with planned oral surgical procedures. It is also equally as important to document in the chart if the patient chooses not to follow through with a recommended oral surgical procedure, and this often referred to as the "informed refusal process."

FOLLOW-UP

After any significant oral surgical office procedure is performed, it makes for good patient management to follow up with a phone call 1 to 3 days later. If the patient

---

Box 3
Key elements of informed consent for oral surgical procedures

- Consent should always be obtained by the treating doctor, ideally at a separate consultation visit; it should only be obtained at the time of care if an emergent surgical procedure is required

- Additional educational materials, videos, textbooks, and picture brochures should be used, if available, to help educate the patient about the prepared treatment plan

- When the patient does not understand English, a translator must be present and that fact documented in the patient's chart

- Consent for minors (under age 18 in most states) must be obtained by a parent or legal guardian; however, if urgent care is needed, telephone consent is often acceptable if the parent cannot leave work or is out of town. Patients who are under 18 and are married or have children are able to give consent

- If the patient refuses treatment that the doctor believes is vitally important to his or her future health, this fact should be documented in the patient's chart; many doctors use a special "refusal care" form

- The patient should be advised of the risks of the proposed treatment and the risks of no treatment

- The patient should be advised of alternatives to the proposed treatment

- The patient should be advised of the cost of treatment

- No guarantees of results or outcomes should be made

- Consent should be discussed at separate time from the planned surgical procedure; the patient should be allowed to take the consent form home, which allows time to think about the procedure

- Informed consent forms for surgical procedures performed by oral and maxillofacial surgeons are the standard of care, though this is not the national standard among general dentists and other dental specialists

---

states he or she has a problem the nature and extent of which cannot be clearly appreciated over the phone, the patient should be recommended to visit the practitioner as soon as possible. If no phone call is made the patient should be scheduled for a follow-up office visit, especially following a complex oral surgical procedure. If the patient selects not to attend the follow-up, the critical elements of the conversation should be documented in the patients' record. If a biopsy was performed, the treating doctor should review the findings, inform the patient, and document the results in the patient's charts.

COMPLICATIONS

If a patient does develop a complication during or directly following an office oral surgical procedure, the treating dentist should immediately inform the patient of the problem and either treat the complication if he or she is able to, or make the necessary referral. The treating dentist should make it clear that the patient must follow up with the specialist, or help arrange the appointment if necessary. If the patient refuses to follow the treating doctor's recommendation, this must be documented in the patient's chart. Complications happen and can occur to anyone at any time; it is the lack of timely acknowledgment and treatment, or lack of appropriate referral that can lead to poor clinical outcomes and potential lawsuits.

TERMINATING THE DOCTOR-PATIENT RELATIONSHIP

Health care providers are not legally obligated, nor do they have a duty, to treat all patients who enter their office, unless they agree to do so. This statement is generally true, but dentists on call for their hospital emergency medicine department, or who are managed by care panels, may be bound by hospital bylaws or state laws to accept all such patients; inquiries to their hospital medical board or managed care program should be made if one decides not to treat such a patient. However, once a doctor-patient relationship is established, treatment continues until (1) the patient's condition no longer warrants attention, (2) the patient leaves the practice, (3) a mutual doctor-patient decision is made to terminate care, or (4) the doctor chooses to end the relationship.

Financial disagreement should not have a bearing on the doctor-patient relationship. Those patients who are not compliant with instructions and thus may jeopardize the outcome of care, who continuously fail to meet their appointments, or who are verbally or physically abusive to the doctor or staff may be discharged from care. Certain legal protocols, however, should be followed when terminating the doctor-patient relationship to avoid charges of patient abandonment:

- The doctor should send a letter to the patient by certified mail informing the patient of his/her intention to end the doctor-patient relationship
- The doctor does not need to state a reason, but one should avoid stating "incompatibility" as a reason or discussing any personal issues in the letter
- The doctor should be sure that the patient's condition at the time of termination is stable and not emergent
- The patient should be given the address or name of a colleague who has agreed to see the patient, the name of a dental school, or the dental society referral services number
- The patient's missed appointments should be documented; failure to comply with office recommendations of care, and any abusive behavior, should be recorded in the patient's chart
- The doctor should inform the patient that all records will be available for transfer
- The doctor should inform the patient that he/she will be available for emergency care for a 2- to 3-month period, depending on the demographics and the patient's ability to find a new dentist.

SUMMARY

With dental practitioners performing more surgical procedures in their office, the exposure to possible malpractice litigation increases significantly. It is not enough to possess good skills and techniques; dentists must actively and diligently adhere to risk-reduction strategies to help minimize or eliminate future lawsuits (**Box 4**).

Lay people often measure the clinical competency of a doctor by nonclinical measures, such as:

- Were my phone calls taken and did the doctor get back to me promptly?
- Were my questions answered?
- Were the office staff kind and considerate?

It is often these "service-related" issues that cause patients to lose confidence in their doctor and ultimately convince them to begin down the road of litigation.

If dentists are to incorporate more complicated oral surgical procedures into their everyday practice they must be prepared to deal with postsurgical complications, which may also include a malpractice lawsuit.

Box 4
Risk reduction checklist

- Always attempt to develop rapport and communication with the patient
- Before performing any oral surgical procedures, obtain informed (preferably written) consent
- Document clearly, fully, legibly
- Always have all necessary equipment (and backups) before beginning surgical procedure
- Have correct clear and diagnostic radiographs available
- Never minimize planned surgical procedures—learn to manage patient's expectations
- Always provide emergency contact after-hours number and respond timely when called
- Know when to refer the patient for a second opinion
- Review all diagnostic laboratory and radiographic studies ordered; if a complication occurs (such as retained root tip, opening into maxillary sinus, patient fracture of adjacent tooth amalgam), tell the patient and document the findings
- Be knowledgable in the recognition and treatment of common postsurgical complications

---

The dental profession can mitigate possible lawsuits by paying better attention to detail, by following good medical practice, and by better managing patients' expectations and outcomes.

REFERENCES

1. Dym H, Ogle OE. Risk management techniques for the general dentist. Handbook of dental practice. Dent Clin North Am 2008;52:3.
2. Holmes SM, Odey DK. Risk management in oral and maxillofacial surgery, vol. 2. St Louis: Saunders (Elsevier); 2009. p. 373–86.

Endodontic Surgery

Stuart E. Lieblich, DMD[a,b,*]

KEYWORDS

• Endodontic surgery • Retrograde preparation • Biopsy

PREOPERATIVE PLANNING

Although endodontic care is typically successful, in approximately 10% to 15% of cases[1] symptoms can persist or spontaneously reoccur. Many endodontic failures are caused by the failure to place an adequate coronal seal. Therefore there is the competing interest of observing the tooth after endodontic treatment to ascertain successful treatment versus placing a definitive restoration. Many endodontic failures occur a year or more after the initial root canal treatment, often creating a situation in which a definitive restoration has already been placed. This situation creates a higher value for the tooth because it now may be supporting a fixed partial denture. A decision is then needed to determine if orthograde endodontic retreatment can be accomplished, should periapical surgery be recommended or consideration of extraction of the tooth with loss of the overlying prosthesis.

Causes of endodontic failures can often be separated into biologic issues such as a persistent infection or technical factors such as a broken instrument in the root canal system (**Fig. 1**), transportation of the apex, perforation, and ledging of the canal. Failure of endodontic treatment is most commonly caused by lack of an adequate coronal seal, with the presence of bacteria within the root canal system and apical leakage. Continued infection may also result from debris displaced outside the apex during the initial endodontic treatment. Technical factors alone are a less common indication for surgery, comprising only 3% of the total cases referred for surgery,[2] yet it is this author's opinion that there is a higher success rate in these cases.

Before surgery, discussions with patients are critical in order for the patient to give appropriate informed consent. The particular risks of surgery based on the anatomic location (sinus involvement or proximity to the inferior alveolar nerve) need to be reviewed and documented. It is important to stress the exploratory nature of periapical surgery to the patient. Depending on the findings at surgery, a limited root resection with retrograde restoration may be placed. However, the patient and surgeon must also be prepared to treat fractures of the root or the entire tooth. Plans must be

a Oral and Maxillofacial Surgery, University of Connecticut Health Center, Farmington, CT, USA
b Avon Oral and Maxillofacial Surgery, 34 Dale Road, Suite 105, Avon, CT 06001, USA
* Avon Oral and Maxillofacial Surgery, 34 Dale Road, Suite 105, Avon, CT 06001.
E-mail address: slieblich@avonomfs.com

Dent Clin N Am 56 (2012) 121–132
doi:10.1016/j.cden.2011.08.005
0011-8532/12/$ – see front matter © 2012 Elsevier Inc. All rights reserved.

dental.theclinics.com

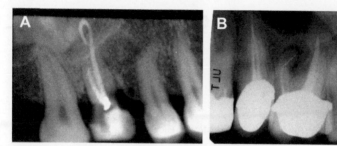

Fig. 1. Two examples of technical factors requiring apical surgery. Although less frequent in occurrence, the success rate is usually high because the canal system is likely well obturated. (A) Overfill of gutta percha causing symptoms including chronic sinusitis. (B) Broken endodontic instrument in apical third with pain and drainage.

made preoperatively on how such situations will be handled should they be noted intraoperatively.

Surgical endodontics success rates have dramatically improved over the years with the developments of newer retrofilling materials and the use of the ultrasonic preparation. Previously cited success rates of 60% to 70% have now increased to more than 90% in many studies,[3–5] because of the routine use of ultrasonic retrograde preparation and the use of mineral trioxide aggregate (MTA) as a filling material. This significant improvement makes apical surgery a more predictable and valuable adjunct in the treatment of symptomatic teeth. Most significantly, studies[6,7] show once the periapical bony defect is considered healed (reformation of the lamina dura or the case has healed by scar) the long-term prognosis is excellent. These studies reported 91.5% of healed cases still successful after a follow-up period of 5 to 7 years. Therefore with adequate radiographic follow-up the surgeon should be able to predict the long-term viability of the tooth and its usefulness to retain a prosthetic restoration.

The primary option for the treatment of symptomatic endodontically treated teeth is that of conventional retreatment versus the surgical approach. An algorithm for a decision regarding retreatment versus surgery versus extraction is presented in **Fig. 2**. In discussions with patients the option of conventional retreatment should be discussed. However, clinical studies have not shown retreatment to be more successful than surgery, and 1 prospective study found surgical treatment to have a higher success rate.[8,9] Although endodontic retreatment seems more conservative, the removal of posts, reinstrumentation of the tooth, and removal of tooth structure increase the chance of fracture. Surgical treatment of failures also provides the opportunity to retrieve tissue for histologic examination to rule out a noninfectious cause of a lesion (**Fig. 3**).

The option of extraction with either immediate or delayed implant placement must also be discussed as an alternative to periapical surgery. There is no debate in dentistry that implants can outlast tooth-supported restorations. It is valuable therefore to have data to predict the expected success of the endodontic surgery so the patient can use that in their decision-making process. Factors that improve success are noted in **Box 1**. In cases of an expected poorer success rate such as the presence of severe periodontal bone loss (especially the presence of furcation involvement), the decision to extract the tooth and place an implant may be a more efficacious and clinically predictable procedure.

There is a body of literature that supports the duration of restorations fabricated on endodontically treated teeth. Basten and colleagues[10] reported a 92% 12-year

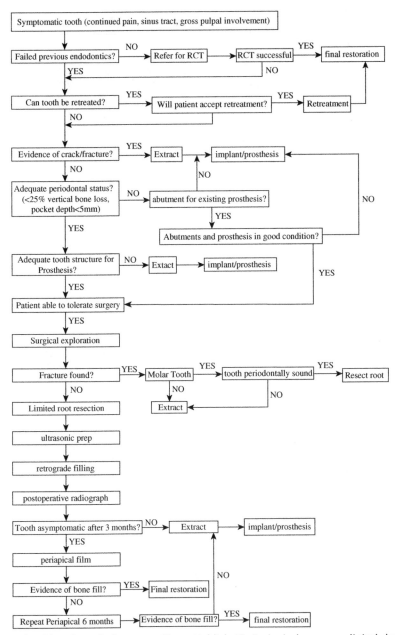

Fig. 2. Algorithm for apical surgery. (*From* Lieblich SE. Periapical surgery: clinical decision making. Oral Maxillofac Surg Clin N Am 2002;14:181.)

survival rate, and Blomlof and Jansson[11] found surgically treated molars with healthy periodontal status had a 10-year survival rate of 89%. The factors most associated with failures are long posts in teeth with little remaining coronal structure. Thus, the condemnation of a tooth because it can be replaced with an implant is not clear.

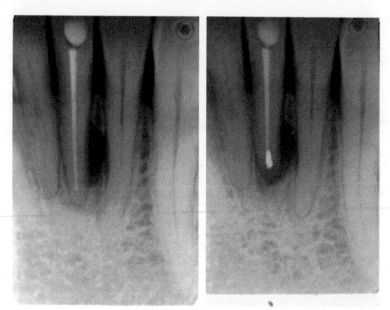

Fig. 3. Atypical radiolucency along the lateral aspect of the root and not truly involving the apex. Although correctly treated at the time of referral because of the nonresolving radiolucency with periapical surgery, the suspicious nature of the lesion warranted submission of the tissue for histologic examination. Confirmation with the original treating dentist revealed the indication for the endodontic treatment was solely the incidental finding of a radiolucency, and vital pulp tissue was noted. The final pathologic diagnosis was a cystic ameloblastoma.

An economic analysis may be indicated to guide the patient's decision. If the case has a final prosthetic restoration already in place it is usually easier to recommend surgical intervention. If the symptoms do not resolve the patient has only expended the additional time, operative risk, and expense of the surgical portion of their care because they have already have a definitive restoration. The surgeon should review the factors in **Box 1** to help predict the likelihood of the surgical intervention being successful. If the tooth has multiple factors that indicate the success of the surgical intervention would be compromised or the tooth has a poor expectation for 10-year survival, then extraction with implant placement is a more efficacious means of care.

The surgeon may be called on to treat teeth that cannot be negotiated for conventional orthograde endodontics. The treatment of teeth with calcified canals may be appropriately managed with apical surgery alone with a retrograde filling if the tooth is critical to a restorative treatment plan. Danin and colleagues[8] showed at least a 50% rate of complete radiographic healing and only 1 failure in 10 cases over a 1-year observation period in cases treated surgically only and without endodontic treatment. Bacteria still remained in the canals of the tooth in 90% of these cases, which may lead to a later failure.

DETERMINATION OF SUCCESS

More complicated decisions are involved with teeth that have not been definitively restored. In that situation not only does the surgeon have to consider the preoperative potential for the apical surgery to be successful, but often must determine when the

---

Box 1
Factors associated with success and failures in periapical surgery

SUCCESS:

Preoperative factors

1. Dense orthograde fill

2. Healthy periodontal status

    a. no dehiscence

    b. adequate crown/root ratio

3. Radiolucent defect isolated to apical one-third of tooth

4. Tooth treated

    a. Maxillary incisor

    b. Mesiobuccal root of maxillary molars

Postoperative factors

5. Radiographic evidence of bone fill after surgery

6. Resolution of pain and symptoms

7. Absence of sinus tract

8. Decrease in tooth mobility

FAILURE:

Preoperative factors

1. Clinical or radiographic evidence of fracture

2. Poor or lack of orthograde filling

3. Marginal leakage of crown or post

4. Poor preoperative periodontal condition (furcation involvement)

5. Radiographic evidence of post perforation

6. Tooth treated

    a. Mandibular incisor

Postoperative factors

7. Lack of bone repair after surgery

8. Lack of resolution of pain

9. Fistula does not resolve or returns

---

case is deemed successful and the case can proceed to the final restoration. Once a final restoration is placed, considerable more time and expense have been invested and subsequent failure is more troublesome to the patient.

Rud and colleagues[12] retrospectively reviewed radiographs after apical surgery to determine radiographic signs of success. Their work showed that with a retrospective review of cases more than at least 4 years after surgery, once radiographic evidence of bone fill occurs (noted as successful healing in their classification scheme), the tooth was stable throughout the remainder of their study period (up to 15 years). A waiting period of more than 4 years is not acceptable in contemporary practice, but these investigators' classification scheme has been validated over shorter observation times. They found that if radiographic evidence of bone fill of the surgical defect is noted, then the tooth remained a radiographic success over their observation periods. Many of the partially healing cases, noted as "incomplete healing" in their study, tended to move into the complete healing group during the 2 years after surgery, with few changes throughout the next 4 years of observation.

An appropriate follow-up protocol is to obtain a repeat periapical film 3 months after surgery, with critical comparison with the immediate postoperative film. If significant bone fill has occurred, mobility has decreased, pain is resolved, and no fistula is present, the case can proceed to the final restoration. However, if significant bone fill has not been noted, the patient should be recalled again at 3 months for a new film. Rubinstein and Kim[6] found complete healing in 25.3% of cases in 3 months, 34% took 6 months, 15.4% 9 months, and 25.3% 12 months. Small bony defects healed faster than large, which showed significant differences in their prospective study. In contrast any increase in the size of the radiolucency or no improvement should caution the dentist about making a final restoration. If the situation is not clear at that time (6 months postsurgically) a temporary restoration, loaded for a least 3 months, is often a good litmus test of the success of the surgery and predictive as to whether the final restoration will last for some time.

THE CRACKED OR FRACTURED TOOTH

Preoperative radiographs and a careful clinical examination should be performed with a high index of suspicion of a vertical root fracture (VRF) before undertaking surgery. Mandibular molars and maxillary premolars are the most frequent teeth to present with occult VRFs. Although surgical exploration may be needed to definitively show the presence of a fracture (**Fig. 4**), subtle radiographic signs may alert the surgeon that a fracture is present and the surgery is unlikely to be successful. Tamse and colleagues[13] looked at radiographs of maxillary premolars for comparison with the clinical findings at the time of surgery. Few (1 of 15) teeth with an isolated, well-corticated periapical lesion had a VRF. In contrast, a halo-type radiolucency was almost always associated with a VRF (**Fig. 5**). This type of radiolucency is also known as a J type, in which a widened periodontal ligament space connects with the periapical lesion, creating the J pattern.

It is critical in patient discussions to review the exploratory nature of the surgery, and this author routinely uses that as a descriptor of the planned surgery. In cases of root fracture a decision during surgery may need to be made to either resect a root or extract a tooth if a fractured root is found. Obtaining the appropriate preoperative consent as well as determining how the extracted tooth site will be managed (with or without a temporary removable partial denture) must be established before surgery commences.

CONCOMITANT PERIODONTAL PROCEDURES

The use of guided tissue regeneration, alloplastic or allogenic bone grafting, and root planing in conjunction with periapical surgery can be considered. In cases of severe bone dehiscence the likelihood of success is known to be substantially compromised and may lead to the intraoperative decision to extract the tooth. Periodontal probing, before surgery, often detects the presence of significant bony defects. Sometimes the amount of bone loss cannot be appreciated until the area is flapped (**Fig. 6**). Thus, the exploratory nature of the surgery needs to be stressed preoperatively with the patient.

The placement of an additional foreign body, such as a Gore-Tex membrane, to an area already infected is more likely to lead to failure of the surgery. Membrane

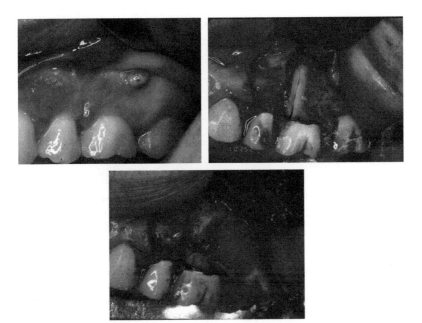

Fig. 4. VRF that was not diagnosed until explored at the time of surgery. The use of a sulcular flap permitted a resection of the mesiobuccal root and preservation of the tooth with its existing restoration.

stabilization and adequate mobilization of soft tissues to cover the membrane may increase the complexity of the surgical procedure. Nonresorbable membranes also require a second procedure for their removal that may not be tolerated by the patient as well as lead to an increase in scarring. A recent review by Tsesis and colleagues[14] seems to show a trend toward higher success with the use of resorbable membranes in cases of large defects and through and through lesions.

SURGICAL PROCEDURES

Various steps are involved in the periapical surgical procedure. Initial exposure of the apical region is needed. This procedure must allow access to the apex for the root resection. Approximately 2 to 3 mm of the root apex is resected. The root resection

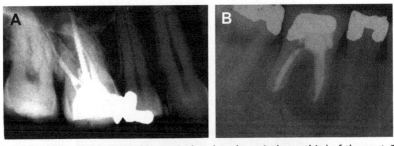

Fig. 5. (A) Example of a periapical lesion isolated to the apical one-third of the root. These lesions are rarely associated with a VRF. (B) In contrast, this type of radiographic lesion, known as a halo or J type of radiolucency, has ill-defined cortical borders and is most likely associated with a VRF.

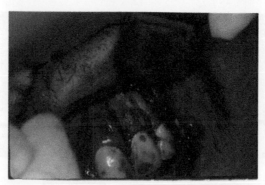

Fig. 6. A combination endodontic and periodontal lesion has a low likelihood of success. The decision was made preoperatively to treat the tooth surgically because an adequate final restoration had already been placed. Otherwise extraction with consideration of local bone grafting is indicated.

removes the end of the root containing the aberrant canals. Also, the further from the coronal portion of the tooth, the less dense the endodontic filling is likely to be.

After the root resection a thorough curettage of the periapical region is accomplished; the surgeon should be cognizant of local structures such as the maxillary sinus or the inferior alveolar nerve. Curettage removes periapical debris that may have been forced out of the apex during the previous preparation of the root canal system. Tissue may be recovered at this time for histologic examination if indicated (see later discussion). A retrograde filling is then prepared with the use of the ultrasonic device (**Fig. 7**). This filling creates a microapical restoration that is retentive because of

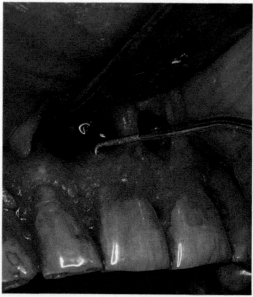

Fig. 7. The use of the ultrasonic tips allow a precise and retentive retrograde preparation. A minimal to no bevel is needed, which exposes less of the dentinal tubules in the apical aspect of the tooth.

the parallel walls. The ultrasonic device creates a conservative preparation and often finds unfilled canals or an isthmus of retained pulpal tissue connecting 2 canals, particularly in the mesiobuccal roots of maxillary first molars. The ultrasonic preparation has been shown to be advantageous to the rotary drills because it centers the preparation along the long axis of the canal and significantly reduces the tendency to create root perforations.[15]

The retrograde filling is important to hermetically seal the root canal system, preventing further leakage of bacteria into the periapical tissues. Many filling materials have been used throughout the years and many do work well. The most contemporary material is MTA and has been shown histologically to deposit bone around it. Its handling characteristics are different from other dental materials because it is hydrophilic and does not reach a full firm set for 2 to 4 hours. This characteristic is not clinically significant because the region is not load bearing, at least for some time after the apical surgery. MTA has been shown to produce regeneration of cementum, something not seen with other root end filling materials.

SURGICAL ACCESS

Surgical access is a compromise between the need for visibility and the risk to adjacent structures. Many surgeons use the semilunar flap to access the periapical region. Although it provides rapid access to the apices of the teeth it substantially limits the surgery to only a root resection and periapical seal. Proponents of this flap claim that it prevents recession around existing crowns, which could lead to a metal margin showing postoperatively.

The semilunar flap is placed entirely in the nonkeratinized or unattached gingiva. By definition this tissue is constantly moving during normal oral function, leading to dehiscence and increased scarring. Incisions placed in unattached tissues tend to heal slower and with more discomfort.

Once a semilunar incision is made, the surgeon has access limited to only the periapical region. If the root is noted to be fractured, extraction via this flap may lead to a severe defect. With a multirooted tooth, a root resection of one of the fractured roots may not be possible. In addition, localized root planing or other periodontal procedures cannot be accomplished. The size of the bone defect may be greater than that anticipated based on the preoperative radiographs, and the possibility of the suture line being over the defect might cause the incision to open up and heal secondarily. Many cases of periapical surgery on maxillary molars and premolars involve an opening into the sinus cavity,[16] and the incision line with this type of flap might contribute to a postoperative oral-antral fistula.

In contrast, a sulcular incision with 1 or 2 vertical releases keeps the incision primarily within the attached gingival, promoting rapid healing with less pain and scarring. Healing of the incision is facilitated by curetting the adjacent teeth and any exposed root surfaces before closure. The incision permits full observation of the root surface, leading to more accurate apical localization and treatment of a fractured root should it be discovered on flap reflection (see **Fig. 4**). By keeping the incision as far away from the sinus opening as possible and over healthy bone (vs a sulcular incision) the chance of an oral-antral communication is significantly reduced.

Concerns about sulcular incisions have revolved primarily around the concern for an esthetic defect that may be created with the shrinkage or loss of the interdental papilla. Jansson and colleagues[17] found the greatest predicator of papilla loss was the presence of a continued apical infection and found no difference in the attachment whether a semilunar or trapezoidal flap was used. Recent publications by Velvart[18] have proposed the use of a papilla-based incision, in which the triangle of interdental papilla is not incised and not mobilized during reflection of the flap. Velvert reported maintenance of the papilla with little to no recession in contrast to mobilization of the papilla. Von Arx and colleagues[4] (**Fig. 8**) reviewed the papilla-based incision with the intrasulcular type and found less recession with this type of flap design.

TO BIOPSY OR NOT?

A clinical controversy has ensued over the consideration as to whether all periapical lesions treated surgically should have soft tissue removed and submitted for histologic evaluation. An editorial by Walton[19] questioning the rationale of submitting all soft tissue recovered for histologic examination then provoked a series of letters to the editor. Organizations such as the American Association of Endodontists have stated in their standards that if soft tissue can be recovered from the apical surgery then it must be submitted for pathologic evaluation.

On cursory review it seems that it is easier to make this recommendation than to have the surgeon determine if there is anything unusual about the case that warrants histologic examination. Walton[19] makes a convincing argument against the submission of all tissues, because similar appearing radiolucencies that are not treated surgically do not have tissue retrieved for pathologic identification. It is also accepted that the differentiation between a periapical granuloma or periapical cyst has no direct bearing on clinical outcomes and therefore cannot be used as a rationalization for the submission of tissue.

The dilemma falls back to the surgeon that if a rare lesion should present itself in the context of a periapical lesion, and is not biopsied in a timely manner, the surgeon may face a malpractice suit. Many surgeons have a case or two in their careers that have

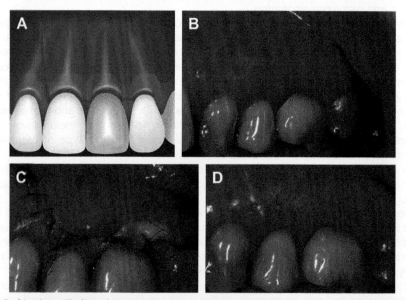

Fig. 8. (*A–D*) Papilla-based incision has been shown to have less recession than the intrasulcular incision. (*From* von Arx T, Vinzens-Majaniemi T, Bürgin W, et al. Changes of periodontal parameters following apical surgery: a prospective clinical study of three incision techniques. Int Endod J 2007;40(12):959–69; with permission.)

> **Box 2**
> **Indications for nonsubmission of periapical soft tissues for histologic review**
>
> 1. Clear evidence of preexisting endodontic involvement of a tooth
>   a. Pulpal necrosis was present, not just a periapical radiolucency
> 2. Unilocular radiolucency associated with apical one-third of the tooth
> 3. Lesion is not in association with an impacted tooth
> 4. No history of malignancy that could represent spread of a metastasis
> 5. Patient will return for follow-up examinations and radiographs
> 6. No tissue recovered at the time of surgery

surprised them based on the final pathologic diagnosis. However, careful review of these cases usually depicts a clinical situation inconsistent with a typical periapical infection (see **Fig. 3**).

An approach more logical than a purely defensive one is to set up guidelines on which it is determined that submission of tissue was not indicated. These guidelines are listed in **Box 2**. It is recommended that the surgeon have documented in the record the rationale for electing not to submit tissue in each specific case. At a recent meeting of the American Association of Oral and Maxillofacial Surgeons only 8% of those attending a symposium on endodontic surgery "always" submit tissue for histologic examination.

REFERENCES

1. Kerekes K, Tronstad L. Long-term results of endodontic treatment performed with a standardized technique. J Endod 1979;5:83–90.
2. El-Siwah JM, Walker RT. Reasons for apicectomies. A retrospective study. Endod Dent Traumatol 1996;12:185–91.
3. Von Arx T, Kurl B. Root-end cavity preparation after apicoectomy using a new type of sonic and diamond-surfaced retrotip: a 1-year follow-up study. J Oral Maxillofac Surg 1999;57:656–61.
4. Von Arx T, Vinzens-Majanemi T, Bürgin W, et al. Changes of periodontal parameters following apical surgery: a prospective clinical study of three incision techniques. Int Endod J 2007;40:959–69.
5. Zuolo ML, Ferreira MO, Gutmann JL. Prognosis in periapical surgery: a clinical prospective study. Int Endod J 2000;33(2):91–8.
6. Rubinstein RA, Kim S. Short term observation of the results of endodontic surgery with the use of a surgical operation microscope and Super-EBA as root-end filling material. J Endod 1999;25:43–8.
7. Rubinstein RA, Kim S. Long-term follow-up of cases considered healed one year after apical microsurgery. J Endod 2002;28:378–83.
8. Danin J, Linder LE, Lundqvist G, et al. Outcomes of periradicular surgery in cases of apical pathosis and untreated canals. Oral Surg Oral Med Oral Pathol Oral Radiol Endod 1999;87(2):227–32.
9. Danin J, Stromberg T, Forsgren H, et al. Clinical management of nonhealing periradicular pathosis. Surgery versus endodontic retreatment. Oral Surg Oral Med Oral Pathol Oral Radiol Endod 1996;82(2):213–7.
10. Basten CH, Ammons WF, Persson R. Long term evaluation of root-resected molars: a retrospective study. Int J Periodontics Restorative Dent 1996;16:206–9.

11. Blomlof L, Jansson L. Prognosis and mortality of root-resected molars. Int J Periodontics Restorative Dent 1997;17:190–201.
12. Rud J, Andreasen JO, Jensen JE. A follow-up study of 1,000 cases treated by endodontic surgery. Int J Oral Surg 1972;1:215–28.
13. Tamse A, Fuss Z, Lustig J, et al. Radiographic features of vertically fractured, endodontically treated maxillary premolars. Oral Surg Oral Med Oral Pathol Oral Radiol Endod 1999;88:348–52.
14. Tsesis I, Rosen E, Tamse A, et al. Effect of guided tissue regeneration on the outcome of endodontic treatment: a systematic review and meta-analysis. J Endod 2011;37(8):1039–45.
15. Wuchenich D, Meadows D, Torabinejad M. A comparison between two root end preparation techniques in human cadavers. J Endod 1994;20:279–82.
16. Feedman A, Horowitz I. Complications after apicoectomy in maxillary premolar and molar teeth. Int J Oral Maxillofac Surg 1999;28:192–4.
17. Jansson L, Sandstedt P, Laftman AC, et al. Relationship between apical and marginal healing in periradicular surgery. Oral Surg Oral Med Oral Pathol Oral Radiol Endod 1997;83:596–601.
18. Velvart P. Papilla base incision: a new approach to recession free healing of the interdental papilla after endodontic surgery. Int Endod J 2002;35:453–60.
19. Walton RE. Routine histopathologic examination of endodontic periradicular surgical specimens–is it warranted? Oral Surg Oral Med Oral Pathol Oral Radiol Endod 1998;86(5):505.

Local Anesthesia: Agents, Techniques, and Complications

Orrett E. Ogle, DDS[a],*, Ghazal Mahjoubi, DMD[b,c]

KEYWORDS

- Local anesthesia • Topical anesthetics
- Cain allergy • Techniques for dental anesthesia

Local anesthesia is a reversible blockade of nerve conduction in a circumscribed area that produces loss of sensation. The chemical agents used to produce local anesthesia stabilize neuronal membranes by inhibiting the ionic fluxes required for the propagation of neural impulses. Today's anesthetics are safe, effective, and can be administered with negligible soft-tissue irritation and minimal concerns for allergic reactions. Indeed, no aspect of office oral surgery is as important as good pain control. Excellent local anesthesia permits the dental surgeon to perform the necessary surgical procedure in a careful, unhurried fashion that will be less stressful for both the operator and the patient. The achievement of good local anesthesia requires knowledge of the agents being used, the neuroanatomy involved, and adherence to good techniques.

This article reviews the widely used local anesthetic agents and common techniques for obtaining local anesthesia, and also discusses some frequently seen complications.

AGENTS
Topical Anesthetics

Topical anesthetics are substances that can cause surface anesthesia of skin or mucosa. In dentistry these agents are used to temporarily anesthetize the tiny nerve

The authors have nothing to disclose.

[a] Oral and Maxillofacial Surgery, Department of Dentistry, Woodhull Medical and Mental Health Center, 760 Broadway, Brooklyn, NY 11206, USA

[b] Department of Dentistry, Woodhull Medical and Mental Health Center, 760 Broadway, Room 2C:320, Brooklyn, NY 11206, USA

[c] Department of Oral and Maxillofacial Surgery, Woodhull Medical and Mental Health Center, 760 Broadway, Room 2C:320, Brooklyn, NY 11206, USA

* Corresponding author.

E-mail address: orrett.ogle@woodhullhc.nychhc.org

Dent Clin N Am 56 (2012) 133–148

doi:10.1016/j.cden.2011.08.003

0011-8532/12/$ – see front matter © 2012 Elsevier Inc. All rights reserved.

dental.theclinics.com

endings located on the surfaces of the oral mucosa, with the aim of reducing the discomfort of dental injections and other minimally invasive procedures. The agents are supplied in various forms—gels, ointments, sprays, and solutions—and can be obtained in flavors such as strawberry, mint, cherry, banana, and bubble gum. The concentrations of topical anesthetic solutions are higher than those of injectable anesthetics but take longer for the full effect in comparison with the injectable anesthetics. In general, 1 to 5 minutes of contact time is required for topical anesthetics to reach their full effectiveness (up to 2–3 mm from the surface) so patience is required on the part of the dentist. For maximum effectiveness, the area of the mucosa where the topical anesthetic is to be placed should be dry.

Most of the widely used topical anesthetics use 20% benzocaine in either a gel or liquid form. The 20% benzocaine has virtually no systemic absorption. Compound topical anesthetics are used to relieve pain and discomfort in minimally invasive or noninvasive procedures (orthodontic bands application, root planing, and scaling). These combination agents are neither regulated nor unregulated by the US Food and Drug Administration (FDA).[1] Studies have shown that combination topical anesthetic products are considerably more efficacious than topical benzocaine when used as the sole anesthetic. One widely used combination topical anesthetic is One Touch (Hager Worldwide, Inc, Odessa, FL, USA), which is composed of 18% benzocaine and 15% tetracaine.

Benzocaine

Benzocaine is one of the ester local anesthetics (the ethyl ester of p-aminobenzoic acid [PABA]) and is poorly soluble in water. It is poorly absorbed into the cardiovascular system, and will remain at the site of application, giving it a long duration of action. In comparison with amide anesthetics, ester anesthetics are more allergenic because of the PABA structure. Benzocaine is available in 5 different forms: aerosol, gel, gel patch, ointment, and solution. These different forms can be used for different cases. For instance, aerosol can be used to administer palatine anesthesia to decrease gag reflex in patients during impressions; gel forms can be used before application of local anesthetic injection to minimize the discomfort of injection; and ointment and solutions usually are used to provide comfort in cases that a patient has oral aphthous ulcer.

Benzocaine is a well-known cause of methemoglobinemia, and should never be used on patients who have had methemoglobinemia in the past or on children 2 years or younger. Because most dental preparations are used in a concentration of 20%, it will not be difficult to administer a dose sufficient to cause this problem. Methemoglobinemia may occur after only one application or even after the patient has had several uneventful applications. The signs and symptoms may occur within minutes or up to 2 hours after the use of benzocaine topical in the mouth or if it is sprayed into the throat to prevent gagging. The FDA still maintain notification to health care professionals and patients that methemoglobinemia associated with benzocaine products is still being reported, and that it may be a serious and potentially fatal adverse effect.[2]

Combination topical anesthetics

Compounding is the process by which drugs are combined or the ingredients altered to create a custom-made medication. In the case of topical anesthetics the aim is to produce a strong topical anesthetic that can be used for minimal to moderately painful procedures. These preparations contain higher concentrations of topical anesthetics, making them stronger and capable of maintaining their efficacy for longer durations after application. Compound topical anesthetics are used on children by pediatric

Table 1 Topical anesthetics		
Trade Name	**Composition and Form**	**Flavor**
CaineTips	Individually wrapped, disposable swabs prefilled with 20% benzocaine	Cherry flavored
Comfortcaine	20% benzocaine	Available in 6 flavors
Gingicaine	20% benzocaine	Available in 7 flavors
Hurricaine	20% benzocaine in gel and liquid formulations	Gel is available in 4 flavors and liquid in 2 flavors
LolliCaine	20% benzocaine gel on a single-use clean swab applicator	Available in 3 flavors
Topex	20% benzocaine	Available in 7 flavors
Cetacaine	Benzocaine 14%, aminobenzoate 2%, and tetracaine 2%. Spray	
One Touch	18% benzocaine and 15% tetracaine as a gel	Available in 5 flavors
Profound	Tetracaine, lidocaine, and prilocaine as a gel	

dentists for restorative procedures, by periodontists and hygienists for scaling and root-planing procedures, and by orthodontists for the placement of orthodontic temporary anchorage devices.

These combination preparations of local anesthetics are commonly referred to as eutectic mixtures of local anesthesia (EMLA). When mixed together in certain ratios they form a "eutectic mixture" in which the melting point of the mixture is lower than the melting point of the individual components. This blending allows the mixture to be more in a liquid state that will allow the agents to be better absorbed through the oral mucosa. In 2004, the FDA approved an EMLA product called Oraqix for use in dentistry. Oraqix (Dentsply Pharmaceutical, Philadelphia, PA, USA) is a gel that can be inserted into the gingival sulcus to produce sufficient anesthesia to permit deep-cleaning procedures such as scaling and root planing. Two compound topical anesthetics used during placement of orthodontic appliances are TAC 20% Alternate Anesthetic Gel (tetracaine 4%, phenylephrine 2% and lidocaine 20%; Professional Arts Pharmacy, Lafayette, LA, USA) and Profound (lidocaine 10%, prilocaine 10% and tetracaine 40%; Stevens Pharmacy + Compounding, Costa Mesa, CA, USA). **Table 1** gives a more complete list of topical anesthetic agents.

To date, there have not been many problems reported with these agents and they appear to be relatively safe. The most common adverse reactions seem to be tissue irritation (usually after prolonged application) and transitory taste alterations. The maximum recommended dosage of these topical anesthetics is unknown, but they are thought to have a low therapeutic index. Because some may contain several active anesthetics, often resulting in a mixture of esters and amides, they may pose the risk of allergic reactions. Ester-type anesthetics (benzocaine, tetracaine) are contraindicated in patients with PABA allergy or atypical pseudocholinesterase activity. Tetracaine is associated with a higher incidence of allergic reactions than are other local anesthetics.

Injectable Anesthetics

Lidocaine

Lidocaine hydrochloride (HCl) is the first amino amide type of local anesthetic, and has been in use for more than 60 years. It is considered as the prototype for amide local anesthetics, and is very familiar to dentists (**Table 2**). As a local anesthetic, lidocaine

Table 2
Injectable local anesthetics

Short Acting	Intermediate Acting	Long Acting
Lidocaine 2% 30–45 min	Mepivicaine 3% 90–120 min	Bupivacaine 0.5% with
	Prilocaine 4% (nerve block)	epinephrine 1:200,000
	120–240 min	240–720 min
	Prilocaine 4% (infiltration)	
	60–120 min	
	Articaine 4% with epinephrine	
	1:200,000 180–240 min	
	Mepivicaine 2% with	
	epinephrine 1:200,000	
	120–240 min	
	Lidocaine 2% with	
	epinephrine 1:50,000	
	180–300 min	
	Lidocaine 2% with	
	epinephrine 1:100,000	
	180–300 min	
	Mepivicaine 2% with	
	levonordefrin 1:20,000	
	180–300 min	
	Articaine 4% with epinephrine	
	1:100,000 180–300 min	
	Prilocaine 4% with	
	epinephrine 1:200,000	
	180–480 min	

is characterized by a rapid onset of action and intermediate duration of efficacy, making it suitable for infiltration and nerve block anesthesia, and the "perfect" local anesthetic for dentistry. The maximum recommended dose of lidocaine with epinephrine is 3.2 mg/lb or 7 mg/kg of body weight for adult patients, and should not exceed 500 mg in total. The dose of lidocaine without epinephrine is 2 mg/lb or 4.4 mg/kg, not to exceed 300 mg in total. It must be noted, however, that as with all local anesthetics, the dose will depend on the area to be anesthetized, the vascularity of the tissues, and individual tolerance.

Lidocaine is metabolized by the liver via microsomal fixed-function oxidases and is converted to monoethylglycerine and xylidine. It is excreted through the kidneys with 10% unchanged and 80% as their metabolites. It has pregnancy classification of B. Allergic reaction to lidocaine is virtually nonexistent and has not been documented.[3] Adverse drug reactions (ADRs) are rare when lidocaine is used as a local anesthetic and is administered correctly. Most of the ADRs have been related to administration techniques—mainly intravascular injections resulting in systemic exposure.

Some contraindications for the use of lidocaine include[4]:

- Heart block, second or third degree (without pacemaker)
- Serious adverse drug reaction to lidocaine or amide local anesthetics
- Concurrent treatment with Class I antiarrhythmic agent
- Severe hepatic disease.

Mepivicaine
Mepivicaine is another of the amide class of local anesthetics, and has been available in the United States since 1960. It has a reasonably rapid onset (2–3 minutes

after infiltration in the maxilla and about 5 to 8 minutes for inferior alveolar nerve block for full effect) and medium duration of action. The duration of action of mepivacaine without vasoconstrictor when infiltrated is about 20 to 40 minutes and about 2 hours for regional anesthesia. Its half life is 1.9 hours. Mepivacaine 3% causes slight vasoconstriction, and this effect will give it a longer duration of action, as the anesthetic will remain at the site of injection. Mepivacaine 2% with levonordefrin or epinephrine provides anesthesia of longer durations. Levonordefrin is a sympathomimetic amine used as a vasoconstrictor in local anesthetics. It has pharmacologic activity similar to that of epinephrine, but is more stable. In equal concentrations, levonordefrin is less potent than epinephrine in raising blood pressure and as a vasoconstrictor.[5]

The maximum recommended dose of mepivacaine is 3.0 mg/lb or 6.6 mg/kg of body weight, and should not exceed 400 mg in an adult patient. In children the recommended dose is 3.0 mg/lb up to a maximum of 5 cartridges of form 2% to 3%. The maximum recommended dose of mepivacaine without a vasoconstrictor is 2 mg/lb or 4.4 mg/kg, not to exceed a total dose of 300 mg.

Like lidocaine, the clearance of mepivacaine is almost entirely due to liver metabolism, and depends on the liver blood flow and the activity of the metabolizing enzymes. It is metabolized by hepatic microsomal fixed-function oxidases, hydroxylation, and N-demethylation reactions. Mepivicaine is pregnancy category C and therefore should not be used for pregnant patients.

Local anesthetics exist in both an ionized (cation) and un-ionized (base) form. The un-ionized form of local anesthetic can pass through the nerve membrane and take effect. During infection, local tissue becomes acidic and therefore anesthetic remains mainly in cation (ionized) form. Mepivacaine has a higher pH than lidocaine; therefore when it is used in an acidic environment it has more base form and thus will pass through nerve membrane, and is more effective. This characteristic makes mepivacaine a good choice of local anesthetic when there is infection.[6]

Prilocaine

Prilocaine is another amide local anesthetic that is currently most often used for infiltration anesthesia in dentistry.[7] It differs from lidocaine and mepivacaine because it is a secondary amide. Prilocaine is available in two formulations, prilocaine 4% plain and prilocaine 4% with 1:200,000 epinephrine. The recommended dose of prilocaine both with and without epinephrine is 2.7 mg/lb or 6.0 mg/kg of body weight for adult patients. The maximum total dose for adult patients should not exceed 400 mg. Prilocaine is pregnancy category B and therefore it is safe for use in pregnant women.

When used for infiltration anesthesia in dental patients, the time of onset of prilocaine 4% with epinephrine 1/200,000 (Citanest Forte; Dentsply Pharmaceutical, York, PA, USA) averages 2 minutes with a duration of soft-tissue anesthesia of approximately 2 hours. Operative anesthesia lasts up to 45 minutes. When used for infiltration anesthesia, prilocaine 4% (Citanest 4% Plain) has a rapid onset time of approximately 2 to 3 minutes, and a duration of approximately 1 to 1.5 hours for soft-tissue anesthesia. Prilocaine 4% plain has a short duration for operative anesthesia of approximately 15 minutes. When used for inferior alveolar nerve block, the time of onset of the Forte solution averages approximately 2 to 4 minutes with an average duration of soft-tissue anesthesia of approximately 3 hours, providing 1.5 hours of operative anesthesia. Prilocaine 4% plain requires 5 minutes or more to take full effect. The duration of soft-tissue anesthesia is approximately 2.5 hours while the operative anesthesia has a duration of 1 to 1.5 hours.[8]

Prilocaine is metabolized in both the liver and the kidney and is excreted via the kidney, thus hepatic and renal dysfunction may alter prilocaine kinetics. Most of it is metabolized and only a small fraction of intact prilocaine is secreted in urine. Hydrolysis of prilocaine by amidases yields orthotoluidine and N-propylalanine. Both of these compounds may undergo ring hydroxylation.

In some patients, the metabolite orthotoluidine may cause the unusual side effect of methemoglobinemia when large doses of prilocaine are used. The formation of methemoglobin will reduce the blood's oxygen-carrying capacity, and this can lead to cyanosis. The total dose of prilocaine should be limited to 600 mg to eliminate symptomatic cyanosis. Because prilocaine can decrease the oxygen-carrying capacity of blood, it should be avoided in patients with idiopathic or congenital methemoglobinemia, sickle cell anemia, chronic anemia, and cardiac or respiratory failure with hypoxia. Its use should also be avoided in patients who take acetaminophen or phenacetin, as these both elevate levels of methemoglobin.[6]

Articaine

Articaine is the most recently introduced local anesthetic, approved by the FDA in 2000. It is a member of the amino amide class of local anesthetics, but its structure is unique among this group in that it does not contain a benzene ring like the others but instead contains a thiophene ring. This thiophene ring increases its liposolubility, making it more effective in crossing lipid barriers. It also contains an additional ester group, which enables articaine to undergo biotransformation in the plasma (hydrolysis by plasma esterase) as well as in the liver (by hepatic microsomal enzymes). Articaine HCl is available in 4% strength with 1:100,000 or 1:200,000 epinephrine.

Articaine has very low systemic toxicity, and with its wide therapeutic range it may be used in higher concentrations than other amide-type local anesthetics. Also, because it is hydrolyzed very quickly in the blood, the risk of systemic intoxication seems to be lower than with other anesthetics, especially if repeated injection is performed.[9] The maximum recommended dose of 4% articaine HCl should not exceed 7 mg/kg or 3.2 mg/lb of body weight. It is pregnancy category C and should not be used in pregnant patients.

The main quality of articaine that makes it an attractive local anesthetic is the fact that it diffuses through bone and soft tissue better than other local anesthetics. The concentration of articaine in the alveolus of a tooth in the upper jaw after extraction was about 100 times higher than that in systemic circulation.[10] This higher ability to diffuse through bone and soft tissue has made articaine useful in giving profound anesthesia via infiltration without the need for mandibular block.

Persistent paresthesia of the lips, tongue, and oral tissues have been reported with the use of articaine HCl, with slow, incomplete, or no recovery. These adverse events have been reported chiefly following inferior alveolar nerve blocks, and seem to involve the lingual nerve most often. Such reports have caused some early and persistent controversy concerning articaine. However, this is no longer considered as a complication of articaine 4%. In a detailed review of paresthesia cases due to nerve blocks evaluated by the Oral and Maxillofacial Surgery Department of the University of California at San Francisco, Pogrel and colleagues[11,12] reported that 35% of the cases involved the use of lidocaine and 30% involved the use of articaine. The investigators concluded that nerve blocks can cause permanent damage to the nerves, independent of the local anesthetic used, and that they did not find any disproportionate nerve involvement from articaine but that articaine is associated with this phenomenon in proportion to its usage.

Bupivacaine

Bupivacaine is another amino amide type of local anesthetics that is 4 times as potent as lidocaine, mepivacaine, and prilocaine. It has a longer duration of action than lidocaine—approximately 6 to 8 hours as opposed to 1 to 2 hours for lidocaine. Bupivacaine is often administered after the extraction of impacted third molars to reduce pain for up to 12 to 20 hours after the surgery. It is also commonly injected into surgical wound sites to achieve long-term postoperative pain control.

Bupivacaine is available in concentrations of 0.25%, 0.5%, and 0.75%, either plain or combined with epinephrine (1:200,000) The 0.25% form is the concentration most widely used in dentistry. The maximum recommended dose is 0.6 mg/lb or 1.3 mg/kg for adult patients, and the total maximum dose should not exceed 90 mg. Bupivacaine is pregnancy category C and should not be used in pregnant patients. Compared with other local anesthetics, bupivacaine is markedly cardiotoxic and should be used with caution in patients taking β-blockers (eg, atenolol) or digoxin because the risk of side effects such as abnormal heartbeat may be increased. Bupivacaine is metabolized in liver by amidases and is excreted via kidneys.

Epinephrine

Epinephrine or adrenaline is a sympathomimetic amine that is added to local anesthetic to cause vasoconstriction. Some of the adverse effects of local anesthetic use such as tachycardia and tremor are caused by epinephrine. It is added to local anesthetics to oppose the vasodilating effects of local anesthetics and therefore increase their duration of action. Furthermore, the vasoconstriction effect decreases systemic absorption of local anesthetics and therefore lowers systemic toxicity. Another purpose of adding epinephrine to local anesthetics is to achieve hemostasis at the surgical site, as it causes vasoconstriction by stimulating α and β2 receptors in vessels supplying skeletal muscles.

The action of epinephrine on β1 receptors in the myocardium is to increase the heart rate and the contractility. It can trigger ventricular tachycardia and premature ventricular contractions, due to stimulation of cardiac pacemaker cells. The overall effect of epinephrine on the cardiovascular system is to increase cardiac efficiency. Epinephrine has a bronchodilatory effect on the respiratory system, due to its action on β2 receptors.

Epinephrine action is terminated mainly by reuptake in the adrenergic nerve terminals. The remainder of epinephrine will be inactivated by catechol-O-methyltransferase and monoamine oxidase, and only 1% of epinephrine is excreted unchanged in urine.

Adverse reactions to epinephrine include palpitations, tachycardia, arrhythmia, anxiety, headache, tremor, and hypertension. Patients with coronary artery disease are usually more sensitive to epinephrine and can have episodes of angina due to the increase in heart rate. The administration of epinephrine will not cause heart failure by constricting coronary arteries, because coronary arteries only have β2 receptors, which cause vasodilation in the presence of epinephrine.[13] As a general rule, use of epinephrine in patients with cardiovascular disease should be limited to 2 carpules of local anesthetic with epinephrine. All patients with cardiovascular disease and elderly patients at risk for cardiovascular disease need to have their blood pressure taken before administration of local anesthetics with epinephrine.

Patients with a heart transplant have a heart that has been surgically denervated. Loss of adrenergic nerve terminals that control both release and reuptake of epinephrine will make a transplanted heart more sensitive to epinephrine. Therefore, in this special class of patients epinephrine use should be minimized and heart function should be continuously monitored for any changes in rhythm.

Caine Allergy

When a patient gives a history of being "allergic" to local anesthetics it will be very difficult for the clinician to dismiss the claim, even in the absence of proper documentation. It must be noted, however, that true allergic reactions to the commonly used local anesthetics are rare, and adverse reactions are more common. Differentiating between allergic and adverse reactions is often difficult because of the similarity of the symptoms, and physicians may label patients as "allergic" to "-caine" drugs even when the signs and symptoms are consistent with an adverse reaction.

Local anesthetics are grouped, depending on their chemical structure, into two categories: esters and amides. The esters are derivatives of *para*-aminobenzoic acid, which is known to be allergenic, hence a certain percentage of the population will demonstrate allergic reactions to this group of drugs. True allergic reactions to amides are extremely rare. In a study conducted to determine the incidence of true local anesthetic allergy in patients with an alleged history of local anesthetic allergy, the researchers concluded that "a history of allergy to local anesthesia is unlikely to be genuine and local anesthetic allergy is rare."[14] Other investigators have also concluded that a true immunologic reaction to a local anesthetic is rare, and that patients who are allergic to ester local anesthetics can be treated with a preservative-free amide local anesthetic.[15]

When a patient presents with a history of allergy to a local anesthetic, the first step should be to ascertain the signs and symptoms of the reaction and to try to determine, by history, whether it could have been an allergic reaction. The quantity of anesthetic that was used should also be questioned, as the reaction may have been toxic arising from either large amounts of local anesthetic (as used in liposuction or extensive facelift procedures) or an intravascular injection. Question also if the individual underwent any dental procedures since being told of the allergy. If doubt persists, the patient may be sent to an allergist to do a progressive challenge with dilute solutions and then undiluted intradermal injection of local anesthetics, to diagnose allergy to the agent.

RELATIVE ANATOMY AND TECHNIQUES

Local anesthesia can be achieved by infiltration (field anesthesia) or by conduction anesthesia (nerve block). For maxillary surgical procedures, in the vast majority of cases infiltration anesthesia is all that is required because the cortical plate of the alveolus of the upper jaw is almost always thin and porous enough to make infiltration anesthesia effective. Procedures on the lower jaw will most often require nerve-block anesthesia of the inferior alveolar, lingual, and buccal nerves.

In the maxilla it is the network of nerves within the spongy bone that is anesthetized, along with nerve endings in the adjacent soft tissues and the mucosa of the maxillary sinus. This network is a part of the dental plexus, which is derived from the superior alveolar nerves. After infiltration of the local anesthetic in the buccal vestibule, the anesthetic fluid diffuses uniformly through the spongy bone of the maxilla to produce anesthesia of the adjacent tooth and its periodontal ligament, the gingiva on the buccal surface, the adjacent soft tissue, and the bone itself. For extraction of teeth, infiltration on the palatal aspect will also be needed.

As mentioned previously, surgical procedures on the lower jaw will require nerve-block anesthesia of the inferior alveolar, lingual, and buccal nerves. These nerves are all accessible in the pterygomandibular space (**Fig. 1**). This space is an inverted triangularly shaped cleft between the pterygoid musculature and the ramus of the

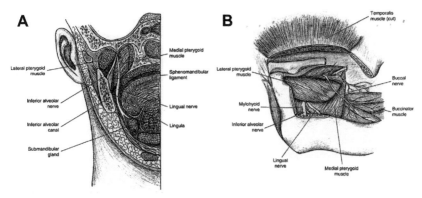

Fig. 1. (*A, B*) Anatomy of the pterygomandibular space. (*From* Dym H, Ogle O. Atlas of minor oral surgery. Philadelphia: W.B. Saunders Company; 2010. p. 34; with permission.)

mandible. The contents of the pterygomandibular space include the inferior alveolar and lingual nerves, and the inferior alveolar artery and vein, which converge with the inferior alveolar nerve as it enters the mandibular foramen. The buccal nerve also travels for a short distance through the upper and anterior part of the space (see **Fig. 1**B).

With regard to nerve block of the inferior alveolar nerve, two anatomic entities should be clearly understood. The first is the position of the lingula and the second is the anatomy of the sphenomandibular ligament. The sphenomandibular ligament, which is actually a broad sheet of fibrous tissue, extends from the sphenoid bone, spreading downward and outward to attach to the mandible at the lingula, the inferior margin of the mandibular foramen, and above the attachment of the medial pterygoid muscle.[16] Its zone of attachment continues posteriorly and superiorly to the posterior border of the ramus and extends up to the condylar neck, where it blends into the stylomandibular ligament. The sphenomandibular ligament has a very important influence on the diffusion of anesthetic solution injected into the area.[17] Anesthetic solutions deposited low in the pterygomandibular space will not diffuse up to where the inferior mandibular nerve enters the mandibular canal.

The lingula is a ledge of bone that guards the mandibular foramen, which is located near the center of the ramus. The position of the mandibular canal is extremely variable, however. Research by Bremer[18] showed that:

- In 16% of mandibles, the lingula was less than 1 mm above the occlusal plane
- 48% were from 1 to 5 mm above the occlusal plane
- 27% were from 9 to 11 mm above the occlusal plane
- 4% were from 11 to 19 mm above the occlusal plane.

Using this as a guide, one can see that a needle inserted 5 mm above the occlusal plane and parallel to it would lie above the lingula in 64% of mandibles and below it in 36%. A needle placed 11 mm above the occlusal plane would be above the lingula in 96% of mandibles (**Fig. 2**).[17] To obtain profound anesthesia, at least 6 mm of the nerve must be bathed by the anesthetic solution.

In the growing child (ages 10–19 years), the lingula is more posterior and superior on the ramus than in the adult.[19] To perform an inferior alveolar nerve block in the growing

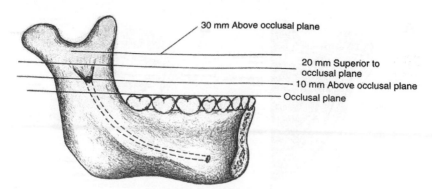

30 mm Above occlusal plane

20 mm Superior to occlusal plane

10 mm Above occlusal plane

Occlusal plane

Fig. 2. Position of the lingula relative to the occlusal plane. (*From* Dym H, Ogle O. Atlas of minor oral surgery. Philadelphia: W.B. Saunders Company; 2001. p. 32; with permission.)

mandible, the tip of the needle must reach an area that is high and far back on the ramus.[17]

Techniques for performing an inferior alveolar nerve block are as follows. (1) The Halstead method, in which the nerve is blocked as it enters the mandibular foramen. This technique has a success rate of between 71% and 87%. The method does not deposit the solution high enough to anesthetize the buccal nerve, and another injection may be required for the buccal nerve. (2) The Akinosi technique, which makes use of a higher level of injection and anesthetizes the inferior alveolar nerve, the lingual nerve, and the buccal nerve by a single injection (**Fig. 3**). It is very useful in patients with limited jaw opening, particularly in patients with trismus from infection, or in fearful patients who will not open their mouth to permit the use of the standard Halstead technique. The Akinosi technique has a 96% success rate in producing inferior alveolar nerve block. (3) the Gow-Gates technique uses external landmarks that direct the needle to a higher puncture point, thus ensuring an adequate height for depositing the solution above the lingula. This technique has a reported success rate of 98%.[20]

Maxillary Nerve Blocks

In rare cases when field anesthesia is contraindicated because of an infection in the area, or when it is necessary to anesthetize several teeth, a block of the posterior

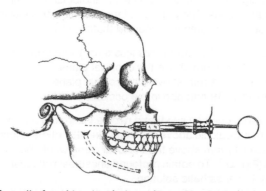

Fig. 3. Position of needle for Akinosi technique. (*From* Dym H, Ogle O. Atlas of minor oral surgery. Philadelphia: W.B. Saunders Company; 2010. p. 33; with permission.)

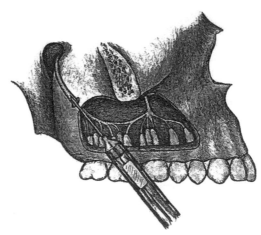

Fig. 4. Posterior superior alveolar nerve block. (*From* Dym H, Ogle O. Atlas of minor oral surgery. Philadelphia: W.B. Saunders Company; 2010. p. 38; with permission.)

superior alveolar or infraorbital nerve may be required. The posterior superior alveolar nerve may be blocked before it enters the bony canals located on the zygomatic aspect of the maxilla above the third molar.[21,22] The puncture is made high in the mucobuccal fold above the distobuccal root of the second molar, and the needle is directed upward and inward to a depth of about 20 mm, keeping the point of the needle close to the periosteum of the tuberosity. Doing so will minimize the chance of entering the pterygoid venus plexus.[17] This block provides anesthesia on the lateral maxilla from the pterygomaxillary fissure to the distobuccal root of the first molar (**Fig. 4**).

The infraorbital nerve block is indicated when inflammation or infection contraindicates the use of infiltration anesthesia in the anterior portion of the maxilla. The general position of the infraorbital foramen is estimated (5 mm below the infraorbital rim on the midpupillary line or 4 mm lateral and 5 mm below the infraorbital notch). After the area

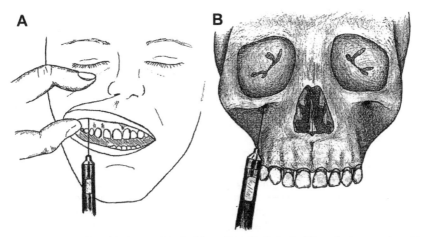

Fig. 5. (*A, B*) The infraorbital nerve block. (*From* Dym H, Ogle O. Atlas of minor oral surgery. Philadelphia: W.B. Saunders Company; 2010. p. 35; with permission.)

is estimated, a finger should be placed over the site. The cheek is then retracted as far laterally as possible and the needle (a long dental needle should be used) is introduced 5 to 7 mm away from the buccal surface of the alveolus. The needle is directed parallel to the long axis of the second premolar, and is advanced until it is below the palpating finger. Once in the area of the foramen the content of one anesthetic cartridge should be deposited. This block will anesthetize the skin over the lower eyelid, ala of the nose, and upper lip, and the lateral maxilla from the first molar to the central incisor, including the teeth (**Fig. 5**).[17]

COMPLICATIONS
Allergic Reactions

When exposed to an antigen, the immune system is triggered to produce a hypersensitivity reaction or an allergic reaction. Most allergic reactions are minor but will depend on the person's immune system response, which is sometimes unpredictable. In rare cases, an allergic reaction can be life threatening (anaphylaxis). Symptoms and signs of an allergic reaction may include any or some the following: skin irritation with itching and swelling, welts or bumps on the face and neck, stuffy or runny nose, wheezing, shortness of breath, and headaches.

As previously mentioned, allergic reactions to amide local anesthetics seldom occur. The most common sign of an allergic reaction seen with local anesthetic is skin reactions, but there can be severe reactions such as bronchospasm and systemic anaphylaxis. Again, as mentioned previously, these severe reactions rarely, if ever, occur. An allergic reaction could occur, however, to various compounds that are used in local anesthetic carpules. Sodium bisulfate, which is a preservative for epinephrine, is one such compound that can cause allergic reaction in patients allergic to bisulfites. In patients that are allergic to sulfonamide antibiotics, there is no cross-allergenicity to sulfites.

The earliest treatment for an allergic reaction should be removal of the causative agent (eg, topical benzocaine). An oral antihistamine—diphenhydramine (Benadryl), 25 or 50 mg—should be given. Hydrocortisone cream may be prescribed to relieve skin itching or redness.

Postinjection Pain and Trismus

Persistent pain at the site of injection is the most common complication of local anesthesia in the oral cavity. Some causes of the pain are multiple injections in a short period of time, injection into the belly of one of the adjacent muscles, or muscle tears from too forceful injections. Following maxillary tooth removal or third molar extractions it will be difficult to determine whether pain is from the surgery or the injection. Pain following inferior alveolar nerve block is easily discernible. This condition is almost always self-limiting and will improve in 5 to 10 days, and no definitive therapy is necessary. A nonsteroidal anti-inflammatory drug (NSAID) should be taken every 4 hours until the pain is tolerable. NSAIDs are best used continuously rather than on an "as necessary" basis.

Trismus is also a relatively common complication following local anesthetic administration. Several factors may play a role in causing the trismus. Injection into the temporalis, masseter, or medial pterygoid muscles may damage the muscle fibers and cause limitations in opening. The most common muscle to be the source of trismus is the medial pterygoid, which can be penetrated during an inferior alveolar nerve block using any of the 3 main techniques. When any one of the muscles is damaged, the muscle fibers engender pain when they are stretched. The pain causes the muscles to contract, resulting in loss of range of motion. Bleeding into the muscle following the injection may also cause muscle spasm and trismus. Hematoma formation in the pterygomandibular space may also occur secondarily to an injury of the inferior alveolar artery or vein.

NSAIDs should be used for the first 48 hours and the condition observed. If no improvement in jaw opening is noted then treatment of the trismus should begin. It should be noted that although the duration of symptoms and their severity are both variable, improvement should be noted within 3 to 5 days following the initiation of management. It must be stressed, however, is that in treating this condition it is important to avoid rapid motion or the use of powerful forces. Rapid motion or force may worsen the injury and increase the reflex that causes muscles to contract, thereby making subsequent stretching of connective tissue difficult or even impossible. The main aim of therapy is to gently get the jaw functioning early to avoid fibrosis, which would make the condition difficult to reverse. Passive motion applied several times per day is significantly more effective than static stretching in reducing inflammation and pain. Passive motion is aimed to constantly move the jaw through a controlled range of motion to prevent fibrous scar tissue formation, which would tend to decrease the range of motion over time. Chewing gum at short intervals should be the first management technique, followed by gentle stretching exercises using the thumb on the upper teeth and middle finger on lower teeth to exercise the jaw muscles. Additional opening can be achieved by the use of stacked tongue depressors. These devices are stacked, forced, and held between the teeth in an attempt to push the mouth open over time by adding additional tongue blades while the stack is between the teeth.

Trismus occurring 2 or 3 days after the injection is most likely a needle tract infection, and should be treated with antibiotics.

Facial Nerve Paresis

Facial nerve (cranial nerve VII) gives motor innervations to the muscles of facial expression. The nerve exits the skull from the stylomastoid foramen. After exiting the foramen it enters the parotid gland, divides, and exits the parotid as 5 major branches. Facial nerve paralysis can occur if local anesthetic is injected close to the "deep lobe" of the parotid. This paralysis can occur if during administration of local anesthetic for inferior alveolar nerve block the needle goes posterior and the anesthetic solution is deposited within the substance of the parotid; this will consequently paralyze the muscles of facial expression, causing a unilateral Bell palsy. The mouth will deviate to the affected side and the individual will be unable to close the eye on the affected side. The paralysis usually lasts a few hours, depending on the type of anesthetic used. There is no treatment to reverse the effect of local anesthesia other than waiting until the anesthetic wears off. If paralysis of facial muscles happens, the patient should be reassured that this is transient and that the effect of local anesthesia will wear off in a few hours. In patients who wear contact lenses these should be removed, as the lenses may cause damage to the cornea. An eye patch should be placed on the affected eye to maintain eye moisture. Although the effect is transient, the authors have seen cases in which the palsy lasted for a week.

Broken Needle

Local anesthetic needle breakage is rare and because there are few reports, the mechanism and best treatment options are undetermined. The vast majority of cases (94%)[21] of broken needles occurs in connection with an inferior alveolar nerve block, often with 30-gauge needles.[21] Incidents of broken needle are associated with prior bending of the needle, unexpected patient movement, and defective needles. If the needle breaks during an inferior alveolar nerve block, the dental surgeon should immediately advise the patient to keep the mouth open, insert a bite block to prevent closure, inform the patient, and try to retrieve the needle with a hemostat if possible. If the needle is not visible, the patient should be immediately referred to an oral and maxillofacial surgeon. If the surgeon is not immediately available a microradiograph should be obtained if possible, an antibiotic prescribed, and the patient advised not to open his or her mouth widely so as to limit the needle's movement. Three-dimensional computed tomography scanning to identify the position of the needle will most likely be necessary, and the patient will need to be hospitalized to have the needle removed in the operating room under general anesthesia. If the broken needle is left in situ, there is a risk that over time the needle may migrate and injure major blood vessels, or damage other vital structures of the head and neck.

To prevent needle breakage the following important points should be considered:

- Do not deliberately bend the needle before inserting it into the tissue
- Avoid using a short or a 30-gauge needle to administer inferior alveolar blocks
- Do not bury the needle in the tissue all the way to the hub.

Lingual Nerve Injury

Anesthesia, paresthesia, or dysesthesia of the lingual nerve occur on rare occasions with inferior alveolar nerve blocks. Although both the inferior alveolar and lingual nerves can be damaged during an attempted inferior alveolar nerve block, most studies show that it is the lingual nerve, rather than the inferior alveolar nerve, that is predominantly affected and that the lingual nerve may be affected in up to 80% of cases.[12] Pogrel and colleagues[23] believe that the lingual nerve may be predominantly affected because of its fascicular pattern. In their studies they found that just above the lingula, where an inferior alveolar nerve block is normally deposited, the lingual nerve was unifascicular in one-third of cases, and a unifascicular nerve may be injured more easily and permanently than a multifascicular nerve, which may have greater powers of recovery. The lingual nerve is also more likely to be injured by a needle because of its position (5–6 mm below the surface mucosa) and because it is exposed below the mandibular foramen.

The mechanism of nerve damage is believed to be caused by direct needle trauma, hemorrhage inside the epineurium, or a neurotoxic effect from the local anesthetic. There is no known way to avoid the possibility of nerve damage resulting from an inferior alveolar nerve block, and lingual nerve injury will always be an unavoidable risk of the procedure. If the patient feels an "electric shock" in the tongue, stopping the injection, backing the needle out a few millimeters, and repositioning it may minimize the incidence of permanent nerve damage. This contact does not always cause paresthesia, so it is uncertain what should be done. If after 24 hours the patient continues to experience residual loss of sensation, this is a paresthesia. Although not proved to be effective, high-dose corticosteroids to reduce immune inflammatory reaction may be considered. Most paresthesias resolve within 10 to 14 days, but may take up to 6 months. On rare occasion, however, it may be permanent.

SUMMARY

Local anesthesia is possibly the most important aspect of oral surgery practice. Without it, none of the surgical procedures discussed in this issue would have been possible. This article has given an overview of local and topical anesthetics, their mechanism of action, indications, and contraindications, as well as the techniques of administering local anesthetic. Commonly occurring and known complications associated with local anesthesia and possible treatment modalities have been discussed.

Local anesthetics have made a great advancement in dentistry and have changed patients' perspectives of dental procedures to a great extent. There is still room for the improvement of painless techniques in administrating local anesthetics. It is important for clinicians to be familiar with all the local anesthetics available for dental procedures, their mode of action, and their adverse reactions and how to treat them.

REFERENCES

1. Kravitz N. The use of compound topical anesthetics. J Am Dent Assoc 2007; 138(10):1333–9.
2. Available at: http://www.drugs.com/fda/benzocaine-topical-products-gels-liquids-risk-methemoglobinemia-12941.html. Accessed March, 2011.
3. Jackson D, Chen AH, Bennett CR. Identifying true lidocaine allergy. J Am Dent Assoc 1994;125(10):1362–6.
4. Available at: http://en.wikipedia.org/wiki/Lidocaine. Accessed April, 2011.
5. The Comprehensive Resource for Physicians, drug and illness information. Available at: http://www.rxmed.com/b.main/b2.pharmaceutical/b2.1.monographs/CPS-%20 Monographs/CPS-%20(General%20Monographs-%20P)/POLOCAINE.html. Accessed April, 2011.
6. Malamed SF. Handbook of local anesthesia. 5th edition. St Louis (MO): Elsevier Mosby; 2004. p. 68–73.
7. Department of Drugs, Division of Drugs and Toxicology, American Medical Association. AMA drug evaluations annual. Chicago: American Medical Association; 1992. p. 16.
8. Citanest Drug Insert, Dentsply Pharmaceutical.
9. Oertel R, Ebert U, Rahn R, et al. Clinical pharmacokinetics of articaine. Clin Pharmacokinet 1997;33(6):417–25.
10. Vree TB, Gielen MJ. Clinical pharmacology and the use of articaine for local and regional anesthesia. Best Pract Res Clin Anaesthesiol 2005;19: 293–308.
11. Pogrel MA, Bryan J, Regezi J. Nerve damage associated with inferior alveolar nerve blocks. J Am Dent Assoc 1995;126(8):1150–5.
12. Pogrel MA, Thamby S. Permanent nerve involvement resulting from inferior alveolar nerve blocks. J Am Dent Assoc 2000;131(7):901–7.
13. Sun D, Huang A, Mital S, et al. Norepinephrine elicits beta2-receptor-mediated dilation of isolated human coronary arterioles. Circulation 2002;106(5):550–5.
14. Fisher MM, Bowie CJ. Alleged allergy to local anaesthetics. Anaesth Intensive Care 1997;25(6):611–4.
15. Eggleston ST, Lush LW. Understanding allergic reactions to local anaesthetics. Ann Pharmacother 1996;30(7–8):851–7.
16. Barker BCW, Davis PL. The applied anatomy of the pterygomandibular space. Br J Oral Surg 1972;10:43–55.
17. Ogle O. Local anesthesia. In: Dym H, Ogle O, editors. Atlas of minor oral surgery. Philadelphia: W.B. Saunders; 2001. p. 30–40. Chapter 3.
18. Bremer G. Measurements of special significance in connection with anesthesia of the inferior alveolar nerve. Oral Surg Oral Med Oral Pathol 1952;5: 966–88.
19. Kaban LB. Surgical correction of the facial skeleton in childhood. In: Kaban LB, editor. Pediatric oral and maxillofacial surgery. Philadelphia: W.B. Saunders; 1990. p. 425.

20. Gow-Gates GA, Watson JE. The Gow-Gates mandibular block: further understanding. Anesth Prog 1977;24:183–9.
21. Manual of local anesthesia in general dentistry. New York: Cook-Waite Laboratories. p. 12.
22. Pogrel MA. Broken local anesthetic needles: a case series of 16 patients, with recommendations. J Am Dent Assoc 2009;140(12):1517–22.
23. Pogrel MA, Schmidt BL, Sambajon V, et al. Lingual nerve damage due to inferior alveolar nerve blocks: a possible explanation. J Am Dent Assoc 2003;134(2): 195–9.

Diagnosis and Treatment of Temporomandibular Disorders

Harry Dym, DDS[a],*, Howard Israel, DDS[b]

KEYWORDS

- Temporomandibular disorders • Temporomandibular joint
- Diagnostic imaging • Masticatory muscles

Temoporomandibular disorders (TMDs) are defined as clinical problems involving the masticatory musculature, the temoporomandibular joints (TMJs) and associated structures, or both.[1] The abbreviation MPD (myofascial pain dysfunction) has been used to describe those disorders that involve only the muscles of mastication and associated fascia, which are the result of excessive muscle activity causing muscle pain.[2]

TMD is considered the most common musculoskeletal disorder that causes orofacial pain. The cardinal presenting signs of TMD that the patient may present with include the following:

1. Limitation of jaw opening or function
2. Pain with jaw opening or function
3. Joint sounds.

TMDs occur disproportionately in women of childbearing age in a female to male ratio of between 4:1 and 6:1; the prevalence drops off significantly for males and females after age 55 years. One study has estimated that approximately 12% of the adult population in the United States suffers from temoporomandibular symptoms every 6 months.[3]

Current concepts and recommended treatment for TMDs and TMJ pain and dysfunction have evolved over time. This article attempts to distill the current information for this often confusing topic into relevant clinical issues that will allow the general dental practitioner to be better able to diagnose and interpret clinical findings, and institute a therapeutic regimen that will provide needed relief to patients suffering

[a] Department of Dentistry/Oral and Maxillofacial Surgery, The Brooklyn Hospital Center, 121 DeKalb Avenue, Brooklyn, NY 11201, USA
[b] Division of Oral & Maxillofacial Surgery, Weill-Cornell Medical College, Cornell University, New York, NY 11021, USA
* Corresponding author.
E-mail address: DrHowardIsrael@yahoo.com

Dent Clin N Am 56 (2012) 149–161
doi:10.1016/j.cden.2011.08.002
0011-8532/12/$ – see front matter © 2012 Published by Elsevier Inc.

from TMD dysfunction. A review of some basic TMJ anatomy and physiology is needed to better understand the current treatment philosophy and objectives.

RELEVANT TMJ ANATOMY

The mandible and cranium make up the craniomandibular articulation, made up of a mandibular condyle below and the temporal bone above. The articular space of the TMJ inside the glenoid fossa is divided into upper and lower quadrants by an avascular fibrous disc (**Fig. 1**). The disc condyle complex and the mandibular fossa are enclosed within a temoporomandibular ligament. The lateral pterygoid muscle attaches to the disc, and the disc is firmly attached to the medial and lateral poles of the mandibular condyle and moves in tandem with the lower jaw bone.

The mandible on maximal opening undergoes two basic movements:

A. A rotary or hinge movement
B. A translatory or sliding movement, which involves a bodily movement of the mandible in an anteroposterior/mediolateral direction.

The normal jaw opening is to 40 to 50 mm, and is caused by the relaxation of the masticator elevator muscles and the combined action of lateral pterygoid, geniohyoid, mylohoid, and digastric muscles (**Box 1**). The elevators of the mandible contract to close the jaw bone with the disc gliding along with the condyle in synchrony. When the disc fails to move in tandem with the condylar head, the joint is said to have an internal derangement. The most common disc disorder includes anterior disc displacement with and without reduction.

Anterior disc displacement without reduction is the state in which the anteriorly displaced disc is maintained in this position throughout rotational translation. The condyle fails to translate down the articular eminence, limiting mouth opening to about 25 mm; this is referred to as a closed lock. In a TMJ that suffers from anterior disc displacement with reduction, there is no limitation in jaw opening but as the condyle moves down the articular eminence sometimes there is pain and deviation of the mandible, concluding with a click as the displaced disc returns to its normal position. This movement is then often followed by a closing click as the condyle moves

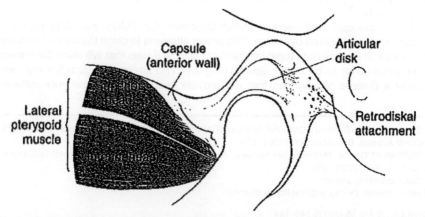

Fig. 1. The disc and other temoporomandibular components. (*From* Fonseca RJ. Oral and maxillofacial surgery. vol. 2. 2nd edition. Elsevier; p. 816; with permission.)

Box 1
Main actions of muscles in groups

Elevating Muscles

   Temporalis

   Masseter

   Medial pterygoid

Depressing Muscles

   Digastric

   Mylohyoid

   Geniohyoid

Protracting Muscles

   Lateral pterygoid

Retracting Muscles

   Digastric

---

backward into the fossa. A major point that must be emphasized is that the altered biomechanics associated with disc displacement is the end result of biochemical and tissue changes within the joint. All intra-articular structures that are not cartilaginous are lined with the synovial membrane, which in vascular tissue and responsible for the production of synovial fluid.

EVALUATION TECHNIQUES

It is critical that the treating dentist or physician arrives at the correct diagnosis and cause of the patient's chronic facial pain/TMD so that the correct treatment will be rendered. It is not unusual for patients who have facial pain due to a TMD to have sought numerous opinions or treatments from various physicians (ear/nose/throat specialist, neurologist, internist, and so forth) before finally visiting the office of the dentist/oral surgeon. The key components in a thorough facial/TMJ examination that clinicians must perform include the following:

- Chief complaint
- History of present illness
  - Chronology of onset
  - Description of any trauma
  - Factors that increase symptoms
  - Factors that improve symptoms
- Patient's medical and dental histories
  - Prior history of joint dysfunction
  - Has this individual ever been treated for a similar problem
  - What were the results of that treatment?
  - Are any comorbid systemic disorders present?
- Findings of the clinical examination include the following:
  - Muscles of the neck and shoulders
  - Conditions found within the oral cavity that might be contributing to the patient's pain complaints (ie, an evaluation of the soft tissues, periodontium, and teeth)

○ Myofunctional and/or parafunctional habits
○ Mandibular range-of-motion measurements
○ Auscultation of the TMJs during movement
○ Radiologic findings.

DIAGNOSTIC IMAGING

TMDs often are associated with displacement of the disc along with arthritic and inflammatory changes in the components of the TM joint. The panoramic radiographic study must be performed in all patients who present with possible TMDs. This basic study can help identify gross arthritic changes, or other hard-tissue abnormalities such as tumors, bone cysts, or malformations of the mandibular condyle and surrounding glenoid fossa. However, the panoramic radiograph is only as good as screening modality that does not show soft tissue pathology.

Cone beam computed tomography (CT) is increasingly being used as an imaging modality in the assessment of the TMJ, and has been reported to provide superior reliability and greater accuracy than panoramic projections in the detection of condylar cortical erosions.[4,5] Moreover, it offers a low-dose alternative to conventional CT imaging for visualization of the osseous structures.

Axial CT scanning has the capability to image both hard and surrounding soft tissue. The disc usually is difficult to visualize with CT, especially if it is thin and small. The gold standard for TMD/TMJ studies is magnetic resonance imaging (MRI). This modality does not expose the patient to ionizing radiation and provides the most detail of the articular disc and muscles of mastication, permitting visualization of inflammatory changes and the presence of effusions.

Imaging studies beyond the basic panoramic screening film should be reserved only for those patients with abnormal pain and jaw dysfunction, or both, and who have failed to respond to conservative short-term treatment such as nonsteroidal anti-inflammatory drugs (NSAIDs) and physical therapy.

HISTORY OF TMD/TMJ TREATMENT APPROACHES

Recognition and treatment of TMD/TMJ disorders is more than a century old, and a variety of differing treatment philosophies has evolved over that time. Thomas Annandale[6] is credited with the first published description of TMJ disc repair in 1887. He described a surgical approach to treating patients with jaw locking and painful clicking by surgical disc repositioning. In 1936[7] an otolaryngologist, James Costen, thought that loss of posterior dental occlusal support was the primary cause of TMJ disorders, and subsequent to his publication on the matter, patients who presented with headaches, ear pain, or abnormal jaw movements were said to have "Costen's syndrome" and were treated with dental prosthesis reconstruction.

In 1959, Laszlow Schwartz[8] applied the newly described concepts of myofascial pain, myalgia, and trigger areas to too stiff, sore muscles in the masticatory system, and thus an era of nonsurgical medical therapy ensued. He introduced the new therapies of local anesthetic injection and vapor coolant therapy. In 1969, Daniel Laskin published an article in the *Journal of the American Dental Association* in which he proposed a shift in thinking about TMJ disorders from joint pathology to an emphasis on muscle pathology. He presented his findings linking a strong psychological origin to the muscle disorder in TMJ/TMD disorder, and coined the term myofascial pain dysfunction (MPD).

The 1970s and 1980s brought the dental profession full circle, back to a purely surgical approach for the treatment of TMD/TMJ. Dolwick and colleagues[9] postulated that in almost all patients with classic TMJ/TMD symptoms, (pain in the preauricular area, inability to open jaw maximally, joint clicking) there was to disc function or lack of function, and all treatment was then focused on open surgical procedures to reposition or repair the TMJ articular disc.

Following the introduction of joint arthroscopy in 1975 by Ohnishi, it soon proved to be a successful treatment modality of TMJ/TMD disorders despite the fact that it failed to reduce the articular disc to the "normal" position. In 1991 Nitzan and colleagues[10] published an article in which they questioned the direct primary role of disc displacement as causative in TMJ symptoms.

The current understanding of TMDs is more complex and nuanced. Abnormal TMJ disc position is now felt to be the result of abnormal joint physiology (joint inflammation secondary to macrotrauma or microtrauma is thought to cause changes in synovial fluid viscosity,[11] which also leads to disc adhesions that result in abnormal disc position) rather than the direct cause of TMJ pain and dysfunction. Consequently, surgery purely directed to disc repositioning would be both futile and nonproductive. Treatment objectives are now directed toward first dealing with the causes of joint pathology that lead to joint inflammation and arthritis and tackling temporomandibular pain with nonsurgical methods, using invasive techniques only if the previously attempted nonsurgical approaches fail to improve the clinical situation.

PATHOPHYSIOLOGY OF TMJ DYSFUNCTION AND PAIN

Current thinking on the etiology of TMJ pain and dysfunction has moved on from disc position and disc shape to biochemical processes involved within the TMJ itself. Today there exists overwhelming evidence that internal joint derangement and abnormal disc position is not the cause but the end result of changes in joint biochemistry.[3] Biochemical changes in the TMJ occur as a response to joint overloading, due to chronic clenching and grinding as well as immobilization. These biochemical changes include elevation in inflammatory mediators[3] resulting in morphologic changes in the tissues including the synovial inflammation and cartilage degradation, which then result in altered biomechanics and impaired joint mobility.[3] Inflamed synovial tissues then lead to alteration of the lubricating properties of the synovial fluid. Therefore a vicious cycle takes place in the joint, which feeds on itself. Constant overloading of the joint (due to bruxism) then leads to biochemical changes in the synovial fluid and painful inflammation, which then causes adhesions and immobilization of the joint, further leading to altered joint tissue responses. The chronic clenching will also possibly lead to muscle inflammation and spasm, which will further exacerbate the TMJ problem by causing and joint immobilization, impeding the joint healing process.

The principles currently recommended in the management and treatment of TMDs is based on our understanding of the pathogenesis of TMJ and MPD.

PRINCIPLES OF NONSURGICAL MANAGEMENT OF TMD

Nonsurgical therapeutic interventions are a necessary part of the treatment of common TMJ conditions, and represent the initial management interventions by clinicians (**Box 2**). These treatment modalities are effective for the common TMJ disorders (synovitis, osteoarthritis, adhesions, displaced disc, acute closed lock) as well as the common muscle disorders seen in TMD (myalgia, myospasm, tendonitis).

The treating general dentist or oral surgeon must be able to examine and diagnose the patient's primary problem. Is the pain or problem coming from the patient's musculature, or is the cause emanating from the pathologic changes (inflammation and degeneration) of the intra-articular tissues, or is it a combination of both?

Box 2
Management of acute TMD

1. Soft diet
2. Behavior modification (ie, reduce stress levels, develop exercise program, nutritional eating, increase sleep times)
3. Muscle relaxants
4. NSAIDs
5. Interocclusal splint
6. Moist heat
7. Muscle trigger-point injections
8. Ultrasound massage/cool spray and stretch therapy for relief of trismus
9. Botox injections

Recognizing and Treating Masticatory Muscle Disorders

It is important for the clinician to evaluate the relative impact of masticatory muscle disorders on the degree of orofacial pain. Masticatory muscle spasm is common in patients with orofacial pain and represents a natural response to immobilize injured tissues. Patients who have severe pain from intra-articular TMJ pathologic conditions will often have significant masticatory muscle spasm and myalgia (muscle pain). Because joint overload from a parafunctional masticatory activity is a common factor leading to joint inflammation and pathologic conditions, it is often difficult for the clinician to determine whether the main pathologic condition is intra-articular, with secondary masticatory muscle spasm, or if the main pathologic condition is masticatory muscle spasm and myalgia, with secondary joint inflammation.

Although there are some patients who clearly have primary joint or muscle joint pathologic conditions, these individuals are relatively rare. Most patients have both muscle and joint components that contribute significantly to their orofacial pain. In this scenario, when the clinician is unsure of relative contributions of joint and muscle pathologic conditions to the overall pain condition, it is helpful to treat the muscle component of the pain with muscle relaxants and muscle-trigger injections to address the masticatory myalgia component of the pain. If the myalgia component improves with persistent intra-articular pain then the clinical picture becomes clearer, with the focus being shifted to treating the intra-articular pathologic condition. Unfortunately, there are many patients in whom the intra-articular pathologic conditions and myalgia components are so severe that it is difficult if not impossible to determine the relative contributions of each to the overall orofacial pain condition. These patients are quite challenging, and often require prolonged treatment to manage both the masticatory myalgia and the intra-articular pathologic condition.

Reduction of Joint Loading

Because chronic joint overload leads to cartilage degradation and the production of inflammatory components, the clinician must be aware of parafunctional masticatory activities and control their deleterious effects. Furthermore, a synovial joint that is undergoing osteoarthritic and inflammatory changes requires a reduction in joint loading to give the tissues a chance to recover and repair. A soft no-chew diet for a specified period of time is necessary. Unfortunately, many patients adhere to this regimen for too short a period of time, and as soon as the symptoms subside they immediately return to a diet that their joint tissues cannot tolerate, contributing to a relapse of symptoms.

Education of patients on the deleterious effects of clenching and making them aware of episodes whereby their teeth come together during times of stress are important. It is common for individuals to spend hours in front of the computer, studying for examinations, or enduring job stress while unaware of their teeth being in a clenched position. Simply making patients aware of times when they are susceptible to clenching will often help them reduce this deleterious habit. Occlusal splint appliances that distribute the forces equally between the maxillary and mandibular teeth can be used at night to reduce the deleterious effects of clenching and bruxism. These appliances can also be used during the daytime hours, usually in nonsocial settings, to help reduce joint overloading. The clinician must carefully evaluate the patient's response to these appliances because there are some individuals who tend to clench more when there is an appliance in their mouth.

There are a variety of splints recommended and written about in the literature that are available for use. The "stabilization" type covers all the teeth of either the mandible or maxilla, and is balanced so that all teeth are in occlusion when the patient closes. It is a flat plane and can be soft or hard. There are also those proponents of "repositioning" splints, which are made of hand acrylic and attempt to alter the occlusion by guiding the jaw to a predetermined position in an attempt to recapture the disc. Studies have shown that this is often not the case,[12] and such splints are not recommended by the author.

Improving Sleep

Obtaining adequate, uninterrupted sleep is very important in the management of patients suffering from TMD. Sleep is necessary for joints and muscles to undergo a period of physiologic rest, recovery, and repair. Individuals who have difficulty falling asleep or who have interrupted sleep are much less likely to have the ability to reduce joint loading and permit the natural process of joint repair. In addition, the increased muscle activity without a period of physiologic rest makes individuals more prone to masticatory myospasm and myalgia.

The clinician should consider prescribing a muscle relaxant before bedtime to assist in sleep and reduce muscle activity. Benzodiazepines at a dose adequate to promote sleep are often beneficial in the management of these patients. Because most muscle relaxants cause some degree of sedation, these are usually avoided during the daytime hours.

Pharmacotherapy

The one drug class that is central to the treatment of TMDs is the NSAID group (**Box 3**). Inflammation of synovial tissues must be controlled for the TMJ to recover normal joint function. NSAIDs should be prescribed for a minimum of 14 days, though the author often starts with at least 30 days recommended in patients who have a long history of TMD prior to seeking relief. NSAIDs are prescribed both for their analgesic and anti-inflammatory properties (see **Box 3**). Careful monitoring for side effects, usually gastrointestinal must be undertaken. Patients with altered kidney or liver function should be monitored carefully and often NSAID's should not be used in those cases.

NSAIDs act by preventing the binding of arachidonic acid to cyclooxygenase enzyme.

Box 3
Commonly used NSAIDs in treatment of TMD

Most Commonly Used Medication (NSAIDs)		
	Brand Name	Dosage
Diclofenac	Voltaren	50 mg-3x/day
Diflunisal	Dolobid	250 mg-2x/day
Etodolac	Utradol	300 mg-2x/day
Fenoprofen	Nalfon, Naprofen	200-600 mg-3-4x/day
Flurbiprofen (Systemic)	Ansaid	100 mg-2x/day
Ibuprofen	Motrin, Advil	600 mg-3x/day
Indomethacin	Indocin	25 mg-3x/day
Ketoprofen	Orudis	50 mg-3x/day
Ketorolac	Toradol	10 mg-4xday (po)
Meclofenamate	Meclomen	50 mg-4x/day
Mefenamic Acid	Ponstel	250 mg-4x/day
Nabumetone	Relafen	1 g-4x/day
Naproxen	Aleve	250-500 mg-q12hr(po)
Oxaprozin	Daypro	600 mg
Piroxicam	Feldene	20 mg-4x/day
Sulindac	Clinoril	150 mg-2x/day
Tolmetin	Tolectin	200-600 mg-3x/day

Muscle Relaxants

Muscle relaxants have been used for many years in the treatment of TMDs.[13] Of course they have no effect on disc position and joint inflammation, and function only to reduce the muscle spasms caused by the hyperactivity of the masticatory musculature. There are many such muscle relaxants (**Table 1**) available; the author most often prescribes cyclobenzaprine (Flexeril), 5 to 10 mg twice a day to 3 times a day.

Botox

A relatively new method recently approved by the Food and Drug Administration is the use of botulinum toxin A (Botox) for the use of muscle relaxation in the treatment of TMD.[14] Botox functions by inhibiting the release of acetylcholine, which decreases

Table 1
Muscle relaxants

Drug	Dosage
1. Chlorzoxazone (Parafon Forte)	250–500 mg 3 times daily Poorly tolerated in elderly

2. Cyclobenzaprine (Flexeril)
   Do not use with monoamine oxidase
   inhibitors
	10 mg at bedtime initially; 10 mg 3 times
	daily (usual adult dosage); do not use
	longer than 2–3 weeks

3. Methocarbamol (Robaxin)	1500 mg four times daily for 2-3 days then decreased to 1000 mg 3 times daily
4. Orphenadrine (Norflex)	100 mg 2 times daily

Like all medications these drugs have possible adverse effects, so prescribing doctors must be familiar with all information.

the transmission after neural stimulus to the muscles. Administration of Botox is directly into the muscles of mastication. Botox should only be considered in those patients who get some level of relief from trigger point injections of local anesthetics into the masticatory muscles.

Antidepressants/Minor Tranquilizers

Low doses of (10–50 mg) of tricyclic antidepressants such as amitriptyline have been shown to be effective in treating chronic pain related to TMD/TMJ disorders **(Table 2)**.[15] When given at these low doses these drugs fail to reach their therapeutic levels to achieve any significant antidepressant effect, but do have analgesic properties at these low levels.

Disc Displacement

As discussed earlier, it was previously postulated that the temporomandibular disc displacement was in itself a pathologic condition, and directly responsible for TMD/TMJ pain and dysfunction. Once such a diagnosis was made, by either clinical or radiologic studies; internal joint disc repositioning surgery was then advised to definitively treat the patient's problem. This surgical approach is no longer considered to be acceptable, as many studies have shown that 30% to 50% of populations have reducing discs and clicks.[16]

Most of these patients with TMJ clicks have no history of TMJ pain or dysfunction. Clinical studies reporting on long-term follow-up of patients with disc displacement show the vast majority to be asymptomatic 30 years later.[16] However, if the patient does have an persistent pain and limitation of function due to intra-articular pathology (synovitis/osteoarthritis), it can and should be addressed.

PRINCIPLES OF SURGICAL MANAGEMENT OF TMJ DISORDERS

The indications for performing TMJ surgery in the patient population are as follows:

1. The patient has severe TMJ pain and mandibular dysfunction
2. The cause of the pain and or mandibular dysfunction is attributable to a diagnosis consistent with a significant intra-articular pathologic condition (synovitis, osteoarthritis, adhesions) leading to disc displacement
3. A full course of nonsurgical therapy has failed to improve the patient's symptoms

The surgical options that are available to treat the more common TMJ disorders are arthrocentesis, arthroscopy, and open joint surgery when indicated.

Table 2
Tranquilizer/anxiolytics medications

Drug	Dosage
Common Minor Tranquilizers	
Alprazolam (Xanax)	0.25–0.5 mg 3 times daily; maximum dosage 4 mg/d
Diazepam (Valium)	2–10 mg 2–4 times daily
Lorazepam (Ativan)	1–2 mg 2 times daily
Tricyclic Antidepresssants	
Amitriptyline (Elavil)	10–50 mg at bedtime: start at low dose and increase slowly
Tofranil (Imipramine)	10–50 mg at bedtime: start at low dose and increase slowly

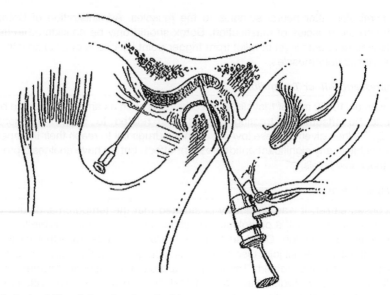

Fig. 2. Lysis of fibrotic bands using the blunt trocar in sweeping movements from anterior to posterior. (*From* Fonseca RJ, Marciani RD, Turvey TA. Oral and maxillofacial surgery. 2nd edition. Trauma, surgical pathology, temporomandibular disorders, vol. 2. Saunders, Elsevier; 2009; with permission.)

Arthrocentesis, Arthroscopy, Open Joint Surgery

Arthrocentesis is the insertion of usually two needles into the superior TMJ space followed by irrigation of the space with copious saline solution (**Fig. 2**). It has been reported to be highly successful for the treatment of TMJ synovitis (**Box 4**) and limited opening due to an anterior displaced disc without reduction, as found in the closed-lock patient.[17] Caravaja and Laskin[18] reported an 88% success rate for their patients who underwent arthrocentesis. These investigators state that arthrocentesis can reduce pain and dysfunction in patients with anterior disc displacement over both the long and short term.

Box 4
Management of internal joint derangement (synovitis, capsulitis)

1. NSAIDs
2. Muscle relaxants
3. Soft diet
4. Moist heat compress
5. Interocclusal splint
6. Behavior modification
7. Arthrocentesis
8. Arthroscopy
9. Open joint surgery

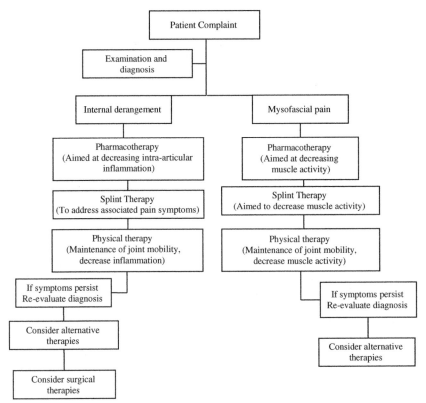

Fig. 3. Nonsurgical treatment algorithm of TMJ disorders. (*From* Fonseca RJ, Marciani RD, Turvey TA. Oral and maxillofacial surgery. 2nd edition. Trauma, surgical pathology, tempo- romandibular disorders, vol. 2. Saunders, Elsevier; 2009; with permission.)

The objective of arthrocentesis is to wash out the inflammatory mediators respon- sible for inflammation in the joint. It is also thought that irrigation and lavage under high pressures can also potentially remove adhesions to improve joint mobility.[19] Arthroscopy can now be performed with extremely small-diameter endoscopes, allowing for direct visualization and diagnosis as well. Arthroscopic therapy is mini- mally invasive and permits direct removal and treatment of pathologic intra-articular tissues with proper patient selection, the success rate for arthroscopy that this author has seen in 85–90%. Open joint surgical procedures are also an option for the treat- ment of intra-articular joint pathology, but they should be used only if there is pathology that is obliterating the joint space and the previously mentioned procedures prove ineffective. The type of open joint surgery to be performed is decided by the clinician, with numerous surgical options currently available, from alloplastic TMJ reconstruction to autogenous reconstruction.

SUMMARY

General dentists will, over the course of their career, see may patients who seek their help in treating facial pain of nondental origin. Knowledge of the diagnosis and management of MPD and TMJ disorder (**Fig. 3**) is essential in order for the treating doctor to offer the necessary help and assistance for this most common ailment.

Most patients will achieve significant reduction in symptoms if offered the treatment regimens discussed in this article. In fact Okeson[20] found in a review of multiple studies a 70% to 90% success rate in the nonsurgical treatment of TMJ disorders.

If patients fail to improve sufficiently, referral to an oral maxillofacial surgeon for consideration of minimally invasive techniques. The least invasive procedure with the maximum potential, such as arthrocentesis should be the surgical treatment of choice.

REFERENCES

1. Heir GM. Assessing temporomandibular disorders. In: Fonseca RJ, Marciani RD, Turvey TA, editors. Oral and maxillofacial surgery, vol. 2. 2nd edition. St Louis (MO): Elsevier; 2009. p. 815.
2. Israel HA. The essential role of the oral and maxillofacial surgeon in the diagnosis, management, causation and prevention of chronic orofacial pain: clinical perspectives. In: Fonseca RJ, Marciani RD, Turvey TA, editors. Oral and maxillofacial surgery, vol. 1. St Louis (MO): Saunders, Elsevier; 2009. p. 126.
3. Lipton JA, Ship JA, Larach-Robinson D. Estimated prevalence and distribution of reported orofacial pain in the United States. J Am Dent Assoc 1993;129:115–21.
4. Honey OB, Scarfe WC, Hilgers MJ, et al. Accuracy of cone-beam computerized tomography imaging of the TM joint: comparisons with panoramic radiology and linear tomography. Am J Orthod Dentofacial Orthop 2007;132(4):429–38.
5. Westesson PL, Yamamoto M, Sano T. Temporomandibular joint. In: Som PM, Curtain HD, editors. Head and neck imaging. 4th edition. Philadelphia: Mosby; 2002.
6. Annandale T. Displacement of the inter-articular cartilage of the lower jaw and its treatment by operation. Lancet 1887;8:411.
7. Costen JB. Neuralgias and ear symptoms associated with disturbed function of the TM joint. J Am Dent Assoc 1936;107:252–8.
8. Schwartz LL. Ethyl chloride treatment of limited painful mandibular movement. J Am Dent Assoc 1954;48:497–507.
9. Dolwick MF, Reid R, Sanders B, et al. 1984 Criteria for TMJ meniscus surgery. Chicago: American Association of Oral and Maxillofacial Surgeons; 1984. p. 30.
10. Nitzan DW, Dolwick MF, Heft MW. Arthroscopic lavage and lysis of the TM Joint: a change in perspective. J Oral Maxillofac Surg 1990;48:798–811.
11. Nitzan DW. Friction and adhesive forces- possible underlying causes for TM joint derangement. Cells Tissues Organs 2003;174:6–16.
12. Simmons HC III, Gibbs SJ. Anterior repositioning appliance therapy for TMJ disorders: specific symptoms relieved and relationship to disk status on MRI. Cranio 2005;23(2):89–99.
13. Indresano TA, Acplia CX. Non-surgical management of temporomandibular disorders. In: Fonseca RJ, Marciani RD, Turvey TA, editors. 2nd edition, Oral and maxillofacial surgery, vol. 2. St Louis (MO): Elsevier; 2009. p. 887.
14. Schwartz M, Freund B. Treatment of temporomandibular disorders with botulinum toxin. Clin J Pain 2002;18(Suppl 6):S196–203.
15. Sharav Y, Singer E, Schmidt E, et al. The analgesic effect of amitriptyline on chronic facial pain. Pain 1987;31(2):199–209.
16. Goddard G. Temporomandibular disorders. In: Lalwani A, editor. Current diagnosis and treatment in otolaryngology. Head and neck surgery. New York: Lange Publication; 2009.
17. Brennan PA, Ilankovan V. Arthrocentesis for temporomandibular joint pain dysfunction syndrome. J Oral Maxillofac Surg 2006;64:949–51.

18. Carvaja WA, Laskin DM. Long term evaluation of arthrocentesis for the treatment of internal derangement of the TM joint. J Oral Maxillofac Surg 2000;58:852–5.
19. Ziccardi VB. Arthrocentesis of the temporomandibular joint. Temporomandibular disorders. In: Fonseca RJ, Marciani RD, Turvey TA, editors. Oral and maxillofacial surgery, vol. 2. 2nd edition. St Louis (MO): Elsevier; 2009. p. 912, 48.
20. Okeson J. Management of TMJ disorders and occlusion. 4th edition. St Louis (MO): CV Mosby; 1998.

Preoperative Evaluation of the Surgical Patient

Stephen Petranker, MD, MBA[a],*, Levon Nikoyan, DDS[b],
Orrett E. Ogle, DDS[c]

KEYWORDS

• Preoperative evaluation • Dental anesthesia • Surgical patient

A thorough preoperative evaluation to identify correctable medical abnormalities and understand the residual risk is mandatory for all patients undergoing any surgical procedure, including oral surgery. Routine preoperative evaluation will vary among patients, depending on age and general health. This article addresses the preoperative evaluation of surgical patients in general, and the evaluation for general anesthesia in the operating room.

PART 1

In evaluating a patient for any surgical procedure, surgeons must consider two aspects: (1) the necessary workup that must be performed for the surgical procedure itself, and (2) whether the patient can safely undergo the planed surgical procedure.

In the preoperative evaluation of a patient for oral surgery, regardless of the clinical setting, a good medical history is undoubtedly the most important aspect. A detailed medical history will identify potential management problems (physiologic and pharmaceutical) and allow the dental surgeon to formulate an oral surgical treatment plan in light of the medical status. Patients will present with one or multiple established medical diagnoses, which may alter how dental care is delivered. The role of the dentist is to determine how these medical problems will influence care, or how dental care may affect medical treatment. Medical illness may predispose to acute physiologic decompensation under stress or failure to do well posttreatment, or lead to drug interactions. Dentists must be aware of what potentially can occur and what precautions must be taken to minimize risks. They must identify issues that should

---

[a] Department of Anesthesia, Woodhull Medical and Mental Center, 760 Broadway, Brooklyn, NY 11206, USA
[b] Department of Oral and Maxillofacial Surgery, Woodhull Medical and Mental Center, 760 Broadway, Brooklyn, NY 11206, USA
[c] Oral and Maxillofacial Surgery, Department of Dentistry, Woodhull Medical and Mental Health Center, 760 Broadway, Brooklyn, NY 11206, USA
* Corresponding author.
E-mail address: Stephan.Petranker@woodhullhc.nychhc.org

Dent Clin N Am 56 (2012) 163–181
doi:10.1016/j.cden.2011.06.003
0011-8532/12/$ – see front matter © 2012 Elsevier Inc. All rights reserved.

dental.theclinics.com

addressed pretreatment (eg, insulin, warfarin, aspirin use), such as illnesses that may cause physiologic decompensation during surgery (eg, angina, seizure disorders, asthma) and conditions that may affect the posttreatment phase (eg, diabetes [infection and delayed wound healing], aspirin use [impaired hemostasis]) (**Tables 1** and **2**).

Review of the dental history should reveal the patient's reason for seeking oral surgery, because the procedure will be irreversible. The patient's previous experience with oral surgery should also be determined because this will aid in the decision to use sedation and in determining how to manage postoperative pain. Surgeons should get to know the patient; the old adage "never treat a stranger" should be applied to the normal preoperative evaluation.

The preoperative evaluation for oral surgery will almost always require imaging studies for proper diagnosis and treatment planning. A panographic radiograph is the gold standard, because it will show the entire dentition of both jaws and adjacent structures, and will permit early and accurate identification of dental aberrations and disease. Other radiographs that could be needed are periapical films for endodontic surgery or to provide greater clarity of detail; localizing films for issues such as impacted canines; and cone beam CT three-dimensional radiographic imaging for implantology or pathology cases.

The initial evaluation should help the general dentist decide on the complexity of the procedure and whether the case should be referred to an oral and maxillofacial surgeon. Both the clinical and radiographic examinations should inform the operator if a tooth extraction will be possible through simple forceps delivery, whether the tooth should be sectioned for ease of removal, or whether a surgical flap is necessary.

PART 2
Preoperative Anesthesia Evaluation

Preoperative evaluation is the foundation for maximizing the chances of the desired outcome, from both the surgical and anesthesia perspectives, because during this process risks are identified and mitigated, and a plan is developed that best balances the risks, benefits, and alternatives available. The products of preoperative evaluation process are diminished patient anxiety and accomplishment of the first steps of risk mitigation and the essential first phase of the informed consent process. Ultimately, the sum of the work product leads to a plan that encompasses the pre-, intra-, and postoperative periods, and establishes the pain management plan and where the patient will go after surgery.

As seen in **Fig. 1**, the preoperative evaluation is a truly iterative process. As information is gathered and decisions made in one aspect of the evaluation, upstream and downstream elements may change, and may require starting over from the beginning, until the full picture is elucidated. The preoperative evaluation is a highly dynamic process, requiring frequent thoughtful pauses and reconsiderations as information is gathered and the needs of the patient and surgeon and the abilities of the organization are considered in the development of a perfect plan.

The Perfect Plan

The perfect plan is one that melds the patient's needs, the care team's capabilities (knowledge, experience), and the ability of the organization to support (bits, pieces) the contemplated procedure. For completeness sake, the perfect procedure is the one that maximizes the patient's desired outcome. Occasionally the perfect procedure is so far from what is being offered that no procedure at all should be performed, and other times a procedure should be performed elsewhere. The patient and care team must collaboratively decide how close to perfection is acceptable, when perfection itself is elusive. During the preoperative evaluation process is when this "go/no go" decision must be made.

Elements of an anesthesiologist history and physical

Each member of the clinical care team must perform an evaluation. Unquestionably, each member can use the information obtained by another, and independently verify the information as needed. The team must acknowledge that each specialty has its own perspective, albeit overlapping, to bring to the evaluation table. For example, the surgeon may consider gender from the point of view of disease prevalence and function, the nurse from the vantage point of social issues, and the anesthesiologist may be thinking about the need for a pregnancy test. Each specialty has its own anxiety points that must be addressed during the evaluation period, and therefore each specialty must, in some measure, perform its own assessment. **Table 3** lists some of the common historical questions that most practitioners explore, and how an anesthesiologist would consider the information.

Similarly, the unique point of view each specialty brings to the evaluation of historical data is what is brought to the physical examination. Physicians are taught early on that pertinent positive and negative findings are the drivers of not only the history but also the physical examination. The anesthesiologist's point of pride is the airway examination, with a focus on trying to discern whether difficulty will be encountered on ventilating or intubating the patient. No one best airway examination component exists; rather, the anesthesiologist must integrate the totality of the examination to reach a conclusion.[8] One commonly adopted algorithm of airway evaluation is the LEMON approach (**Fig. 2**).[9]

The Mallampati classification (**Fig. 3**), which relates tongue size to pharyngeal size, is a common component of a thorough airway examination. The examination is performed with the patient in the sitting position, the head held in a neutral position, the mouth wide open, and the tongue protruding to the maximum. The subsequent classification is assigned according to the pharyngeal structures that are visible:

Class I: visualization of the soft palate, fauces, uvula, and anterior and posterior pillars
Class II: visualization of the soft palate, fauces, and uvula
Class III: visualization of the soft palate and the base of the uvula
Class IV: soft palate not visible at all.[10]

The anatomic considerations in determining whether the patient can be intubated revolve around mouth-opening ability, relative sizes of the oral structures, and the ability of the mobile parts of the airway axes to align in a "sword swallower" sniffing position. Although the Mallampati classification evaluates soft tissue sizes and relationships, along with mouth opening, 13 other examination features should also be considered as part of the airway evaluation, as listed in **Box 1**.

Other particular parts of the physical examination, beyond the basic heart and lung examination, are directed by the contemplated surgery and anesthetic technique, along with the patient's presentation. For example, a patient undergoing a carotid endarterectomy would require a more concerted neurologic examination. The fine art of history and physical examination must embrace documenting the pertinent positive and negative findings after integrating large quantities of information from the surgeon, patient, and other sources.

The history and physical examination work product

The history and physical examination contribute to several follow-on activities, such as ordering consultations and laboratory investigations, along with the initial steps in risk

Table 1
Diagnoses and suggestions for preoperative assessment

Disease	Suggested Preoperative Evaluation
Allergies	Allergies to drugs or latex should be determined
Asthma	Emotional factors may trigger an attack Evaluate wheezing and do not treat if patient is wheezing Have rescue inhaler available Do not prescribe nonsteroidal anti-inflammatory drugs or aspirin for pain if the patient has aspirin-induced asthma
Cerebral vascular disease	Evaluate blood pressure No elective oral surgery within 6 months of the cerebrovascular accident Patients who have had a stroke are usually on anticoagulation therapy; if so, review method and obtain satisfactory recent International Normalized Ratio (INR) from physician
Chronic obstructive pulmonary disease	Only the most severe respiratory compromise is a contraindication to routine outpatient dental/oral and maxillofacial surgical care with local anesthesia Determine the patient's functional capacity (eg, able to walk a block or two on level ground at 2 to 3 miles per hour [mph]; climb a flight of stairs [five metabolic equivalent tasks]) Plan on not performing long or extensive surgical procedures and do not administer 100% oxygen if the patient is suspected to be on carbon dioxide drive
Coagulopathy	Consult hematologist for individuals with definitively diagnosed coagulopathies In the absence of a history of bleeding diathesis, abnormal bleeding following exodontia is rare Prothrombin time or partial thromboplastin time is not indicated
Coronary artery disease	Stratify patients based on symptoms and exercise capacity according to history Determine the patient's functional capacity (eg, able to walk a block or two on level ground at 2 to 3 mph, climb a flight of stairs, do light house work) Patients who can perform these functions are at low risk for cardiac decompensation during oral surgery (see **Table 2**)
Diabetes mellitus	Diabetes is only associated with higher perioperative risks in vascular surgery and coronary artery bypass grafting Patients with well-controlled diabetes pose no problem Review symptoms such as excessive thirst, nocturia, malaise, and hunger to assess control
Epilepsy	Patients with well-controlled epilepsy are no different from average patients Review compliance with therapy

Hypertension	• Stage 1: 140–159/80–99 • Stage 2: 160–179/100–109 • Stage 3: >180/>110 • Stage 1: minimal risk • Stage 2 and 3: delay nonemergency treatment until pressure can be controlled, attempting to decrease risk to stage 1 and 2 levels, respectively • Stage 2: moderate risk of cardiac complication; emergency procedures only; infections • Stage 3: high risk of cardiac complication
Liver disease	Screen for hepatitis B and C Patients being treated with Interferon for hepatitis C virus will be anemic and easily fatigued, and platelets may also be low Chronic severe liver disease may increase INR Check history of ethanol use
Medication	Medication history will provide information on what conditions the patient is being treated and how severe the condition may be Avoid drug interactions
Outpatient treatment with warfarin	Check current INR with treating physician Values of the INR at the therapeutic dose <3.5 does not significantly influence the incidence of postoperative bleeding[1–3] Dental extractions can be performed without modification of oral anticoagulant treatment INR of up to 3.4 is acceptable for extraction of up to three teeth Local hemostasis with gelatin sponge and sutures seems to be sufficient to prevent postoperative bleeding[4]
Renal insufficiency	Consult with nephrologist if patient history is inadequate Compensated renal disease is not a contraindication to office oral surgery and simple extraction of teeth in the office under local anesthesia is not generally a problem For patients undergoing dialysis: perform oral surgery on nondialysis day to avoid problems with anticoagulation In emergency: treat patient more than 4 hours after dialysis; do not use penicillin with potassium (Pen VK) because K^+ is difficult to eliminate through dialysis and may cause electrocardiogram changes

Table 2
Cardiac stratification

Major Heart Diseases to be Treated in Hospital Setting	Heart Diseases That May be Treated in Office Setting
Myocardial infarction within 6 month; delay surgery if possible; consult with cardiologist	Previous myocardial infarction (more than 6 months prior); determine the patient's functional capacity.
Unstable or severe angina (class III or IV)	Mild angina pectoris (class I or II)
Decompensated heart failure (class III or IV; ejection fraction <30%)	Compensated or prior heart failure (class I or II)
Significant arrhythmias	Low functional capacity (eg, inability to walk three city blocks)

mitigation, anesthesia plan development, and the informed consent process. As areas of concern become unmasked, more tests or consultations and different approaches to mitigating the risks may become necessary. As the evaluation telephoto lens is brought from near to far, and back again, changes in the anesthesia plan and consent must be kept in mind.

Consultations are necessary when questions remain that are beyond the evaluating physician's knowledge base. The basic questions that are asked of the consultant are (1) is the patient in optimal condition, (2) does the patient have reversible disease, and (3) where is the patient in the continuum of disease. Simply sending a request to a consultant to clear a patient for surgery is likely to yield an equally noninformative response of "patient cleared," and must be avoided. The consultant is a key member of the preoperative evaluation team. Referral patterns are frequently in place with consultants who are sensitive to preoperative evaluation needs; this type of network should be encouraged. Basic required tests can be ordered in advance of the consultant appointment, such as an echocardiogram, before the internist or cardiologist sees a patient with known heart disease. The need for quality communication cannot be overstated, especially with consultant interactions. Calling the consultant before sending the patient over for evaluation can speed the preparation process tremendously, with the invested time yielding substantially greater insight when the final report comes back. The request to the consultant should include the three basic questions mentioned earlier, laying the groundwork for answers.

Laboratory guidelines

A few considerations must be addressed before a laboratory investigation is ordered, and which routine tests, other than pregnancy testing, should be avoided must be determined. First, the physician should determine whether the laboratory results will make a difference in treatment. If the results of the laboratory investigation will make no difference, then it should not be performed. Second, whether the disease is prevalent in the patient population should be determined, and then the laboratory investigation may be considered a screening tool, such as an echocardiogram in the elderly to screen for ischemic heart disease.[11–13] Otherwise, laboratory investigations should answer the same basic questions for which consultations are sought: (1) is the patient in optimal condition, (2) does the patient have reversible disease, and (3) where is the patient in the continuum of disease. An example of this approach is to order a pre- and post-bronchodilator pulmonary function test for a patient with asthma. **Fig. 4** highlights a suggested rational thought process in ordering laboratory tests, and **Fig. 5** highlights supporting information.

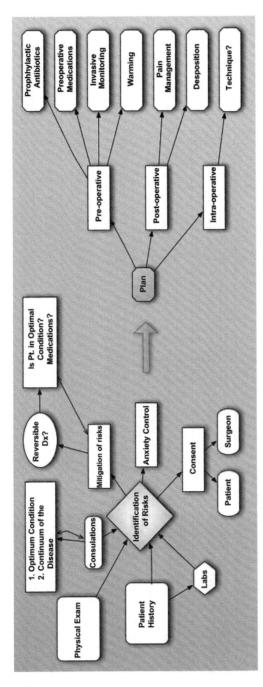

Fig. 1. Preoperative evaluation.

Table 3
Common history considerations with representative anesthesiologist concerns

Historical Area	Anesthesia Import
Proposed procedure	Patient positioning, possible anesthetic techniques, fluid shifts, blood loss, invasive monitoring, prophylactic antibiotic requirement
Past medical history	Possibility of recrudescence, psychological (anxiety) impact, lingering physical impact
Concurrent medical history	End-organ damage, where the patient is in the continuum of disease, whether the patient is in optimal condition, whether the disease processes be reversed, need for full stomach prophylaxis, need for prophylactic beta-blockade
Medications	Indication of disease severity, drug interactions
Surgical history	Psychological impact, increased complexity if returning to the same area, disease severity, difficult airway previously, history of postoperative complications, such as nausea and vomiting or delayed awakening
Family history	Malignant hyperthermia and other genetic disorders
Gender	Proper approach, pregnancy testing, increased sensitivity to nausea and vomiting postoperatively
Age	Pharmacokinetic and dynamic impact, patient interaction/communication, different equipment/skills for pediatric age group, associated ischemia risks
Smoking	Carboxyhemoglobin level, reactive airway disease, postoperative intubation increased, pulmonary disease, diminished postoperative nausea and vomiting[5–7]
Sleep apnea	Need for postoperative respiratory monitoring until narcotics are no longer needed, increased intubation risks, associated cardiovascular disease
Height and Weight	Obesity is linked to full stomach risks, and the need to base most medication dosing on lean body weight, with airway and pulmonary issues Body positioning and equipment consideration go along with morbid obesity In patients with markedly low body mass index, the pharmacokinetic impact of low protein state must be considered

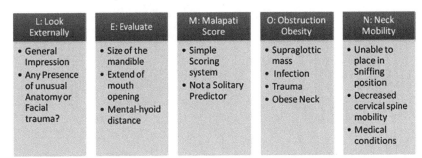

Fig. 2. LEMON approach. (*Data from* Emergency airway management. 3rd edition; *From* Monson J, Weiser M. Sabiston textbook of surgery: the biological basis of modern surgical practice. 18th edition. 2007. p. 1154.)

The marriage of patient- and surgery-specific risks

When the history, physical, consultations, and laboratory tests are completed, the patient-specific risks should be clear, and the surgery-specific risks must now be considered, which together will yield total patient risk. Fluid shifts, blood loss, and surgical site are part of the surgical contribution to the total risk palate. Intrathoracic, cardiac, major intra-abdominal, major vascular, and long bone procedures, and those that are likely to result in 20% blood loss (typical adult, 1000 mL), are all considered to present a major surgical risk (**Fig. 6**).[14]

Total patient risk is determined by patient-specific risk combined with surgical risk. Anesthesia-specific risk is negligible, because it is low in modern practice.[15–17] The first key element of the preoperative evolution is completed once total patient risk is identified and quantified, and then practitioners can proceed to the second element, risk mitigation.

Risk Mitigation

Risk mitigation strategies must be considered and a balance found between the risks and benefits of performing an oral procedure. Alternative approaches and when it is appropriate to perform no intervention should also be considered. The first step in risk mitigation is to ensure that the patient is in as good condition as possible. Disease that can be reversed should be, and the forthcoming surgical and anesthesia procedures that are now being considered must take the patient-specific issues into consideration, always ensuring that the risk/benefit ratio stays in the patient's favor. For example, in a smoker who is a high-risk patient,[18] risk mitigation involving smoking cessation and allowing time for the body to recalibrate to the new state would reduce the risk to almost the same as the general population.[18–22] Medical practice is now effective at getting patients in optimum condition for surgery. Three areas of risk mitigation, beyond selection of the anesthetic technique, are frequently missed by the perioperative team: full stomach prophylaxis, beta-blockade with superior pain management, and avoidance of postoperative nausea and vomiting.

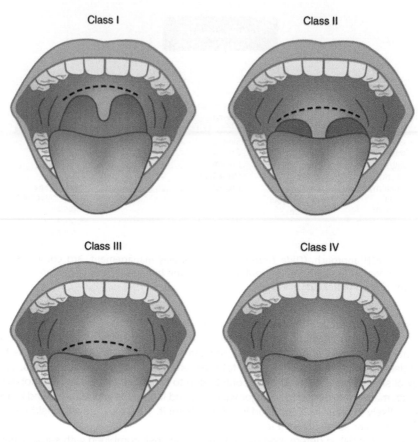

Fig. 3. Mallampati classification. (*From* Townsend CM, Beauchamp RD, Evers BM, editors. Sabiston textbook of surgery, 18th edition. The Biological Basis of Modern Surgical Practice. Philadelphia: WB Saunders, 2007; with permission.)

Full Stomach

A full stomach before surgery is a concern because of the risk of aspiration and the difficulty with intubation if stomach contents are in the posterior pharynx. Once general anesthesia is induced, patients lose their ability to maintain a patent airway and breath and the protective ability to cough. The elements to consider are gastro-esophageal junction tone minus hydrostatic pressure within the stomach, which is equal to barrier pressure. If the barrier pressure is negative, the patient is at high risk for regurgitation or vomiting. Therefore, to ensure a positive barrier pressure, patients are required to fast before surgery in an attempt to lower the hydrostatic pressure. Many articles have been written on what constitutes sufficient time for stomach emptying,[23–25] with modern practice segregating the issues into type of meal and patient age. Based on the body of literature, **Tables 4** and **5** provide somewhat conservative approaches to preoperative fasting. However, these must be regarded as a set of guidelines rather than a firm set of rules.

Practitioners must remember that the data shown in **Tables 4** and **5** pertain to normal patients. Several conditions prevent the nothing by mouth guidelines from providing the margin of safety that practitioners would want. For example, conditions

Box 1
Airway examination and history aspects to consider
Previous complications
Loose teeth or dentures
Buck teeth
Long upper incisors
Cannot prognath
Interincisor distance <3 cm
Nonvisualized uvula
High or arched palate
Thyromental distance <6 cm
Noncompliant submandibular space
Short neck
Thick neck
Not capable of sniffing position
Mallampati classification

that diminish stomach emptying, such as diabetes,[26] morbid obesity[27] (body mass index [BMI] >35, in the authors' organization), pregnancy,[28,29] bowel obstruction, previous upper gastrointestinal surgery, and gastrointestinal disease such as stomach ulcer, along with scleroderma, all increase the risk that a full stomach is present. In addition, patients who are judged to have a difficult airway should also be treated with full stomach prophylaxis, because the time to intubation may be prolonged, exposing them to a longer period with an unprotected airway.[30]

The focus in the preoperative period is to identify patients who are at risk for having a full stomach despite following the nothing by mouth guidelines, and to add a prokinetic and a pH-elevating drug to diminish the caustic nature of untreated gastric acid. The preferred kinetic agent is metoclopramide (Reglan). Caution must be exercised when administering this agent to patients with Parkinson disease, because it may worsen the underlying condition because of its dopaminergic effects. The second agent used is ranitidine (Zantac) to elevate the stomach pH. Some practitioners prefer ranitidine because it does not induce hepatic enzymes like cimetidine (Tagamet), which may affect anesthetic agent metabolism. These two agents should be administered the night before and the morning of surgery. Two doses help ensure that the time needed for agent effectiveness is secured. The third agent, citric acid/sodium citrate (Bicitra), should be administered within 2 hours of surgery. This agent works as a direct buffering material on contact with the low pH stomach acid to help reduce the possibility of chemical pneumonitis if the patient aspirates. Unfortunately, this agent is bitter-tasting, and itself may lead to emesis, and therefore should be administered at least several minutes before the patient enters the operating room.

Beta-Blockade

An organ becomes ischemic when there is a decoupling of oxygen supply versus the demand. Specifically when looking at the heart, as myocardial work diminishes, oxygen demand also diminishes. The critical point at which demand exceeds supply

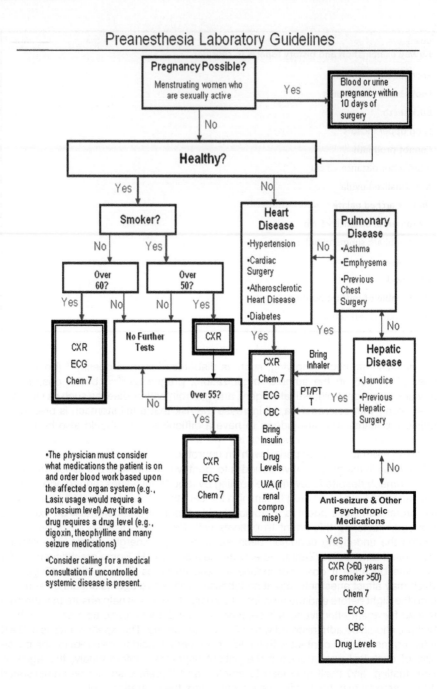

Fig. 4. Preanesthesia laboratory guidelines.

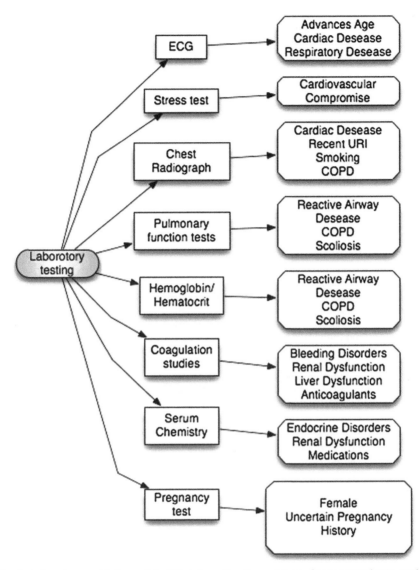

Fig. 5. Laboratory guidelines. (*Modified from* Practice advisory for preanesthesia evaluation: a report by the American Society of Anesthesiologists Task Force on Preanesthesia Evaluation. Anesthesiology 2002;96(2):485–96; with permission.)

is unknown, and therefore the focus of caring for a prone patient with ischemia is to keep the workload low and the supply high. The current state of medicine allows the workload side (demand) of the equation to be addressed more effectively than the supply side. The greatest consumer of myocardial oxygen consumption is tachycardia,[31,32] with increased systemic vascular resistance being second.[33–36] The cornerstone of myocardial protection is beta-blockade (and slow normalization of blood pressure).

Patients at risk for cardiovascular disease (eg, long-standing diabetes, hypertension, elderly, dyslipidemia, smoking, previous myocardial infarction, angina) should

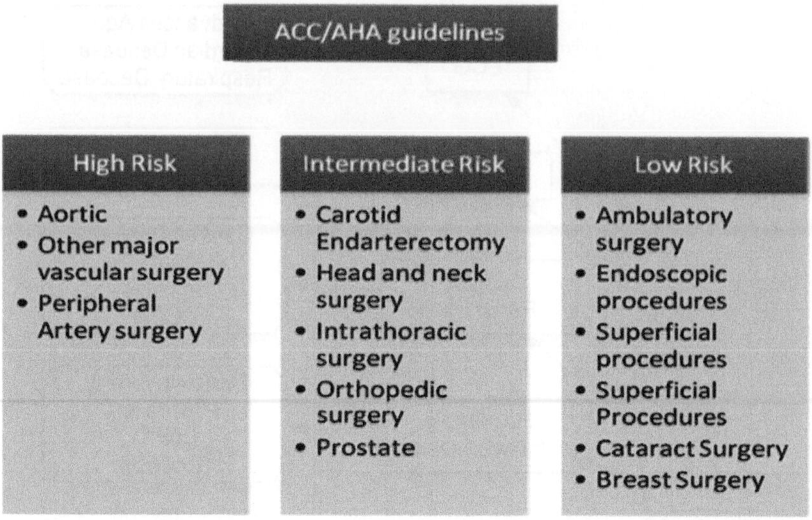

Fig. 6. American College of Cardiology/American Heart Association guidelines. (*Modified from* Fleisher LA, Beckman JA, Brown KA, et al. ACC/AHA 2007 Guidelines on Perioperative Cardiovascular Evaluation and Care for Noncardiac Surgery: executive summary: a report of the American College of Cardiology/American Heart Association Task Force on Practice Guidelines (writing committee to revise the 2002 Guidelines on Perioperative Cardiovascular Evaluation for Noncardiac Surgery): developed in collaboration with the American Society of Echocardiography, American Society of Nuclear Cardiology, Heart Rhythm Society, Society of Cardiovascular Anesthesiologists, Society for Cardiovascular Angiography and Interventions, Society for Vascular Medicine and Biology, and Society for Vascular Surgery. Circulation 2007;116(17):1971–96; with permission.)

be evaluated by an internal medicine specialist for disease, and managed medically. Reversible disease should be addressed before surgery. According to the American College of Cardiology, patients with two or more risk factors, or the presence of a major factor such as previous myocardial infarction, should be treated with beta-blockade if undergoing major surgery. Asking the consultant to specifically evaluate the patient for

Table 4 Adult nothing by mouth guidelines[a]	
Ingested Material	**Minimum Fasting Time (h)**
Clear liquids	2
Breast milk	4
Infant formula	6
Nonhuman milk	6
Light meal	6

Clear liquid examples include water, fruit juices without pulp, clear tea, and black coffee. With nonhuman milk, similar to solids, consider the amount ingested when making a decision. Light meal consists of toast and clear liquids. Fatty foods considerably delay gastric emptying time.

[a] Presumes normal stomach emptying.

Data from American Society of Anesthesiologists Committee. Practice guidelines for preoperative fasting and the use of pharmacologic agents to reduce the risk of pulmonary aspiration: application to healthy patients undergoing elective procedures: an updated report by the American Society of Anesthesiologists Committee on Standards and Practice Parameters. Anesthesiology 2011;114(3):495–511.

Table 5		
Pediatric nothing by mouth guidelines[a]		
<6 mo	No milk or solids 4 h before procedure	[b]No clear liquids 2 h before procedure
6 mo to 3 y	No milk or solids 6 h before procedure	No clear liquids 3 h before procedure
>3 y	No milk or solids 8 h before procedure	

Consider H_2 antagonists (ranitidine), nonparticulate antacids, and gastric motility agents (eg, metoclopramide) for patients at risk for aspiration because of delayed gastric emptying.

[a] Presumes normal stomach emptying.

[b] Consider intravenous hydration if procedure is delayed more than 2 hours.

Data from Ingebo KR, Rayhorn NJ, Hecht RM, et al. Sedation in children: adequacy of two-hour fasting. J Pediatr 1997;131(1 Pt 1):155–8.

the need for beta-blockade is a legitimate request. A typical approach to beta-blockade is metoprolol (Lopressor) titrated to a resting heart rate of 60 to 65 beats per minute (bpm), and maintenance of the heart rate during surgery at no greater than 85 bpm by the anesthesia team. Clearly, beta-blockade should be started well in advance of the contemplated surgery to allow enough time for the medication to be titrated and side effects to be addressed. Under urgent circumstances, beta-blockade can be undertaken on the day of surgery. Beta-blockade is associated with increased incidence of stroke,[37,38] which is an area of research to better refine who would benefit most from therapy.

Tachycardia is the largest consumer of myocardial oxygen. Therefore, postoperative pain management must be considered in the preoperative period, because uncontrolled pain leads to tachycardia and hypertension, probably contributing to preoperative myocardial infarction being particularly elevated up to 72 hours postoperatively.[39–41] Nerve blocks are a highly effective method of analgesia, but also have associated risks and potential to cause discomfort from numbness. The risks, benefits, and alternatives of nerve blocks should be discussed with the patient preoperatively to determine the best course of action. Patient-controlled analgesia is available in the hospital setting for when nerve blocks recede. Practitioners must be careful to select the agent with the desired concentration and duration of action among the various local anesthetics. Mixing of local anesthetic agents should be avoided. One approach to minimizing tachycardia associated with pain is to give a preoperative block, and then reinforce it at the end of the procedure.

The final step in patient assessment is to assign an American Society of Anesthesiologists (ASA) physical status classification (**Table 6**) to inform the anesthesia and surgical teams of the degree of risk the patient's physical aliments constitute; a "worry" meter of sorts. Practitioners must be mindful that patients are classed without regard for the surgical risks, and therefore the patient may be healthy (ASA I) when undergoing an extraordinarily high-risk surgery. Although ASA I is clearly defined, often some confusion occurs in assigning the proper class to a patient. No further information is available other than what is published in **Table 6**. For instance, extremes of age must be regarded as an additional risk (perhaps less than one year old and older than 70), and what BMI or pregnancy estimated date of confinement presents greater risk is unclear. An example of ASA II might be a patient with a history of hypertension that is now controlled. ASA III might be a patient who is stable on dialysis, and ASA IV a patient who had a leg amputated for peripheral vascular disease. An example of ASA V is a patient who is hypotensive from a bowel injury requiring an urgent laparotomy. The "E" designator is added to the classification to denote an emergency, a patient who is at higher risk because of not being able to wait for an elective procedure, and the diminished resources frequently found after

Table 6
American society of anesthesiologists physical status classification

Class	Description
1	A normal healthy patient
2	A patient with mild systemic disease
3	A patient with severe systemic disease
4	A patient with severe systemic disease that is a constant threat to life
5	A moribund patient who is not expected to survive without the operation
6	A declared brain-dead patient whose organs are being removed for donor
E	An emergency case (one that does not appear on the operating room schedule published the day before)

Data from Anesthesiologist ASo. ASA Physical Status Classification. 2011; ASA Classification. Available at: http://www.asahq.org/clinical/physicalstatus.htm. Accessed May 29, 2011.

hours. Centers for Medicare & Medicaid Services, New York State Health Code, and the Joint Commission all require an ASA classification assignment. Beyond documentation, the classification should be regarded as another element in establishing an informed conclusion of physical status that will then segue into an informed conversation with the patient while obtaining consent.

Consent

The last segment of the preoperative evaluation process is the consent. Consent is considered after the risks are identified, quantified, and qualified based on history, examination, and consultation, and a plan has been generated integrating the patient's underlying conditions and the surgical goals, along with a pain management strategy. In essence, this is the composite management approach to the patient residual risks, after mitigation, and the contemplated surgical plan.[42,43] The key

Box 2
Factors to agree on for anesthesiologists and surgeons

- Contemplated surgical procedure
- Blood loss anticipated
- Use of blood conservation techniques (eg, permissive hypotension, induced hypotension, blood sequestration, autologous versus homologous, cell saver)
- How much blood to type and cross/screen
- Need for and type of prophylactic antibiotic
- Need for and type of consultations, beta-blockade, full stomach prophylaxis, and laboratory investigations
- Requirement for postoperative intubation (nasal vs oral intubation)
- Anticipated difficulty with intubation, with backup personnel and equipment availability
- Need for advanced monitoring (eg, central line, Foley, arterial line)
- Turning of the operating table 180° for surgical team ease
- Need for edema-lowering steroid administration
- Postoperative pain management strategy
- Need for intensive care availability

participants in the consent process are typically the surgeon, anesthesiologist, and patient. Any of these players has veto power over the plan that is presented.

Communication is the key component of the united professional face that the typically anxious patient should see. The anesthesiologist and surgeon should caucus, discuss, and ultimately agree on several factors, listed in **Box 2**, with the conversation occurring as early as possible for complex procedures.

Once these issues are collaboratively sorted out between the surgical and anesthesia team, the consensus must be presented to the patient for acceptance. Specifically, the risk, benefits, and alternatives, and the risk and benefits of the alternatives, must be presented. If the patient objects to any component, or all, of the plan, the team must recaucus to address the issues, and return with new alternatives, risks, and benefits. Sometimes no alternative can be offered, in which case the surgery cannot be performed. One must consider whether other practitioners may have different skills, techniques, or equipment that may satisfy the patient, surgeon, or anesthesia requirements better, in which case the case should be performed where the surgical goals can be better met. Obtaining consent is a patient-centric iterative process that most advantageously balances the risks and benefits, while taking into account the patient's informed requirements.

SUMMARY

The preoperative period represents perhaps the most critical time in the surgical timeframe, in during which a patient's risks are identified and mitigated, and anesthesia and surgical plans are crafted and presented to the patient for consent, inclusive of the pain management program. Risks are identified through directed history and physical examination and thoughtful laboratory investigations. Risk identification and mitigation strategies are enhanced by consultations that determine the extent of disease and reversal of disease processes when possible. The patient-specific residual risk after treatment, combined with the contemplated surgery-specific risks, constitutes the composite risk of the patient. Early and frequent communication between the surgical and anesthesia team is the first element of the informed consent process, whether the surgical and anesthesia consent is one or separate documents. The collaborative designed plan is presented to the patient, along with the attendant risks, benefits, and alternatives, who then can accept or require modifications. The interactive process concludes when the collaboratively generated plan is agreed to by all parties, setting the stage for a coordinated team approach to the best possible surgical outcome.

REFERENCES

1. Madrid C, Sanz M. What influence do anticoagulants have on oral implant therapy? a systematic review. Clin Oral Implants Res 2009;20(Suppl 4):96–106.
2. Evans IL, Sayers MS, Gibbons AJ, et al. Can warfarin be continued during dental extraction? results of a randomized controlled trial. Br J Oral Maxillofac Surg 2002;40(3):248–52.
3. Aframian DJ, Lalla RV, Peterson DE. Management of dental patients taking common hemostasis-altering medications. Oral Surg Oral Med Oral Pathol Oral Radiol Endod 2007;103(Suppl):S45.e1–11.
4. Pototski M, Amenabar JM. Dental management of patients receiving anticoagulation or antiplatelet treatment. J Oral Sci 2007;49(4):253–8.
5. Brattwall M, Warren Stomberg M, Rawal N, et al. Postoperative impact of regular tobacco use, smoking or snuffing, a prospective multi-center study. Acta Anaesthesiol Scand 2010;54(3):321–7.

6. Stadler M, Bardiau F, Seidel L, et al. Difference in risk factors for postoperative nausea and vomiting. Anesthesiology 2003;98(1):46–52.

7. Chimbira W, Sweeney BP. The effect of smoking on postoperative nausea and vomiting. Anaesthesia 2000;55(6):540–4.

8. Egan TD, Wong KC. Predicting difficult laryngoscopy for tracheal intubation: an approach to airway assessment. Ma Zui Xue Za Zhi 1993;31(3):165–78.

9. Murphy Michael F, Walls RM. Identification of the difficult and failed airway. In: Walls RM, Michael F, editors. Emergency airway management. 3rd edition. Philadelphia: Lippincott Williams & Wilkins; 2008. p. 82.

10. Mallampati SR, Gatt SP, Gugino LD, et al. A clinical sign to predict difficult tracheal intubation: a prospective study. Can Anaesth Soc J 1985;32(4): 429–34.

11. Daviglus ML, Liao Y, Greenland P, et al. Association of nonspecific minor ST-T abnormalities with cardiovascular mortality: the Chicago Western Electric Study. JAMA 1999;281(6):530–6.

12. De Bacquer D, De Backer G, Kornitzer M, et al. Prognostic value of ischemic electrocardiographic findings for cardiovascular mortality in men and women. J Am Coll Cardiol 1998;32(3):680–5.

13. Knutsen R, Knutsen SF, Curb JD, et al. The predictive value of resting electrocardiograms for 12-year incidence of coronary heart disease in the Honolulu Heart Program. J Clin Epidemiol 1988;41(3):293–302.

14. Fleisher LA, Beckman JA, Brown KA, et al. ACC/AHA 2007 Guidelines on Perioperative Cardiovascular Evaluation and Care for Noncardiac Surgery: executive Summary: a Report of the American College of Cardiology/American Heart Association Task Force on Practice Guidelines (Writing Committee to Revise the 2002 Guidelines on Perioperative Cardiovascular Evaluation for Noncardiac Surgery): developed in Collaboration With the American Society of Echocardiography, American Society of Nuclear Cardiology, Heart Rhythm Society, Society of Cardiovascular Anesthesiologists, Society for Cardiovascular Angiography and Interventions, Society for Vascular Medicine and Biology, and Society for Vascular Surgery. Circulation 2007;116(17):1971–96.

15. Cohen MM, Duncan PG, Tate RB. Does anesthesia contribute to operative mortality? JAMA 1988;260(19):2859–63.

16. Lanier WL. A three-decade perspective on anesthesia safety. Am Surg 2006; 72(11):985–9 [discussion: 1021–30, 1133–1048].

17. Botney R. Improving patient safety in anesthesia: a success story? Int J Radiat Oncol Biol Phys 2008;71(Suppl 1):S182–6.

18. Warner DO. Perioperative abstinence from cigarettes: physiologic and clinical consequences. Anesthesiology 2006;104(2):356–67.

19. Warner DO. Helping surgical patients quit smoking: why, when, and how. Anesth Analg 2005;101(2):481–7.

20. Rodrigo C. The effects of cigarette smoking on anesthesia. Anesth Prog 2000; 47(4):143–50.

21. Barrera R, Shi W, Amar D, et al. Smoking and timing of cessation: impact on pulmonary complications after thoracotomy. Chest 2005;127(6):1977–83.

22. Moller AM, Villebro N, Pedersen T, et al. Effect of preoperative smoking intervention on postoperative complications: a randomised clinical trial. Lancet 2002; 359(9301):114–7.

23. American Society of Anesthesiologists Committee. Practice guidelines for preoperative fasting and the use of pharmacologic agents to reduce the risk of pulmonary aspiration: application to healthy patients undergoing elective procedures:

an updated report by the American Society of Anesthesiologists Committee on Standards and Practice Parameters. Anesthesiology 2011;114(3):495–511.

24. Brady M, Kinn S, Stuart P. Preoperative fasting for adults to prevent perioperative complications. Cochrane Database Syst Rev 2003;4:CD004423.

25. Stuart PC. The evidence base behind modern fasting guidelines. Best Pract Res Clin Anaesthesiol 2006;20(3):457–69.

26. Kadoi Y. Anesthetic considerations in diabetic patients. Part I: preoperative considerations of patients with diabetes mellitus. J Anesth 2010;24(5):739–47.

27. Jackson SJ, Leahy FE, McGowan AA, et al. Delayed gastric emptying in the obese: an assessment using the non-invasive (13)C-octanoic acid breath test. Diabetes Obes Metab 2004;6(4):264–70.

28. O'Sullivan G. Gastric emptying during pregnancy and the puerperium. Int J Obstet Anesth 1993;2(4):216–24.

29. Ewah B, Yau K, King M, et al. Effect of epidural opioids on gastric emptying in labour. Int J Obstet Anesth 1993;2(3):125–8.

30. Ogunnaike BO, Whitten CW. Anesthesia and obesity. In: Barash PG, Cullen BF, Stoelting RK, editors. Clinical anesthesia. 5th edition. Philadelphia (PA): Lippincott Williams & Wilkins; 2006. p. 1040–53.

31. Tardif JC. Heart rate as a treatable cardiovascular risk factor. Br Med Bull 2009; 90:71–84.

32. Fox KM, Ferrari R. Heart rate: a forgotten link in coronary artery disease? Nat Rev Cardiol 2011;8(7):369–79.

33. Chatterjee K, Parmley WW, Ganz W, et al. Hemodynamic and metabolic responses to vasodilator therapy in acute myocardial infarction. Circulation 1973;48(6): 1183–93.

34. Sarnoff SJ, Braunwald E, Welch GH Jr, et al. Hemodynamic determinants of oxygen consumption of the heart with special reference to the tension-time index. Am J Physiol 1958;192(1):148–56.

35. Braunwald E. Control of myocardial oxygen consumption: physiologic and clinical considerations. Am J Cardiol 1971;27(4):416–32.

36. Braunwald E. 50th anniversary historical article. Myocardial oxygen consumption: the quest for its determinants and some clinical fallout. J Am Coll Cardiol 2000; 35(5 Suppl B):45B–8B.

37. Lindholm LH, Carlberg B, Samuelsson O. Should beta blockers remain first choice in the treatment of primary hypertension? A meta-analysis. Lancet 2005; 366(9496):1545–53.

38. Bangalore S, Messerli FH, Kostis JB, et al. Cardiovascular protection using beta-blockers: a critical review of the evidence. J Am Coll Cardiol 2007;50(7):563–72.

39. Beattie WS, Badner NH, Choi P. Epidural analgesia reduces postoperative myocardial infarction: a meta-analysis. Anesth Analg 2001;93(4):853–8.

40. Holte K, Kehlet H. Effect of postoperative epidural analgesia on surgical outcome. Minerva Anestesiol 2002;68(4):157–61.

41. Beattie WS, Buckley DN, Forrest JB. Epidural morphine reduces the risk of postoperative myocardial ischaemia in patients with cardiac risk factors. Can J Anaesth 1993;40(6):532–41.

42. Waisel DB, Truog RD. The benefits of the explanation of the risks of anesthesia in the day surgery patient. J Clin Anesth 1995;7(3):200–4.

43. Whitney SN, Holmes-Rovner M, Brody H, et al. Beyond shared decision making: an expanded typology of medical decisions. Med Decis Making 2008;28(5): 699–705.

Pediatric Dentoalveolar Surgery

Sean W. Digman, DDS[a],*, Shelly Abramowicz, DMD, MPH[b,c]

KEYWORDS

- Children • Dentoalveolar surgery • Dental development

Dentoalveolar surgery in children presents general dentists with unique challenges not encountered in adults. The long-term effects that treatments have on these children must always be taken into consideration. A clear understanding of the growth and development of pediatric patients is necessary to correctly identify dental abnormalities.

The tooth bud is a collection of cells derived from the ectoderm of the first brachial arch and the ectomesenchyme of the neural crest cells. The formation of primary teeth is evident between 6 and 8 weeks in utero and the permanent teeth form in the twentieth week. The initial calcification of the primary teeth ranges from 14 weeks for the incisors to 19 weeks for the second molars. The permanent incisors calcify between age 3 and 4 months and the third molars calcify between 7 and 10 years. If the dentition does not develop at these times or there is an event that disrupts the formation, then tooth development ceases. The most common congenitally missing teeth are the third molars followed by the lateral incisors and the mandibular second premolars.

The eruption pattern of the primary and permanent dentition is of critical importance (**Table 1**). If a tooth or teeth fail to erupt, the cause should be investigated. Possible reasons include but are not limited to tooth malposition, retained primary teeth, arch space/length discrepancies, obstruction by a supernumerary tooth or a cyst (usually seen in teens, such as keratocysts and dentigerous cysts), or tumors (usually seen in childhood, such as compound/complex odontomas and fibro-osseous lesions). An anomaly in dental growth and development may be indicative of a more ominous

This project was in part supported by OMSF/AAOMS Faculty Educator Development Award (SA).

The authors have nothing to disclose.

[a] Department of Oral and Maxillofacial Surgery, David Grant USAF Medical Center, 101 Bodin Cir, Travis AFB, CA 94535, USA

[b] Department of Oral and Maxillofacial Surgery, Harvard School of Dental Medicine, 188 Longwood Avenue, Boston, MA 02115, USA

[c] Department of Plastic and Oral Surgery, Children's Hospital Boston, Enders 115, 300 Longwood Avenue, Boston, MA 02445, USA

* Corresponding author.

E-mail address: sean.digman@us.af.mil

Dent Clin N Am 56 (2012) 183–207

doi:10.1016/j.cden.2011.09.002

0011-8532/12/$ – see front matter Published by Elsevier Inc.

dental.theclinics.com

Table 1
The eruption patterns for both the deciduous and permanent dentitions

Deciduous Dentition			Permanent Dentition		
Tooth	Eruption (Mo)	Root Completion (Y)	Tooth	Eruption (Y)	Root Completion (Y)
	Maxillary			Maxillary	
A	7	1.5–2	1	7–8	10
B	8	1.5–2	2	8–9	11
C	16–20	2.5–3	3	11–12	13–15
D	12–16	2–2.5	4	10–11	12–13
E	21–30	3	5	10–12	12–14
			6	6–7	9–10
			7	12–13	14–16
			8	17–21	18–25
	Mandibular			Mandibular	
A	6.5	1.5–2	1	6–7	9
B	7	1.5–2	2	7–8	10
C	16–20	2.5–3	3	9–10	12–14
D	12–16	2–2.5	4	10–12	12–13
E	21–30	3	5	11–12	13–14
			6	6–7	9–10
			7	12–13	14–15
			8	17–21	18–25

This table uses the Zsigmondy system of classification.

problem. Clinicians must be aware of possible systemic causes, including endocrine, nutritional, and genetic abnormalities. These can be manifested in a combination of oral and extraoral findings, such as those associated with ectodermal dysplasia.

Finally, in 2003, approximately 12 of 1000 children were found victims of child abuse and neglect. Medical professionals (and conscientious providers) are obligated to document and report cases of suspected child abuse and neglect to the appropriate law enforcement agency. It is estimated that more than half of the cases of child abuse involve the head, face, and neck. It is likely that you will encounter such cases while in practice and you must act in the best interest of the victim who is most often helpless.

IMPACTED TEETH

The management of impacted teeth requires an understanding of the cause, treatment options, and outcomes. Open dialog between general practitioners, pediatric dentists, oral surgeons, and orthodontists is critical for a successful outcome. This section reviews the incidence, causes, diagnosis, and management of impacted teeth other than third molars.

Incidence

The most common impacted permanent teeth after third molars are maxillary canines, mandibular second premolars, and maxillary incisors. Rates of impacted permanent teeth vary among populations and range from 1% to 5%. Although any tooth can become impacted, most studies agree that the maxillary canine has the highest rate of impaction followed by mandibular second premolars, maxillary second premolars, mandibular second molars, and maxillary incisors. Eruption failure of mandibular incisors is rare and is often associated with pathologic conditions.

Rates of maxillary canine impaction approach 2% of the general population. Of these, 8% show bilateral involvement. This is greater than 5 times the rate of mandibular canine impactions (0.35%). Female patients are twice as likely to have an impacted canine as males.[1] Jacoby found the rate of palatally impacted canines to labially impacted canines to be more than 6:1.[2,3]

Relative to the permanent dentition, primary teeth rarely become impacted. When it occurs, it is most often a mandibular molar. It is important to distinguish between an impacted primary molar and one that appears "submerged" relative to the normal eruption of the adjacent permanent teeth. A congenitally missing succedaneous tooth allows prolonged retention of the primary tooth and often results in ankylosis. As the adjacent permanent teeth erupt, the retained primary tooth takes on a submerged appearance.

Etiology

Before treatment, the cause of an impacted tooth must be ascertained. In general terms, causes of impacted teeth can be categorized into localized mechanical obstruction or systemic abnormalities. Mechanical obstruction can be attributed to arch length deficiency, premature loss of deciduous teeth, prolonged deciduous tooth retention, supernumerary teeth, odontogenic tumors/cysts, abnormal eruption path, and cleft lip and palate (**Fig. 1**).

Systemic causes include hereditary conditions, such as cleidocranial dysplasia (dysostosis) (CCD) and Down syndrome. Other systemic causes include endocrine dysfunction, febrile diseases, and irradiation. Radiographs of patients with CCD show many retained deciduous teeth with unerupted permanent and supernumerary teeth, frequently with distorted crowns and roots. Extraction of the retained deciduous teeth does not promote eruption of their permanent successors so surgical exposure and orthodontic traction is often necessary.[3]

Evaluation

After determining the cause of an impacted tooth, clinicians must devise a treatment plan. Clinical signs of abnormal exfoliation and eruption sequences necessitate that clinicians act early, thus preventing future problems. The initial radiographic examination should include a panoramic radiograph supplemented with a variety of other modalities to determine the position of the impacted tooth in 3-D. Aside from

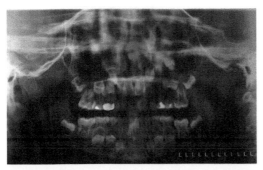

Fig. 1. Radiograph demonstrating an impacted left maxillary first premolar. The premolar was removed with an associated dentigerous cyst. (*From* Fonseca RJ. Oral and maxillofacial surgery. vol. 2. 2nd edition. Philadelphia: Elsevier; with permission.)

determining horizontal and vertical positions of teeth, panoramic radiographs can aid in determining buccal-lingual positions. A tooth that is positioned outside of the radiographic trough appears out of focus and larger or smaller than the adjacent teeth. If positioned palatal to the adjacent teeth (ie, further from the x-ray film), a larger image can be expected (**Fig. 2**). Alternatively, a smaller image can be expected if the tooth is positioned labial to the focal trough.

When the location of an impacted tooth is not obvious, a series of periapical radiographs is used to determine tooth position. This technique is commonly referred to as the tube-shift technique or Clark's rule. To use Clark's rule, an initial periapical radiograph is taken in the standard fashion. A second periapical radiograph is then taken after moving the beam source mesially or distally. If an impacted tooth appears to move in the same direction as the beam, it is located lingual or palatal to the adjacent teeth. If it moves in the opposite direction, the tooth is buccal or labial to the adjacent teeth.[4] The common acronym for this is SLOB (same-lingual, opposite-buccal) (**Figs. 3–5**). Often impacted teeth can be located in the middle of the alveolus or angulated so that half of the tooth is on the buccal side and half on the palatal. In these circumstances, an occlusal radiograph is valuable.

Treatment Options

After determining the location and the cause of an impacted tooth, clinicians should consider the treatment options and determine if referral to a specialist is warranted. Decisions on extraction are based on associated pathologic conditions, tooth position, feasibility of orthodontic alignment, and patient cooperation. Studies by Stivaros and Mandall[5] evaluated the radiographic appearance of teeth and the decision to extract or bring the tooth into the arch. As the angulation of a tooth to the midline increased, it was more likely to be extracted. Palatally impacted teeth were more likely to be retained and brought into the arch than labially positioned teeth. Other treatment options include serial extractions and spontaneous eruption, exposure and spontaneous eruption, exposure with orthodontic traction, autotransplantation, extraction with prosthetic replacement, and no treatment.

Examples

Maxillary canines

To understand the cause of maxillary canine impaction it is important to consider the timing of its development and the surrounding anatomy. The maxillary canine bud is

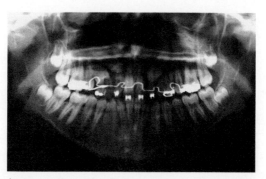

Fig. 2. Radiograph demonstrating palatally impacted maxillary canines. Note the enlarged image of the canines relative to the adjacent teeth. (*From* Fonseca RJ. Oral and maxillofacial surgery. vol. 2. 2nd edition. Philadelphia: Elsevier; with permission.)

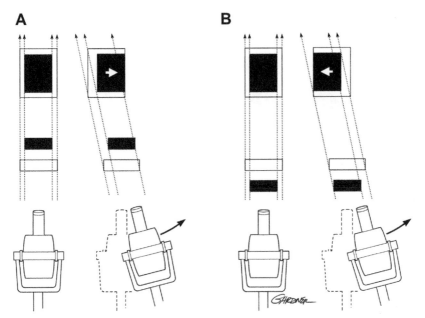

Fig. 3. (*A*) Tube-shift technique demonstrating a palatally impacted object. (*B*) Depiction of a buccally impacted object. (*From* Fonseca RJ. Oral and maxillofacial surgery. vol. 2. 2nd edition. Philadelphia: Elsevier; with permission.)

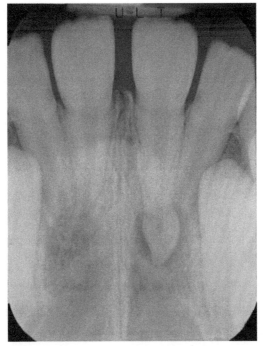

Fig. 4. Periapical radiograph demonstrating an inverted mesiodens. (*From* Fonseca RJ. Oral and maxillofacial surgery. vol. 2. 2nd edition. Philadelphia: Elsevier; with permission.)

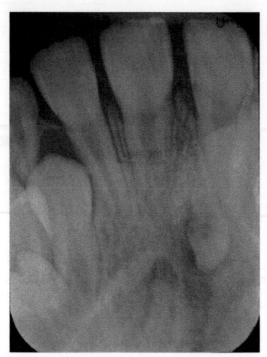

Fig. 5. Periapical radiograph after shifting the x-ray beam source to the patient's left. Note the impacted mesiodens moves in the same direction as the shift in beam source demonstrating palatal location. (*From* Fonseca RJ. Oral and maxillofacial surgery. vol. 2. 2nd edition. Philadelphia: Elsevier; with permission.)

positioned high in the maxilla between the nasal cavity and the orbital rim. Posteriorly, this space is limited by the anterior sinus wall. As root formation progresses, the crown of the canine contacts the roots of the lateral incisor mesially, the first premolar distally, and the resorbing roots of the deciduous canine. Theoretically, these teeth guide the developing canine into its proper position in the arch. When anomalies exist in lateral incisor and premolar form and position, the canine wavers from its expected eruption path and can become palatally or labially impacted.

Palatal impactions are more common because there is more palatal space into which the canine drifts. This is caused by (1) excessive bone growth in the canine area, (2) agenesis or hypodevelopment of the lateral incisor, and (3) stimulated eruption of the lateral incisor or the first premolar.[2] In approximately 13% of cases, the canine becomes labially displaced. This situation, however, probably does not represent a true impaction because these teeth have been shown to spontaneously erupt if given adequate space. Some foretelling signs of maxillary canine impaction include prolonged retention of the deciduous canine (beyond 14 years), presence of a palatal bulge or absence of a labial canine bulge beyond age 11, and abnormal lateral incisor shape or position. Ericson and Kurol[6] found in a study of 505 children between the ages of 10 and 12 that only 5% had nonpalpable canines at age 11.

Treatment In select cases, prevention of canine impaction can be accomplished by extraction of deciduous canines as early as 8 or 9 years of age. These cases are usually limited to dental class 1 patients without crowding. Ericson and Kurol[7] found that the position of the ectopically erupting canine can be normalized in 91% of cases if the canine crown is distal to the midline of the lateral incisor. The success rate decreases to 64% when the canine crown is mesial to the midline of the lateral incisor.

After clinically and radiographically determining the position of a canine, it can be exposed via (1) excisional uncovering, (2) apically positioned flap, or (3) closed eruption techniques. Tooth position and the amount of attached gingiva in the area help determine the correct procedure. Excisional uncovering is usually done after sufficient space is created for eruption of the permanent canine. The procedure is reserved for the palatally impacted canine; however, it can be performed on a labially positioned tooth if there is sufficient attached gingiva in the area to provide 2 mm to 3 mm of gingival cuff after eruption. Without an adequate gingival cuff, the erupting canine is predisposed to future periodontal problems. This procedure is performed when the majority of the crown is above the mucogingival line and there is little alveolar bone to remove. When the impacted tooth is vertically aligned and there is no obstruction, spontaneous eruption usually occurs. Excisional uncovering should not be attempted if the tooth is positioned within the center of the alveolus or apical to the mucogingival line. In this situation, a closed technique or apically positioned flap is indicated (**Fig. 6**).

Exposure of a labially positioned canine is often accomplished using an apically positioned flap. This procedure is indicated if there is insufficient attached gingiva to provide a 2-mm to 3-mm cuff around the erupting tooth and should only be performed if the impacted tooth is near the alveolus. In high impaction cases, the use of an apically positioned flap can result in significant re-intrusion of the impacted tooth after orthodontic therapy.[8] Before surgery, adequate arch space for eruption is usually obtained by an orthodontist. Vertical releasing incisions are made on each side of the edentulous space with the base wider than the apex. A horizontal incision is made over the edentulous alveolar ridge, connecting the 2 vertical incisions and incorporating attached gingiva. A full-thickness mucoperiosteal flap is then reflected apically past the level of the impacted tooth. Bone is removed as necessary from around the crown, and an orthodontic bracket and chain can be attached. The flap is then sutured apically to allow for simultaneous descent of the gingival tissue with the tooth during orthodontic traction (**Fig. 7**).

The closed eruption technique is used for high palatal or labial impactions. In this situation, excisional uncovering or apically positioned flaps is difficult or results in periodontal compromise. The impacted tooth is exposed (in the manner described previously), an attachment with a chain is secured to the tooth, and the chain is sutured to the arch wire for later activation. The flap is replaced with the chain exiting near the

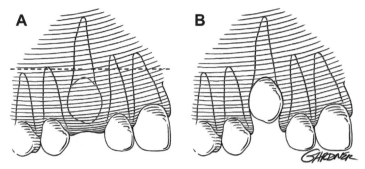

Fig. 6. (A) Impacted canine located above the mucogingival line (*dotted line*). (B) Excisional uncovering of a maxillary canine. (*From* Fonseca RJ. Oral and maxillofacial surgery. vol. 2. 2nd edition. Philadelphia: Elsevier; with permission.)

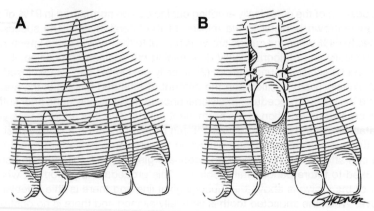

Fig. 7. (*A*) Impacted maxillary canine positioned apical to the mucogingival line (*dotted line*). (*B*) Apically repositioned flap after exposure of maxillary canine. (*From* Fonseca RJ. Oral and maxillofacial surgery. vol. 2. 2nd edition. Philadelphia: Elsevier; with permission.)

alveolar ridge space where the tooth is expected to erupt. The orthodontist then uses the chain to apply traction on the impacted tooth (**Fig. 8**). In a 30-patient study comparing labially impacted teeth treated with apically positioned flaps with those treated with the closed eruption technique, Vermette and colleagues[9] found that more periodontal and esthetic disadvantages can be expected with the apically positioned flap technique. Those treated with apically positioned flaps were shown to have clinically increased crown lengths, gingival scarring, and intrusive relapse when compared with the closed eruption group.

Premolars

Premolar impactions are more common in the mandible than maxilla. They occur more often in the center or lingual aspect of the alveolus. If the impactions are a result of an arch length discrepancy, consultation with an orthodontist should take place (**Fig. 9**).

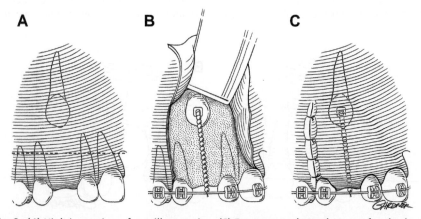

Fig. 8. (*A*) High impaction of maxillary canine. (*B*) Exposure and attachment of orthodontic bracket and chain. (*C*) Repositioned flap for closed eruption. (*From* Fonseca RJ. Oral and maxillofacial surgery. vol. 2. 2nd edition. Philadelphia: Elsevier; with permission.)

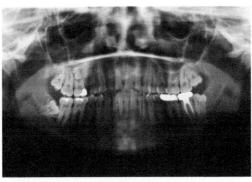

Fig. 9. Radiograph demonstrating an impacted maxillary second premolar with associated resorption of the first molar roots. (*From* Fonseca RJ. Oral and maxillofacial surgery. vol. 2. 2nd edition. Philadelphia: Elsevier; with permission.)

When adequate space exists to accommodate moving the tooth into the arch, the impacted premolar can be treated with the same techniques as for the impacted canine (described previously).

Incisors

Impacted maxillary incisors commonly result from premature loss of the primary incisors or trauma. Radiographs are used to find the location of the impacted tooth and determine root development. If root development is not complete, soft and hard tissue removal is often adequate to promote spontaneous eruption. If root formation is complete or the inclination of the tooth is expected to prevent normal eruption, exposure should include bonding of an orthodontic bracket and chain to allow for orthodontic forces.

Molars

Impactions of permanent first and second molars are rare. If left untreated, the resulting periodontal defects, caries, and resorption can leave a patient without a functioning posterior dentition. Intervention before complete root formation is paramount to a successful outcome. Asymmetric first molar eruption patterns before age 7 should raise suspicion and warrant radiographic examination. After age 7, spontaneous first molar eruption is nearly impossible.[10] Treatment options of unerupted molars include surgical exposure and uprighting, extraction with implant replacement, or a combined surgical and orthodontic correction. Orthodontic correction is often complicated because of limited access and insufficient anchorage, although with the current advances in orthodontic anchorage, this is becoming less of a problem. Patient compliance is also a concern because of the increased treatment time.

Surgical uprighting of a mesially inclined second molar provides a predictable answer if performed at the right time. This procedure is best accomplished when two-thirds of root formation has been completed. If performed after root development is completed, a restricted blood supply from the constricted apical foramen can result in pulpal necrosis. Complications of surgical uprighting include pulpal necrosis, root fracture, dilacerations, internal and external resorption, and periodontal complications. In Dessner's retrospective study[11] of 34 patients treated by surgical uprighting of mandibular second molars, however, 31 molars showed complete bony fill of the space previously occupied by the crown of the uprighted tooth. Only 12 of the 34 teeth showed pulpal changes, and there was no incidence of periapical pathology.

Extraction of Impacted Teeth

The decision to surgically remove an impacted tooth is considered when no other treatment is feasible. When considering removal of an impacted tooth, many factors should be considered, including patient age, associated pathology, severity of impaction, and morbidity associated with the procedure. Anterior teeth are approached from the surface to which they are most closely associated. A full-thickness flap without release is used to expose impacted teeth on the palate.

Extraction of impacted premolars can be challenging because of limited access, adjacent roots, the maxillary sinus, or the mental nerve in the mandible. Extraction of maxillary bicuspids is accomplished in a fashion similar to that of anterior maxillary teeth. Mandibular bicuspids are usually approached from the buccal surface. When access is limited as a result of a lingually impacted premolar, buccal and lingual flaps are used. The lingually impacted premolar is one of the most difficult extractions encountered.

Orthodontic Anchorage

Orthodontic treatment is a complex process that involves the transmission of constant forces to influence tooth movement with the goal of alignment within the alveolus. Anchorage is often the limiting factor when deciding to treat a case with orthodontics alone or in combination with surgery. Specifically, intrusion of posterior teeth to correct an anterior open bite and distal movement of posterior teeth to correct a class 2 or 3 malocclusion presents significant anchorage challenges.

To supplement orthodontic anchorage, various intraoral and extraoral appliances have been used with varying degrees of success. These include headgear, lip bumpers, Herbst appliances, magnets, and multiloop edgewise archwires. Unfortunately, these devices are cumbersome and become ineffective when patient cooperation fades. Surgical correction of skeletal malocclusions is often indicated for these patients with varying acceptance rates. Advances in skeletal orthodontic anchorage over the past 25 years have revealed other options for these patients.

Multiple skeletal anchorage systems exist. Their versatility in size and shape allow them to be placed in anterior and posterior locations of both arches. Common sites for placement include the maxillary buttress and anterior ramus areas. Ease of placement and removal is a clear advantage; however, many clinicians recommend a healing period for osseointegration before applying orthodontic forces. Examples of skeletal fixation for orthodontic anchorage include miniplates fashioned to the posterior mandible or maxilla, microimplants in interdental locations, and palatal implants for distalization of maxillary molars. Miniplates have been used in the posterior maxilla and mandible to intrude molars while closing anterior open bites. In a study by Sherwood and colleagues,[12] anterior open bites were effectively treated by intrusion of maxillary molars using miniplates for anchorage. The miniplates used for fixation proved stable against orthodontic forces, which intruded maxillary molars between 1.45 and 3.32 mm. Miniplate anchorage has also proved effective in the distalization of maxillary and mandibular molars. By fixating miniplates to the anterior ramus, Sugawara and colleagues[13] showed that mandibular molars could be distalized (average of 3.5 mm at the crown level and 1.8 mm at the root level) with minimal relapse (0.3 mm) at 1-year follow-up.

SUPERNUMERARY TEETH

A supernumerary tooth is one found in addition to 20 deciduous teeth or 32 permanent teeth. The cause of these anomalies is controversial. One theory states that there is a dichotomy of the developing tooth bud; another states that the dental lamina becomes hyperactive and produces 2 separate dental follicles. Heredity also seems to play a role because supernumeraries are more common in the relatives of affected children than in the general population.[14] Supernumerary teeth are more common in the permanent dentition (2.1%) than the primary dentition (0.8%).[15] The most common supernumerary tooth is the mesiodens. It is located between the central incisors and most often on the palatal side of the alveolus (**Fig. 10**). Other common supernumerary teeth are fourth molars and mandibular premolars.[16]

Indications for removal of supernumerary teeth include pathology, interference with eruption pattern, and prevention of orthodontic tooth movement. If none of these indications is fulfilled and if access to the impacted supernumerary is limited, observation is a reasonable decision. Patient and parents should be informed, however, that the tooth may need to be removed in the future and that long-term radiographic follow-up is necessary. Timing for surgical removal of a mesiodens is based on the development and the risk of damage to the adjacent roots. Kaban and Troulis[16] recommend removal when one-half to two-thirds of the permanent central incisor roots have been formed. This allows for some stabilization of the permanent teeth while retaining the ability to spontaneously erupt after removal.

ODONTOMAS

The odontoma is the most common odontogenic tumor. It is considered a hamartoma of aborted tooth formation. An odontoma is usually found incidentally during radiographic examination in children and young adults during the ages of tooth development. Others may be discovered after an underlying tooth fails to erupt. It is unlikely that an odontoma forms after the second decade of life. Odontomas can be classified into 2 categories based on morphology. Compound odontomas form multiple tooth-like structures and usually occur in the anterior maxilla or mandible. Complex odontomas contain an amorphous mass of enamel, dentin, and cementum and occur most often in the posterior mandible or maxilla.

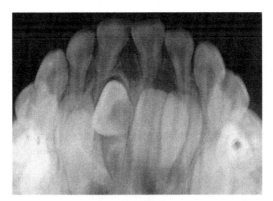

Fig. 10. Occlusal radiograph of an impacted mesiodens preventing the eruption of a central incisor. (*From* Fonseca RJ. Oral and maxillofacial surgery. vol. 2. 2nd edition. Philadelphia: Elsevier; with permission.)

Clinically, most odontomas are asymptomatic. Large odontomas may produce an expansion of bone and can reach up to 6 cm in diameter.[17] Radiographically, compound odontomas appear as multiple malformed teeth surrounded by a radiolucent rim. Complex odontomas appear as a dense amorphous mass with a radiolucent rim. Both forms may have varying degrees of density depending on the maturity of dentin and enamel formation. They are treated by enucleation and curettage, and they do not recur.

SOFT TISSUE ABNORMALITIES
Labial Frenum

The maxillary labial frenum is a band of fibroelastic tissue originating from the upper lip and inserting into the attached gingiva at the midline. It is usually prominent at birth and can be associated with a diastema in the primary and early permanent dentition. As the alveolus grows vertically, the frenum attachment moves apically. Eruption of permanent incisors and canines typically cause closure of the diastema. In some cases, a frenum attachment that crosses over the alveolar ridge and inserts into the incisive papilla can contribute to a persistent diastema. In these cases, a clinical examination reveals an incisive papilla that blanches when the lip is pulled up.[18] Before considering a patient for maxillary labial frenectomy, it is prudent to allow for eruption of all maxillary anterior teeth. Clinicians should rule out other possible causes of diastema, including an impacted supernumerary tooth, behaviors/habits (ie, thumb sucking or tongue thrust), pathology, a midline bony cleft, or notching of alveolar bone between the incisors.

Treatment
When the fibroelastic tissue of the frenum prevents the diastema from closing, it is necessary to completely excise the fibroelastic band rather than simply incising the attachment. The latter results in a high rate of recurrence of the diastema and frenum.[16] After infiltrating with local anesthesia, tension is placed on the frenum by retracting the upper lip. An incision is placed at the base of the frenum attachment to the incisive papilla down to the alveolar bone. A thin margin of attached gingival tissue is left on the mesial aspect of each central incisor, and the incision is carried along the lateral borders of the frenum to its attachment on the labial mucosa. The resultant elliptical defect is undermined with scissors in the unattached labial mucosa. Releasing incisions are made at the mucogingival line. The edges of the labial mucosa are then sutured together and the defect in the attached gingival tissue is left to heal by secondary intention. Sutures should be placed through periosteum at the depth of the vestibule to preserve length (**Fig. 11**).

Lingual Frenum (Ankyloglossia)

A prominent lingual frenum is common among infants. Complaints of limited tongue mobility may initiate consults from concerned parents and pediatricians. Other concerns include sucking and feeding difficulties, airway concerns, future speech difficulty, and periodontal and aesthetic concerns. Parents should be reassured that the lingual frenum usually becomes less prominent during the first 2 to 5 years as the alveolus grows in height and teeth begin to erupt.[16] A tight frenum attachment, however, can lead to oral hygiene problems with the accumulation of plaque on the lingual anterior teeth. A frenectomy is indicated to prevent resulting periodontal disease in these patients. A simple incision to release the tongue should be avoided because of the high rate of relapse and potential for scar formation making future surgery more difficult.

Treatment
Considering the average age of patients and the opportunity for bleeding, lingual frenectomy is best accomplished under conscious sedation and may require an

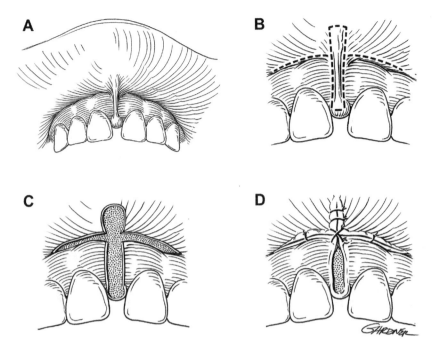

Fig. 11. (*A*) Prominent labial frenum. (*B*) Proposed incisions for labial frenectomy. (*C*) Soft tissue defect after excision of labial frenum and vestibular relaxing incisions. (*D*) Final closure. (*From* Fonseca RJ. Oral and maxillofacial surgery. vol. 2. 2nd edition. Philadelphia: Elsevier; with permission.)

intubated general anesthetic. Special attention is given to location of submandibular ducts. After infiltration with local anesthesia, the tongue is retracted using sutures or a double prong skin hook. The band of fibroelastic tissue is excised from its attachment on the ventral surface of the tongue to its insertion on the attached gingiva of the lingual mandibular alveolus. The margins on the ventral surface of the tongue are undermined. Special attention is given to obtaining good hemostasis to prevent a hematoma on the floor of the mouth. Closure of the wound by a V-Y closure or Z-plasty technique, as described by Kaban and Troulis,[16] is preferable. Both closure techniques result in increased length and mobility of the bound tongue. The V-Y closure begins with a releasing incision at the junction of the floor of the mouth and the ventral tongue. This converts the previous elliptical defect to a V-shaped defect. The wound is closed using 4-0 chromic gut in a Y pattern with the longest arm represented by the ventral surface of the tongue (**Fig. 12**). The Z-plasty closure is begun by creating 2 separate triangles with approximately 45° angles with respect to the initial ventral ellipse (**Fig. 13**). After the flaps have been undermined, the triangles are transposed and sutured to their new locations using 4-0 chromic gut. If required, back-to-back Z-plasties can be used to gain additional length and mobility.

Gingival Hyperplasia

Gingival hyperplasia ranges from mild local to severe generalized gingival enlargement. It can lead to difficulties with oral hygiene, speech, mastication, and tooth eruption. It can be associated with hormonal changes (ie, pregnancy and puberty) or with

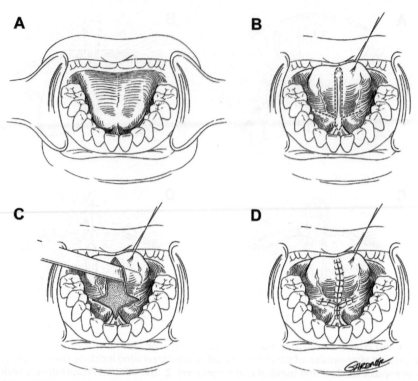

Fig. 12. (*A*) Preoperative depiction of a prominent lingual frenum. (*B*) Proposed incisions for a lingual frenectomy with a V-Y closure. (*C*) Soft tissue defect after excision of a lingual frenum and undermining of the wound margins. (*D*) V-Y closure of a lingual frenectomy. (*From* Fonseca RJ. Oral and maxillofacial surgery. vol. 2. 2nd edition. Philadelphia: Elsevier; with permission.)

leukemia, especially acute myelocytic leukemia, and can be idiopathic in origin. Kimball[19] was among the first to implicate phenytoin as a causative agent in drug-induced gingival hyperplasia. Since then, many other medications have been shown to cause this condition, including anticonvulsants, barbiturates, valproic acid, succinimides, carbamazepine, calcium channel blockers, diltiazem, verapamil, amlodipine, cyclosporine, and certain oral contraceptives.[20]

The mechanism by which drugs cause hyperplasia is still not well understood. It is suggested that some drugs cause the production of an inactive form of collagenase that leads to an imbalance between the production and breakdown of collagen.[21] Other mechanisms include an altered response of collagen to plaque and hypersensitivity to these drugs in certain populations (**Fig. 14**). Pregnancy can result in gingival enlargement by causing a severe inflammatory reaction. It was found that the increase in hormones during pregnancy acted as growth factors for certain bacteria, such as *Prevotella intermedia,* which were present in large amounts during the third and fourth months of pregnancy. This timeline coincided with the development of hyperplastic lesions.[22,23] Di Placido and coworkers[22] also postulated that vascular permeability might be increased, thereby increasing the edema of gingival tissues.

An intraoral finding of gingival hyperplasia in an otherwise healthy patient who is not on any medications likely to cause hyperplasia should raise suspicion of leukemia. The

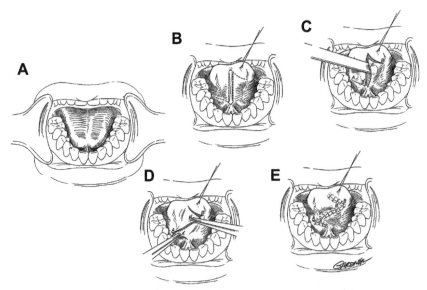

Fig. 13. (*A*) Preoperative depiction of a prominent lingual frenum. (*B*) Proposed incisions for a lingual frenectomy with Z-plasty closure. (*C*) Undermining wound margins. (*D*) Transposition of Z-plasty flaps. (*E*) Final closure. (*From* Fonseca RJ. Oral and maxillofacial surgery. vol. 2. 2nd edition. Philadelphia: Elsevier; with permission.)

most common form of leukemia associated with gingival hyperplasia is acute monocytic leukemia, which is a subtype of acute myelogenous leukemia. The pathogenesis is believed to arise from the infiltration of leukemic cells in the tissues, which causes progressive enlargement of the interdental papillae. With appropriate chemotherapy, partial or complete resolution of gingival enlargement is possible. Gingival enlargement in edentulous leukemia patients has not been shown, suggesting that other local irritants must be present to trigger enlargement.[24]

Treatment
In drug-induced gingival hyperplasia, discontinuation of the medication may allow lesions to regress. This should always be discussed with a patient's physician.

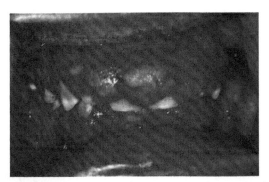

Fig. 14. Drug-induced gingival hyperplasia. The crowns are almost completely covered. This particular patient was taking phenytoin. (*From* Meraw SJ, Sheridan PJ. Medically induced gingival hyperplasia. Mayo Clin Proc 1998;73(12):1196–9; with permission.)

Because poor oral hygiene can exacerbate gingival lesions in susceptible patients, it is recommended that patients see their dentist regularly for dental prophylaxis and practice meticulous home care. In some cases, the only treatment options are gingivectomy or periodontal surgery with scaling and root planing to minimize local irritants. It is recommended that electrocautery or a CO_2 laser be used to minimize bleeding.

Localized Gingival Lesions

There are certain localized gingival lesions commonly seen in the pediatric population. The following is a review of the preponderant lesions found in this population.

An eruption cyst is essentially another type of dentigerous cyst. It usually occurs in young children within the keratinized gingiva as teeth are actively trying to erupt. The cavity contains fluid and, if traumatized (which is common), there is an accumulation of blood that lends the lesion a bluish color. There are 2 main methods of treatment: (1) allowing the tooth to erupt through the cyst, causing it to naturally marsupialize, and (2) performing a small incision over the crest of the ridge, causing the cyst to marsupialize. Both treatments allow the tooth to erupt normally.

Gingival cysts of the newborn appear as multiple white nodules on the maxillary edentulous ridge. Keratin from remnants of dental lamina causes the white color. They can also occur on the palate along the midline as epithelial inclusion cysts (Epstein pearls). Regardless of their location, they spontaneously rupture into the oral cavity. Therefore, monitoring and parent reassurance is the preferred treatment.

The pyogenic granuloma is one of the most common reactive gingival swellings.[25,26] As a result of the rich vascularity, these lesions are red-purple in color and tend to bleed easily. They can be lobular, sessile, and ulcerated (**Fig. 15**). The lesion can occur at any age but is more commonly seen in children and young adults. The precipitating factors are local irritants, such as plaque, calculus, overhanging restorations, and foreign bodies. Because this is an inflammatory process with continuous attempts at healing, the abundant presence of hyperplastic granulation tissue is a characteristic of the pyogenic granuloma. Treatment consists of surgical excision, preferably with

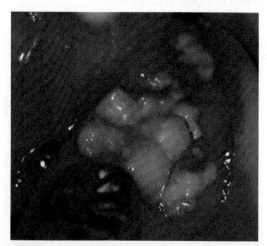

Fig. 15. Pyogenic granuloma, often ulcerated. These lesions are highly vascular and tend to bleed easily. The fibrous connective tissue is not as dense as the peripheral ossifying fibroma. (*From* Oda D. Soft-tissue lesions in children. Oral Maxillofac Surg Clin North Am 2005;17: 383–402; with permission.)

electrocautery or CO_2 laser to minimize bleeding. Depth of the excision should be to the underlying periosteum. Removal of the local irritant is another factor in preventing recurrence. This lesion can resemble other entities, including primary and metastatic malignancies. Therefore, if there is clinical suspicion, prompt biopsy and further work-up may be warranted.

Peripheral ossifying fibroma is a lesion exclusively found on the gingiva. It originates from the periodontal ligament or the periosteum (**Fig. 16**). Unlike the pyogenic granuloma, this lesion makes up only 10% of gingival swellings in children. It has a slight female predilection and rarely involves primary teeth. This mass is more firm and less friable than a pyogenic granuloma and typically has a broad base. Excision including periosteum is the appropriate treatment.

SALIVARY LESIONS
Mucocele

The most common benign salivary gland lesion in children is a mucocele (**Fig. 17A**). It is most often located at the lower lip or along the occlusal plane. The etiology is usually occlusal trauma, self -inflicted accidental bite, or a fall. This causes damage to the minor salivary glands with associated saliva extravagating into the surrounding soft tissue. The body attempts to wall it off and a pseudocyst forms.[27] Patients complain of a clear or blood-tinged circular lesion with intermittent swelling and occasional drainage. When it drains, the fluid is usually thick and viscous (similar to saliva). Drainage causes the lesion to reduce in size or disappear but it usually returns within a few days or weeks. Although the lesion is usually not painful, it can become large and thus unaesthetic (see **Fig. 17B**).

Treatment

Allowing the lesion to drain spontaneously results in a high recurrence rate. Therefore, the definitive treatment is surgical excision. After local anesthesia is administered, an incision surrounding the lesion is made. Blunt dissection to the muscular layer takes place and the lesion is removed with the surrounding associated minor salivary glands (see **Fig. 17C**). Hemostasis is achieved with electrocautery. The wound can be closed with 4-0 gut sutures.[27]

Ranula

The cause of a ranula is congenital or a result of a traumatic incident to the sublingual gland. The lesion is usually blue-tinged and is located in the sublingual space between

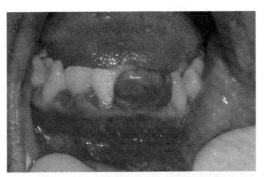

Fig. 16. Peripheral ossifying fibroma. This mass is firm, has a broad base, and contains dense connective tissue. (*From* Oda D. Soft-tissue lesions in children. Oral Maxillofac Surg Clin North Am 2005;17:383–402; with permission.)

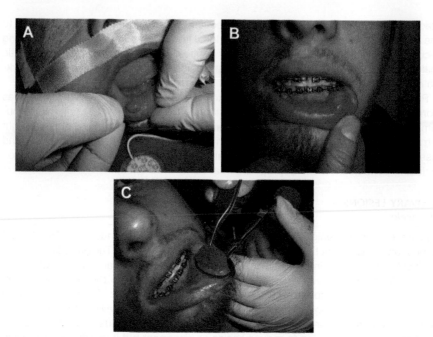

Fig. 17. (*A*) Clinical photo of a mucocele of the lower lip in an infant. (*B*) A 16-year-old boy with mucocele of lower lip resulting from repeated trauma secondary to orthodontic appliances. (*C*) Mucocele and surrounding minor salivary glands is being excised. Note thick and viscous saliva.

the mylohyoid muscle and the lingual mucosa (**Fig. 18**). A plunging ranula dissects through the mylohyoid muscle and can appear as a swelling in the neck. The lesion can elevate the tongue and thus interfere with swallowing, speech, mastication, or respiration. Occasional drainage can cause it to disappear but it usually returns.

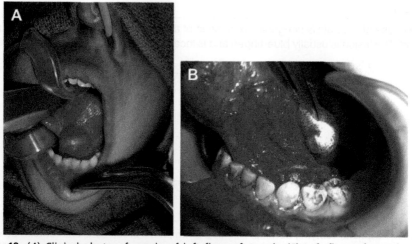

Fig. 18. (*A*) Clinical photo of ranula of left floor of mouth. (*B*) Left floor of mouth and tongue after ranula and sublingual gland have been removed.

Treatment

The 2 main techniques to treat a ranula are marsupialization and excision. A small ranula can be marsupialized or excised with the associated sublingual gland via an intraoral approach. A large ranula or plunging ranula, however, should not be marsupialized. This may lead to recurrence and can make subsequent surgical attempts at excision more difficult.[27] The associated gland must be removed to decrease recurrence.

GENERALIZED DISORDERS OF DENTITION
Cleidocranial Dysplasia

CCD is an autosomal dominant condition affecting growth of the cranial vaults, clavicles, maxilla, nasal, and lacrimal bones. This typically results in the absence of at least one clavicle, a hypoplastic maxilla, delayed closure of cranial sutures and fontanelles, and frontal, parietal, and occipital bossing.[28] The dental characteristics include retained deciduous teeth, supernumerary teeth, and lack of eruption of permanent teeth (**Fig. 19**).[29,30] Patients with CCD may form cysts around unerupted permanent teeth. The jaw relationship in these patients is usually skeletal class III as a result of a deficient maxilla and autorotation of the mandible.[29] The literature describes 3 main treatment algorithms: (1) replacement of teeth with dentures; (2) removal of supernumerary teeth, followed by surgical repositioning and transplantation of the permanent teeth; and (3) surgical and orthodontic treatment aimed at extracting unnecessary teeth and aligning permanent teeth.[30] Extraction of retained primary teeth in these patients does not necessarily stimulate eruption of the permanent teeth. The current trend points toward the surgical and orthodontic combination and typically a staged treatment protocol is used (**Fig. 20**).

The most important aspect in dental and skeletal rehabilitation is staging of extractions. This is followed by exposure of impacted teeth to allow eruption into the oral cavity. These teeth then can serve as vertical stops to maintain dentoalveolar vertical height for the next teeth to be exposed. In the first stage, deciduous and supernumerary teeth are extracted. The intermediate stage is focused on using the erupted permanent first molars as anchors to orthodontically extrude permanent incisors. The final stage consists of surgically exposing and orthodontically extruding permanent premolars and canines.[30–32]

In these patients, chronologic age is different from dental age, so timing of treatment is of the utmost importance. Finally, treatment of CCD occurs over an extended period

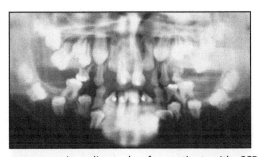

Fig. 19. Pretreatment panoramic radiograph of a patient with CCD showing delayed eruption, impacted teeth, and supernumerary teeth. (*From* Daskalogiannakis J, Piedade L, Lindholm TC, et al. Cleidocranial dysplasia: 2 generations of management. J Can Dent Assoc 2006;72(4):337–42; with permission.)

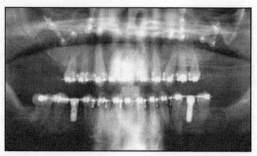

Fig. 20. Posttreatment panoramic radiograph of the same patient after surgical and orthodontic treatment. (*From* Daskalogiannakis J, Piedade L, Lindholm TC, et al. Cleidocranial dysplasia: 2 generations of management. J Can Dent Assoc 2006;72(4):337–42; with permission.)

of time and can be unpredictable.[32] Patients and parents should be educated about the length of treatment, the need for multiple surgical procedures, and continued orthodontic care.

Ectodermal Dysplasia

Ectodermal dysplasia (ED) is a genetic disorder causing aplasia or dysplasia of tissues of ectodermal origin, such as hair, nails, skin, and teeth. This disorder can be further subdivided into 2 categories. An X-linked hypohidrotic form (Christ-Siemens-Touraine syndrome) is characterized by the classic triad of hypohidrosis, hypodontia, and hypotrichosis in addition to dysmorphic facial features. The hidrotic form (Clouston syndrome) usually spares the sweat glands but continues to affect hair, nails, and teeth. This form is autosomal dominant and seems found primarily in Canadian families of French descent (**Fig. 21**).[33] The diagnosis is usually made by the correlation of patient history and physical examination. Classic features include heat intolerance, inability to perspire, abnormal dentition, and sparse hair. As a consequence, one of the main aspects of treatment is to improve a patient's self-image and to preserve psychological health. de Rezende and Amado[34] promote early treatment in these patients because of psychological and physiologic factors.

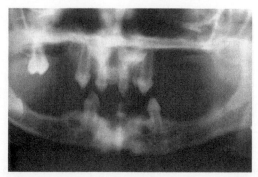

Fig. 21. Panoramic radiograph demonstrating a patient with hereditary ED. Note the hypodontia and the short clinical crowns and roots of the existing dentition. (*From* Fonseca RJ. Oral and maxillofacial surgery. vol. 2. 2nd edition. Philadelphia: Elsevier; with permission.)

The anodontia or hypodontia seen in ED leads to a lack of new appositional bone growth in the vertical dimension. Alveolar bone defects and abnormally shaped crowns reduce tissue support and retention for removable prostheses. This makes conventional prosthodontic treatment difficult because conically shaped teeth and a knife-edged alveolar ridge result in poor retention and instability of a removable prosthesis. The management of these patients requires a multidisciplinary team consisting of a pediatric dentist, orthodontist, prosthodontist, and oral surgeon. The principal aims of dental treatment are to restore missing teeth and bone, establish an appropriate vertical dimension, and provide support for the facial soft tissues. Although implants in children are unpredictable, they aid in dental restorability for children with ED.

Gardner Syndrome

The initial association made between generalized intestinal polyposis, osteomas of the jaws, and multiple sebaceous cysts and lipomas was first described by Devic and Bussy in 1912.[35] It was not until 1953 that Gardner and Richard[36] described a family with a triad of features transmitted in an autosomal dominant fashion consisting of intestinal polyposis, osteomas, and cutaneous lesions. This disorder showed 80% penetrance. Jaw involvement consists of multiple osteomas, complex odontomas, and dental anomalies, including impacted teeth and hypercementosis (**Fig. 22**).[37]

The management of Gardner syndrome is similar to that of CCD and requires a multidisciplinary approach. The goal of treatment is to facilitate the eruption of impacted teeth while removing interferences to normal tooth eruption.

PEDIATRIC IMPLANTS

The use of endosseous implants in adults is accepted and supported in the literature. Alternatively, implant placement in children remains controversial. Implants do not behave like natural teeth because of the absence of a periodontal ligament. One of the periodontal ligament's functions is to facilitate eruption of natural teeth and compensate for the vertical growth of the alveolar process. Implants, however, resemble ankylosed teeth. They can impede vertical dentoalveolar growth when adjacent teeth and alveolus continue to erupt and gain height, causing submersion of the implants.[38,39] Several investigators have shown that implants placed in growing pigs did not move in any single vector and remained ankylosed.[40,41] In the posterior mandible, bony apposition caused the implants to move lingually through the alveolar process. In the maxilla, the implants moved palatally. These implants also seemed to impede the growth of the alveolar process and caused tooth buds to change their path of eruption.

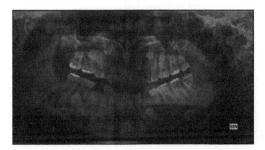

Fig. 22. Panoramic radiograph of a patient with Gardner syndrome. Note the multiple osteomas in the mandible and maxilla, impacted teeth, and odontomas. (*From* Boffano P, Bosco GF, Gerbino G. The surgical management of oral and maxillofacial manifestations of Gardner syndrome. J Oral Maxillofac Surg 2010;68:2549–54; with permission.)

Successful placement of implants in children has been demonstrated in patients with cleft lip and palate and after tumor resections in which bone grafts are used (**Fig. 23**). Kearns and colleagues showed that implants placed in the anterior maxilla of patients resulted in loss of vertical height at the incisal border with the adjacent permanent teeth.[42] This was supported by Thilander and colleagues,[41] who showed that this leads to the prosthesis eventually being out of occlusion, requiring removal and replacement with a longer abutment. Kearns and colleagues[42] were able to demonstrate implants can be successfully placed in these pediatric patients with the realization that functional, aesthetic, and psychological benefits outweigh the need to change or remove abutments.

Ledermann and colleagues[38] state that another possible consideration for implant placement arises from the fact that the most commonly lost teeth as a result of trauma in children are the maxillary incisors (**Fig. 24**). Therefore, immediate implant placement after tooth luxation or avulsion may be indicated to prevent the rapid resorption of the alveolus and help preserve bone. Ledermann and colleagues placed a total of 42 implants in patients aged 9 to 18. Fourteen implants were placed immediately after traumatic luxation of anterior teeth and 28 implants after appropriate healing time was given. Aside from 3 implants failing as a result of additional trauma, the remaining implants osseointegrated. Their study did not show a case of submergence, and implants remained stable despite additional growth of patients.[38]

Although the subject of implants in children requires research, at this time some recommendations can be made regarding the use of implants in growing patients. (1) Implants can be placed with fair predictability in patients with ED, CCD, cleft lip, and palate. (2) Implants do well in areas of tumor resection in which bone grafts are used because these patients do not have the potential for the normal growth patterns of the alveolus. (3) Children who are completely edentulous can have implants placed with a good degree of predictability because of the decreased alveolar growth potential. (4) Caution must be exercised in partially dentate pediatric patients with teeth on either side of a proposed implant because of the risk of submersion and/or eventual compromised restoration, especially when placing an implant in the aesthetic zone. (5) For the most predictable prognosis, implant placement should be delayed until growth is complete. (6) Close follow-up of pediatric implant patients is necessary.

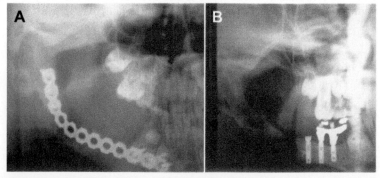

Fig. 23. (*A*) A 6-year-old boy after resection and reconstruction of the right mandible. He was diagnosed with aggressive myofibroma. (*B*) The same patient 5 months after anterior hip graft and implant placement. (*From* Fonseca RJ. Oral and maxillofacial surgery. vol. 2. 2nd edition. Philadelphia: Elsevier; with permission.)

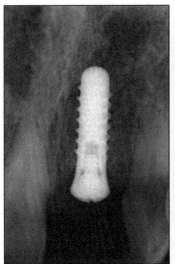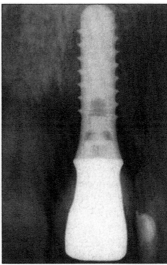

Fig. 24. Series of periapical radiographs taken over 12 years demonstrating submersion of implant with continued growth and eruption of adjacent teeth. (*From* Heij DGO, Opdebeeck H, van Steenberghe D, et al. Facial development, continuous tooth eruption, and mesial drift as compromising factors for implant placement. Int J Oral Maxillofac Implants 2006;21:867–78; with permission.)

ACKNOWLEDGMENTS

The authors would like to thank Samuel L. Hayes, DDS, and Jean-Luc G. Niel, DMD, for their contributions.

REFERENCES

1. Bishara SE. Impacted maxillary canines: a review. Am J Orthod Dentofacial Orthop 2002;101:159–71.
2. Jacoby H. The etiology of maxillary canine impactions. Am J Orthod 1983;84: 125–32.
3. Richardson G, Russell K. A review of impacted permanent maxillary cuspids: diagnosis and prevention. J Can Dent Assoc 2000;66:497–501.
4. Jacobs SG. Radiographic localization of unerupted maxillary anterior teeth using the vertical tube shift technique: the history and application of the method with some case reports. Am J Orthod Dentofacial Orthop 1999;116:415–23.
5. Stivaros N, Mandall NA. Radiographic factors affecting the management of impacted upper permanent canines. J Orthod 2000;27:169–73.
6. Ericson S, Kurol J. Radiographic assessment of maxillary canine eruption in children with clinical signs of eruption disturbances. Eur J Orthod 1986;8:133–40.
7. Ericson S, Kurol J. Early treatment of palatally erupting maxillary canines by extraction of primary canines. Eur J Orthod 1988;10:283–95.
8. Kokich VG. Surgical and orthodontic management of impacted maxillary canines. Am J Orthod Dentofacial Orthop 2004;126:278–83.
9. Vermette ME, Kokich VG, Kennedy DB. Uncovering labially impacted teeth: apically positioned flap and closed-eruption techniques. Angle Orthod 1995; 65:23–32.

10. Frank CA. Treatment options for impacted teeth. J Am Dent Assoc 2000;131: 625–32.
11. Dessner S. Surgical uprighting of second molars: rationale and technique. Oral Maxillofac Surg Clin North Am 2002;14:201–12.
12. Sherwood KH, Burch JG, Thompson WJ. Closing anterior open bites by intruding molars with titanium miniplate anchorage. Am J Orthod Dentofacial Orthop 2002; 122:593–600.
13. Sugawara J, Daimaruya T, Umemori M. Distal movement of mandibular molars in adult patients with the skeletal anchorage system. Am J Orthod Dentofacial Orthop 2004;125:130–8.
14. Garvey TM, Barry HJ, Blake M. Supernumerary teeth—an overview of classification, diagnosis and management. J Can Dent Assoc 1999;65:612–6.
15. Brook AH. Dental anomalies of number, form and size: their prevalence in British schoolchildren. J Int Assoc Dent Child 1974;5:37–53.
16. Kaban LB, Troulis MJ. Dentoalveolar surgery. In: Kaban LB, Troulis MJ, editors. Pediatric oral and maxillofacial surgery. Philadelphia: Saunders; 2004. p. 125–45.
17. Marx RE, Stern D. Odontogenic tumors: hamartomas and neoplasms. In: Marx RE, Stern D, editors. Oral and maxillofacial pathology, a rationale for diagnosis and treatment. Chicago: Quintessence Publishing; 2003. p. 635–703.
18. Edwards JG. The diastema, the frenum, the frenectomy: a clinical study. Am J Orthod 1977;71:489–508.
19. Kimball OP. The treatment of epilepsy with sodium diphenyl hydantoinate. JAMA 1939;112:1244–50.
20. Meraw SJ, Sheridan P. Medically induced gingival hyperplasia. Mayo Clin Proc 1998;73:1196–9.
21. Camargo PM, MElnick PR, Pirih FQ, et al. Treatment of drug-induced gingival enlargement: aesthetic and functional considerations. Periodontol 2000 2001;27:131–8.
22. Di Placido G, Tumini V, D'Archivio D, et al. Gingival hyperplasia in pregnancy. II. Etiopathogenic factors and mechanisms. Minerva Stomatol 1998;47:223–9.
23. Reynolds MA, Aberdeen GW, Pepe GJ, et al. Estrogen suppression induces papillary gingival overgrowth in pregnant baboons. J Periodontol 2004;75: 693–701.
24. Dreizen S, McCredie KB, Keating MJ, et al. Malignant gingival and skin "infiltrates" in adult leukemia. Oral Surg Oral Med Oral Pathol 1983;55:572–9.
25. Regezi J, Sciubba J, Jordan RC. Red-Blue lesions. In: Regezi J, Sciubba J, Jordan RC, editors. Oral pathology: clinical pathologic correlations. Philadelphia: Saunders; 2003. p. 111–2.
26. Oda D. Soft tissue lesions in children. Oral Maxillofac Surg Clin North Am 2005; 17:383–402.
27. Kaban LB, Troulis MJ. Intraoral soft tissue abnormalities. In: Kaban LB, Troulis MJ, editors. Pediatric oral and maxillofacial surgery. Philadelphia: Saunders; 2004. p. 146–68.
28. Angle AD, Rebellato J. Dental team management for a patient with cleidocranial dysplasia. Am J Orthod Dentofacial Orthop 2005;128:110–7.
29. Shaikh R, Shusterman S. Delayed dental maturation in cleidocranial dysplasia. ASDC J Dent Child 1988;65:325–9.
30. Becker A, Lustmann J, Shteyer A. Cleidocranial dysplasia: part 1—general principles of the orthodontic and surgical treatment modality. Am J Orthod Dentofacial Orthop 1997;111:28–33.
31. Becker A. Cleidocranial dysplasia: part 2—treatment protocol for the orthodontic and surgical modality. Am J Orthod Dentofacial Orthop 1997;111:173–83.

32. Daskalogiannakis J, Piedade L, Lindholm TC, et al. Cleidocranial dysplasia: 2 generations of management. J Can Dent Assoc 2006;72:337–42.
33. Lowry RB, Robinson G, Miller J. Hereditary ectodermal dysplasia. Symptoms, inheritance patterns, differential diagnosis, management. Clin Pediatr 1996;5: 395–402.
34. de Rezende ML, Amado FM. Osseointegrated implants in the oral rehabilitation of a patient with cleft lip and palate and ectodermal dysplasia: a case report. Int J Oral Maxillofac Implants 2004;19:896–900.
35. Devic A, Bussy MM. Un cas de polypose adenomateuse generalisée à tout l'intestin. Arch Mal Appar Dig 1912;6:278–89.
36. Gardner EJ, Richard RC. Multiple cutaneous and subcutaneous lesions occurring simultaneously with hereditary polyposis and osteomatosis. Am J Hum Genet 1953;5:139–47.
37. Takeda Y. Multiple cemental lesions in the jaw bones of a patient with Gardner's syndrome. Virchows Arch A Pathol Anat Histopathol 1987;411:253–6.
38. Ledermann PD, Hassell TM, Hefti AF. Osseointegrated dental implants as alternative therapy to bridge construction or orthodontics in young patients: seven years of clinical experience. Pediatr Dent 1993;15:327–33.
39. Björk A. Variations in the growth pattern of the human mandible: a longitudinal radiographic study by the implant method. J Dent Res 1963;42:400–11.
40. Odman J, Gröndahl K, Lekholm U, et al. The effect of osseointegrated implants on dentoalveolar development. A clinical and radiographic study in growing pigs. Eur J Orthod 1991;13:279–86.
41. Thilander B, Odman J, Gröndahl K, et al. Osseointegrated implants in adolescents. An alternative in replacing missing teeth? Eur J Orthod 1984;16:84–95.
42. Kearns GJ, Sharma A, Perrott D, et al. Placement of endosseous implants in children and adolescents with hereditary ectodermal dysplasia. Oral Surg Oral Med Oral Pathol Oral Radiol Endod 1999;88:5–10.

Alveolar Bone Grafting and Reconstruction Procedures Prior to Implant Placement

Harry Dym, DDS, David Huang, DDS*, Avichai Stern, DDS

KEYWORDS

- Alveolar bone grafting • Implantation • Nonunion
- Bone harvest

BONE ANATOMY AND HISTOLOGY

Before implant placement, adequate bone must be present. This step is fundamental to treatment planning for implants. Understanding the basics of bone grafting and reconstruction techniques is critical for successful implant placement.

The maxilla and mandible are derived from the first branchial arch through intramembranous ossification. During embryologic development neural crest cells migrate along the cartilaginous scaffold of the jaws to begin bone formation.[1] Mature bone can be classified into two types, cortical and cancellous. Cortical bone is the dense outer layer of bone, and is minimally porous and rigid. Cancellous (trabecular) is less dense than cortical (compact) bone; it is housed within compact bone and is structurally different. Both types of bone involve a thin connective tissue covering. The periosteum is immediately superficial to cortical bone, whereas endosteum surrounds the trabecular bone. Both the periosteum and endosteum are sources of osteoprogenitor cells, which are capable of differentiation into osteoblasts.

Bone Histology

Cortical bone consists histologically of parallel series of osteons (Haversian systems). Each osteon consists of a central Haversian canal surrounded by concentric layers of bone, or lamellae, interspersed with osteocytes. Osteons are connected to each other and the periosteum by oblique channels called Volkmann canals. Osteocytes, housed in lacunae, are differentiated osteoblasts that exchange nutrients and metabolic waste

Department of Dentistry/Oral & Maxillofacial Surgery, The Brooklyn Hospital, 121 DeKalb Avenue, Box 187, Brooklyn, NY 11201, USA
* Corresponding author.
E-mail address: Ddsdavidhuang@yahoo.com

Dent Clin N Am 56 (2012) 209–218
doi:10.1016/j.cden.2011.09.005
0011-8532/12/$ – see front matter © 2012 Elsevier Inc. All rights reserved.

dental.theclinics.com

through cytoplasmic processes via a network of small canals, or canaliculi. Trabecular bone also forms lamellae, but lacks the arranged systems as in compact bone. Cancellous bone is responsible for hematopoiesis, bone remodeling, and regeneration.

There are largely 4 different cell types responsible for the generation of bone: osteoprogenitor cells, osteoblasts, osteoclasts, and osteocytes. Osteoprogenitor cells, which are derived from mesenchyme, are the precursors to osteoblasts. These cells are found within the periosteum, endosteum, and compact and cancellous bone. Osteoblasts are found within the periosteum and trabecular bone; they are responsible for bone formation and produce osteoid, a collagenous matrix. Once osteoblasts are encompassed by osteoid they have produced, they continue to differentiate into osteocytes, which function in the maintenance of bone. Osteoclasts are derived from monocytes and are responsible for bone resorption.

Bone Healing

Bone heals through either primary or secondary mechanisms. Primary healing involves rigid fixation with close approximation between bone fragments. At the interface of the adjoining ends, osteoclasts form a cutting cone that crosses the gap and resorbs existing bone. Behind them, fibrovascular tissue and osteoblasts begin to secrete osteoid. With maturation these become new Haversian canals. Secondary healing involves the formation of a callus scaffold, within which osteoid is secreted and then mineralized. This process takes place in 3 stages: inflammatory, repair, and remodeling. In the inflammatory stage, a hematoma develops within the fracture site while macrophages, fibroblasts, and other inflammatory cells migrate to the site. The repair stage results in the formation of granulation tissue, ingrowth of vascular tissue, and migration of mesenchymal cells. As vascular ingrowth proceeds, osteoid is secreted and subsequently mineralized, which leads to the formation of a soft callus around the repair site. The callus then ossifies, forming a bridge of woven bone. The remodeling stage extends from months to years, with full functional strength typically achieved in 4 to 6 months.

The physiology of bone graft healing has many similarities to primary or secondary healing. The origin, structure, and size of the graft will dictate how the graft heals. Principally grafts heal through a combination of 3 processes[2]: osteogenesis, osteoinduction, and osteoconduction. Osteogenesis is the formation of new bone from osteocompetent cells, and is the only process whereby the graft itself can produce new bone. Osteoinduction induces formation of bone from the differentiation and stimulation of mesenchymal cells by the bone-inductive proteins. Osteoconduction is the formation of bone along a scaffold from osteocompetent cells of the recipient site.

The structure of the bone harvest affects how the graft will incorporate into the recipient site. Cortical block grafts heal through creeping substitution. Once the graft is fixed to the site, osteoclasts begin to resorb the graft material through existing Haversian systems. This process allows for ingrowth of fibrovascular tissue and the secretion of osteoid by osteoblasts, similar to primary bone healing. The osteoid then proceeds through mineralization and remodeling. Unfortunately, cortical block grafts are not fully resorbed and exist as a mixture of newly formed bone around necrotic centers.[2]

Bone grafts that are particulate in nature share similar processes of secondary bone healing. Unlike cortical block grafts, particulate grafts begin with apposition of osteoid and fibrovascular ingrowth through the existing particulate scaffold. Apposition is then followed by resorption and replacement of graft material by more organized lamellar bone. Due to increased vascularization, particulate grafts have greater resorption of the transfer bone and a larger percentage of newly formed bone in comparison with cortical grafts.

TYPES OF GRAFTS

Bone grafts can be categorized in many different ways. The discussion here classifies grafts based on origin.

Autogenous grafts, taken from a second surgical site in the same patient, are considered to be the gold standard in oral bone grafting. Autogenous bone grafts have been shown to be superior to allogenic bone, xenogeneic bone, bone substitutes, and alloplasts in terms of the function, form, and adaptability.[2] Because the bone is autogenous there is no immunogenic graft rejection. Sites of harvest can be locoregional or distant. Autografts provide the only source of transfer of osteocompetent cells. Healing occurs through osteogenesis, osteoinduction, and osteoconduction. Disadvantages of this graft include increased operating time as well as patient discomfort and morbidity at donor sites.

Allografts are taken from different members of the same species, the most common source being cadaveric. The antigenicity of this bone is reduced through various processes, frequently freeze-drying. Allografts can be used in conjunction with autograft to increase the volume of the autograft. Graft healing occurs through osteoinduction and/or osteoconduction. Advantages of allograft include reduced operative time and no morbidity at the donor site. Though negligible, allografts carry the risk of disease transmission. The risk of human immunodeficiency virus transmission is estimated to be 1 case in 1.6 million.[3] Hepatitis B and C can also be transmitted.[4] Lastly, it is important to discuss the nature of the allograft with the patient to ensure there is no objection for personal, cultural, or religious beliefs.

Xenografts are derived from genetically dissimilar species, mainly bovine or porcine. These grafts are largely osteoconductive and serve as a scaffold for creeping substitution.[5] Though negligible, antigenicity and infectious disease transmission are also issues with these grafts. The advantages of xenografts include reduced operative time and no morbidity at the donor site. By contrast, compared with allografts, xenografts provide less resorption of graft substrate and form less new bone during the first few months.[6]

Alloplastic grafts are derived from inert synthetic materials. Examples include hydroxyapatite crystals, glass ionomer, bioactive glasses, and tricalcium phosphate. There is no cellular or protein material within these grafts. As a group these materials provide variable resorption rates and operate through osteoconduction. Disadvantages of alloplasts include increased resorption time and decreased new bone formation when compared with allografts or xenografts.[5]

Another type of graft that has gained popularity in recent years incorporates the use of bone morphogenic proteins (BMPs). BMPs are a group of 20 proteins found in bone that act as cytokines and metabologens.[7] From this group, BMP2 and BMP7 induce the formation of bone and cartilage. These proteins are produced using recombinant DNA technology, with applications in dentistry and orthopedic surgery. Advantages of BMP include decreased patient discomfort, no risk of disease transmission, and decreased operative time. Disadvantages include localized swelling and increased costs as compared with other bone grafting alternatives.

SURGICAL PRINCIPLES OF GRAFTING

The successful incorporation of bone grafts relies on many different factors. According to Misch[5] these factors are surgical asepsis, soft-tissue coverage, graft immobilization, host site preparation, host bone-regeneration capacity, and optimization of growth factors such as BMP.

The oral cavity, at best, is considered a clean contaminate environment, and sterile placement of any graft is virtually impossible. Surgical asepsis refers to the lack of acute infection to the best of the surgeon's ability. Regardless of the type, grafts can dissolve in pH of 5.5 or less. Infection within bone often results in a pH of 2 and increases the risk of bone loss or insufficient bone volume formation. Antibiotics, such as penicillin or clindamycin, can be mixed with the graft to decrease bacterial contamination.[5]

Tension-free soft-tissue coverage helps maintain the graft by encouraging osteo-competent cell proliferation and healing by primary intention. Proper technique for of onlay grafts includes flap design, adequate releasing incisions, and scoring of the periosteum. Silk or Vicryl sutures provide better strength and adaptability than does chromic suture.

Graft mobilization may result in fibrous encapsulation and nonunion to the host bone. By ensuring stability of the graft, the blood clot and associated growth factors can be maintained and allowed to heal; this will lead to development of granulation tissue with accompanying vascular supply. Without this stability, graft may be jeopardized. Excessive movement disturbs the blood supply and can create a sequestrum of the graft. To this end, it is important to ensure that no contact occurs between any existing dental prosthesis and the soft tissue overlying the membrane or graft.

Misch[5] elaborates on the process of the regional acceleratory phenomenon whereby in response to noxious stimuli, tissue heals faster than during the normal regeneration process. To initiate this phenomenon, holes are drilled into the site of the host cortical bone at low speeds under copious irrigation to minimize thermal necrosis. Perforation of the host cortical bed allows for vascular access from blood vessels within trabecular bone, which increases the release of growth factors and expedites revascularization.

Optimizing revascularization from the host bone provides grafts with adequate growth factors and pluripotential perivascular cells that can differentiate into osteo-blasts. The source of blood vessels affects the type of tissue that forms in and around empty alveolar sockets and graft. Drilling holes in the host cortical bed aids with transfer of osteocompetent cells. Providing a soft-tissue barrier for the graft delays invasion from surface fibroblasts that may inhibit osteogenesis. Application of resorbable or nonresorbable membrane is well established in promoting bone regeneration.[8]

Providing local growth factors such as platelet-derived growth factor, vascular endothelial growth factors, transforming growth factors, and bone morphogenetic proteins can enhance formation and mineralization of bone. Platelet-rich plasma, produced from the patient's whole blood through a double-centrifuge technique, can be utilized to increase the localized growth factors. BMP can be added by including autograft in the site.

BONE HARVEST SITES

Autogenous bone remains the gold standard for bone grafts, its main limitation being increased operative time and possible donor-site complications and morbidity. The choice of donor site depends largely on the size of the defect. Intraoral bone harvesting can be performed in the office under local anesthesia. Small blocks of bone can be harvested from the mandibular symphysis, ramus, maxillary tuberosity, or exostoses. Sittitavornwong and Gutta[9] discuss these techniques. It is important during any harvest procedure to ensure protection of vital anatomy such as mental nerves, maxillary sinuses, and teeth.

For socket or particulate grafting, the maxillary tuberosity can provide approximately 2 cm³ of bone. After local infiltration, a crestal incision is made along the tuberosity. A full-thickness flap is exposed to access the site on both the buccal and palatal aspect. Vital structures to avoid include the maxillary sinus and greater and lesser palatine vessels. The tuberosity can then be removed with rongeurs. Lack of sinus perforation should be verified, before simple closure.

For cortical block graft, the lateral ramus can provide 1.5 × 3 cm². Incision for this harvest is made slightly distal and lateral to the most posterior tooth, and continues along the external oblique ridge (**Fig. 1**). Three complete osteotomies and one partial osteotomy are made, with one complete superior and two complete vertical cuts through cortical bone. The last osteotomy is made by using a round bur to create a horizontal groove along the inferior border. The superior osteotomy is made from the second molar region, and continues posteriorly and vertically along the ascending ramus. The cut is approximately 5 mm medial to the external oblique ridge and extends to the size of the defect or about 3 cm. Next, anterior and posterior vertical cuts 12 to 15 mm in length are made in the superoinferior direction. Lastly, the inferior groove is made with a round bur. The harvest site is then carefully separated with a small chisel. Excessive bleeding can be controlled with pressure and hemostatic agents.

The mandibular symphysis is another harvest site for providing monocortical grafts. The symphysis can be approached through either a sulcular or vestibular incision (**Fig. 2**). Vital structures include the bilateral mental nerves. The vestibular incision is preferred when the anterior mandibular periodontium is less than optimal. This incision is made anterior to the mental nerve, through the mentalis at a beveled angle at the depth of the vestibule. This action facilitates reattachment of the mentalis during closure, which is performed in two layers, mentalis and mucosa. The sulcular incision is made with a bilateral distal releasing incision posterior to the mental foramen.

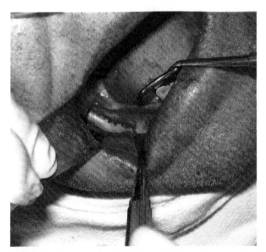

Fig. 1. Osteotomies for lateral ramus graft. (*From* Sittitavornwong S, Gutta R. Bone graft harvesting from regional sites. Oral Maxillofac Surg Clin North Am 2010;22(3):320; with permission.)

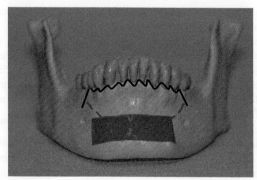

Fig. 2. Incisional approaches to harvesting the mandibular symphysis. Sulcular in black and vestibular in red. (*From* Sittitavornwong S, Gutta R. Bone graft harvesting from regional sites. Oral Maxillofac Surg Clin North Am 2010;22(3):319; with permission.)

Closure is through the mucosa, ensuring reapproximation of interdental papilla. Once exposed the mandibular symphysis harvest can provide about 10×30 mm^2 of monocortical block bone (**Fig. 3**). The superior osteotomy should begin at least 5 mm below the root apices. The vertical osteotomies should be no closer than 5 mm medial to the mental nerves. The final depth of the osteotomies depends on the corticocancellous block required, but is usually no more than 5 to 6 mm. An outline of the osteotomy is marked by creating a series of dots with a small round bur around the periphery

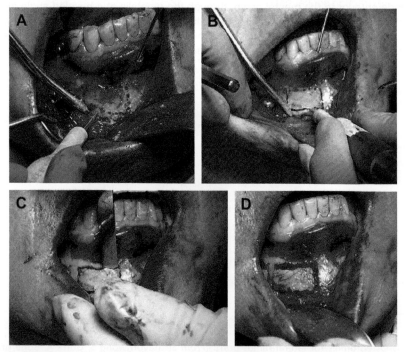

Fig. 3. Osteotomies to outline the harvest are created with a small round bur and then fissure bur (*A, B*). A thin chisel is then used to complete the harvest (*C, D*).

of the proposed site. After verification, the outline is connected with small fissure bur. A thin chisel is then used to complete the osteotomy, freeing a block of corticocancellous bone.

For larger amounts of cortical, corticocancellous, or cancellous bone, distal sites including the tibia, anterior iliac crest, posterior iliac crest, and the calvarium can also be harvested. Zouhary[10] summarizes the amount of bone that can be harvested from each site in **Table 1**.

Although all harvest sites can be safely obtained, the range of potential complications is more serious in distant-site harvests and can include ileus, gait disturbance, fracture, dural tear, epidural or subdural hematoma, stroke, and death. Nonetheless, the risk of complications is relatively small. Tessier and colleagues[11] reported their combined complication rate for major bone graft donor sites in their 20,000 cases; they reported a 0.3% to 0.5% compilation rate for each type of bone harvesting. Cases requiring larger amounts of bone to be harvested from these sites should be referred to an oral surgeon.

BONE GRAFT

One of the important factors in determining application of the bone graft is the type and size of the recipient defect. Misch[12] elaborates on how each type of defect is restored. In a 5-wall defect, as in an empty socket, any graft material will work. Four-wall defects will require a graft with membrane for guided bone regeneration. Two to 3 wall defects are best grafted with autogenous bone that can be mixed with allograft and guided bone regeneration with a rigid membrane. A 1-wall defect should be treated with onlay grafts or other advanced techniques for augmentation.

The extraction socket heals through formation of a blood clot which is replaced by connective tissue. In time, woven bone replaces this tissue and then is remodeled into lamellar bone. The entire process takes 3 to 4 months. While being preferred by patients in the authors' practice, immediate placement of implants is not always possible, given the remaining bony contour after extraction. To make matters worse, waiting for secondary healing to occur may not benefit the patient. Lekovic and colleagues[13] note that 60% of the alveolar width and 40% of the height may be lost in the first 6 months after dental extraction.

To maintain the dimensions of the alveolar ridge, grafting of the empty socket has been shown to help preserve the height and width in comparison with extractions alone.[14] Socket grafting is easier with 4 or 5 wall defects. The procedure begins with an atraumatic extraction. Many instruments such as the periotome, luxator, and physics forceps have been developed to aid preservation of alveolar bone. It is

Table 1		
Typical noncompressed graft volumes available for harvest		
	Noncompressed Corticocancellous (cm³)	**Cortical Block (cm)**
Tibia	25–40	1 × 2
Anterior ilium	50	3 × 5
Posterior ilium	100–125	5 × 5
Calvarium	Minimal	Abundant

Data from Zouhary K. Bone graft harvesting from distant sites: concepts and techniques. Oral Maxillofac Surg Clin North Am 2010;22(3):301–14.

important to plan ahead and section the tooth or bone as needed. Once the extraction is completed, the socket is thoroughly curetted to remove any granulation or fibrous tissue. Active purulent drainage is a general contraindication for socket grafting. If acutely infected, grafting should wait until the infection has resolved.

The graft is then chosen. It is important to remember that autogenous grafts are considered the gold standard and can always be mixed other grafts if the volume is deficient. The material is placed into the socket without forceful compacting. Lastly, the graft is covered with a membrane and possibly relaxed soft-tissue coverage. Membranes are generally classified as resorbable or nonresorbable. Choice of membrane depends on the amount of time needed for socket healing. Resorbable membranes are used when the healing time is approximately 3 months. A minor full-thickness flap is extended beyond the crest of the buccal and lingual/palatal cortical plate. The selected membrane is cut to size and tucked to the depth of the buccal and palatal/lingual flap. Interrupted sutures are then passed to secure the membrane. Alternatively, if adequate relaxation can be obtained, a buccal full-thickness periosteal flap can be exposed and scored to obtain primary closure. The membrane serves two functions: to contain the blood clot and the graft within the socket, and to prevent fibrous ingrowth that would inhibit bone formation. When the alveolar crest height has been compromised, as in loss of buccal cortical plate, a more rigid membrane may aid regeneration of height and width of the alveolar bone. Titanium-reinforced membranes have been used with good success.

Sclar's Bio-Col technique has also been used with good success for socket preservation. The prepared extraction sockets are grafted with Bio-Oss, a natural, porous bone-grafting material. Next, the grafted socket is isolated with an absorbable collagen material. A temporary prosthesis is then fitted over the membrane to provide support to the membrane and help preserve the normal preextraction gingival contour. The technique uses minimal flap elevation for primary closure.[15]

When the alveolar ridge is deficient in the horizontal or vertical direction, implant placement can be problematic. Adequate alveolar height improves the support of dental implants by decreasing the crown-to-implant ratio. Adequate width allows the practitioner to use a larger implant, increasing the surface area of osseointegration. Onlay grafts from either regional or distal sites are often used to resolve these problems. Once the graft is obtained, it is placed in normal saline to preserve vitality. Blood is not a viable solution, as red blood cells lyse and create an acidic environment. The host site is prepared in accordance with optimum surgical principles already described. Next, the graft is shaped to conform to the deficient site, and any sharp ledges of bone are removed with a bur under copious irrigation. Placement of the onlay graft is preformed with a lag-screw technique, ensuring that vital anatomy is maintained. The lag-screw technique involves predrilling holes in the graft and then passing screws that are smaller in diameter than the drilled holes into the recipient bed. Two titanium screws are used to prevent rotation of the graft. Allograft can then be placed around the border of the secured graft and covered with a membrane. The addition of allograft and corresponding membrane to the site is optional, and depends on the size and shape of the defect and graft. The entire site is then closed with tension-free primary soft-tissue coverage. Tissue dissection beyond the releasing incision and scoring the periosteum of the flap will aid in advancing the tissue for closure.

Additional advanced techniques for alveolar ridge reconstruction include interposition bone grafting, alveolar split technique, and distraction osteogenesis. Complete operative details for these various techniques are beyond the scope of this article, but are important options to provide for patients.

Interpositional bone graft, also known as sandwich osteotomy, is used for increasing vertical height in the severe atrophic maxilla and mandible. The advantages of sandwich osteotomy include minimal bone resorption and stability as compared with onlay bone grafting.[16] The procedure entails a vestibular incision with minimal soft-tissue exposure to make a horizontal and two divergent vertical osteotomies. The cut segment is then elevated, the graft inserted, and a miniplate secured to maintain elevation of the initial osteotomized segment. The wound is then closed primarily and allowed to heal for from 4 to 6 months.

Alveolar ridge split osteotomies are used to widen thin ridges of less than 3 to 4 mm and are used to gain to 2 to 3 mm of width, achieved through a crestal incision with minimal reflection. The ridge is then spilt with small osteotomes used in increasing size to force the direction of the split buccally. The site is then grafted and closed primary with split-thickness dissection of the mucoperiosteal flap, or covered with a membrane and closed with sutures. Implants often are simultaneously placed with bone graft.

A variation of the alveolar split is the island flap osteotomy. The two techniques are identical until the buccal bone is split. At this point, to complete an island flap the buccal plate is fractured away from the alveolar ridge to create an island of bone attached to the buccal periosteum. Similar to fracture of the buccal plate is a traumatic extraction. The advantage of this flap is that it provides an environment for vertical and horizontal augmentation. The site is then grafted and closed with a membrane. The buccal plate is not rigidly fixed and is held in place with sutures.

Distraction osteogenesis is often used for severe defects that require more than 5 mm expansion in either horizontal or vertical dimensions. The distraction technique involves creating an osteotomy in a bony segment adjacent to an area of deficiency. Through a distraction device, slow-tension forces are applied between the basal bone and the transport segment, allowing for growth of both bone and soft tissue. McCormick[17] proposes the 5 components of distraction osteogenesis as: (1) osteotomy of the bone site with minimal periosteal stripping; (2) latency period of 3 to 7 days, depending on the surgical site; (3) distraction rate of 1.0 mm per day (range 0.5–2.0 mm); (4) distraction rhythm of distraction twice a day is preferred; and (5) consolidation of usually 6 to 12 weeks.

SUMMARY

Alveolar bone grafting can be very intimidating when first attempted. With careful instruction, education, and practice, grafting can be accomplished by many practitioners. Different methods incorporate similar surgical principles and lead to the development of more advanced grafting techniques.

REFERENCES

1. Olsen B, Reginato A, Wang W. Bone development. Annu Rev Cell Dev Biol 2000; 16:191–220.
2. Wilk RM. Bony reconstruction of jaws. In: Miloro M, editor. Peterson's principles of oral and maxillofacial surgery. 2nd edition. London: BC Decker Inc Hamilton; 2004. p. 783–801.
3. Boyce T, Edwards J, Scarborough N. Allograft bone. The influence of processing on safety and performance. Orthop Clin North Am 1999;30(4):571–81.
4. Conrad E, Gretch D, Obermeyer K, et al. Transmission of the hepatitis-C virus by tissue transplantation. J Bone Joint Surg Am 1995;77(2):214–24.

5. Misch C. Keys to bone grafting and bone grafting materials. In: Contemporary implant dentistry. St Louis (MI): Mosby Elsevier; 2008. p. 839–69.

6. Tolstunov L, Chi J. Alveolar ridge augmentation: comparison of two socket graft materials in implant cases. Comp Cont Educ Dent 2011;32(2):45–8.

7. Reddi AH, Reddi A. Bone morphogenetic proteins (BMPs): from morphogens to metabologens. Cytokine Growth Factor Rev 2009;20(5–6):341–3.

8. Linde A, Alberius P, Dahlin C, et al. Osteopromotion: a soft tissue exclusion principle using a membrane for bone healing and bone neogenesis. J Periodontol 1993;64:1116–28.

9. Sittitavornwong S, Gutta R. Bone graft harvesting from regional sites. Oral Maxillofac Surg Clin North Am 2010;22(3):317–30, v–vi.

10. Zouhary K. Bone graft harvesting from distant sites: concepts and techniques. Oral Maxillofac Surg Clin North Am 2010;22(3):301–14.

11. Tessier P, Kawamoto H, Posnick J, et al. Complications of harvesting autogenous bone grafts: a group experience of 20,000 cases. Plast Reconstr Surg 2005;166: 72–3.

12. Misch C. Tooth extraction, socket grafting and barrier membrane bone regeneration. In: Contemporary implant dentistry. St Louis (MI): Mosby Elsevier; 2008. p. 870–901.

13. Lekovic V, Camargo PM, Klokkevold PR, et al. Preservation of alveolar bone in extraction sockets using bioabsorbable membranes. J Periodontol 1998;69(9): 1044–9.

14. Iasella JM, Greenwell H, Miller RL, et al. Ridge preservation with freeze-dried bone allograft and a collagen membrane compared to extraction alone for implant site development: a clinical and histologic study in humans. J Periodontol 2003;74(7):990–9.

15. Sclar AG. Preserving alveolar ridge anatomy following tooth removal in conjunction with immediate implant placement. The Bio-Col technique. Atlas Oral Maxillofac Surg Clin North Am 1999;7(2):39–59.

16. Jensen J, Sindet-Pedersen S. Autogenous mandibular bone grafts and osseointegrated implants for reconstruction of the severely atrophied maxilla: a preliminary report. J Oral Maxillofac Surg 1991;49(12):1277–87.

17. McCormick S. Distraction osteogenesis. In: Miloro M, editor. Peterson's principles of oral and maxillofacial surgery. 2nd edition. London: BC Decker Inc Hamilton; 2004. p. 1278–95.

Sinus Lift Procedures: An Overview of Current Techniques

Avichai Stern, DDS*, James Green, DMD

KEYWORDS

- Sinus lift • Sinus reconstruction • Bone morphogenic protein
- Osteotomy

For more than 30 years the maxillary sinus augmentation graft has been a mainstay of implant-directed maxillary reconstruction.[1] The purpose of this article is to review the fundamentals of maxillary sinus reconstruction including anatomy and physiology of the sinus, indications for surgery, preoperative evaluation, surgical techniques, and management of complications.

ANATOMY AND PHYSIOLOGY

The paired maxillary sinuses are air-filled spaces lying within the bilateral maxillae, lateral to the nasal cavity, superior to the maxillary teeth, inferior to the orbital floors, and anterior to the infratemporal fossa (**Fig. 1**). These sinuses are the largest of the paranasal sinuses, measuring an average of 12.5 mL in volume.[2] The maxillary sinuses are lined with a thin bilaminar mucoperiosteal membrane known as the Schneiderian membrane, which comprises ciliated pseudostratified columnar epithelium (respiratory epithelium) on the lumen side and a single-cell osteogenic periosteal layer (cambium layer) on the bone side. The infraorbital nerve runs in a posterior-anterior direction in the middle of the maxillary roof. In most cases the canal floor is composed of thick bone; however, in some cases the canal floor is not present, leaving only a thin layer of mucosa between the nerve and the sinus cavity.[3] The sinus ostium, located in the superior aspect of the medial sinus wall superior to the uncinate process, opens into the ethmoid infundibulum located in the middle meatus along the lateral nasal wall. Thin, bony septae that span from the lateral sinus wall to the medial sinus wall may be present in up to 37% of patients with 22.5% of those in the anterior third of the sinus, 45.9% in the middle, and 31.5% in the posterior. One or two septae are present in 89% of patients with septae.[4] The presence and location of septae may

Department of Dentistry/Oral and Maxillofacial Surgery, The Brooklyn Hospital, 121 DeKalb Avenue, Box 187, Brooklyn, NY 11201, USA
* Corresponding author.
E-mail address: Avistern.dds@gmail.com

Dent Clin N Am 56 (2012) 219–233
doi:10.1016/j.cden.2011.09.003
0011-8532/12/$ – see front matter © 2012 Elsevier Inc. All rights reserved.

dental.theclinics.com

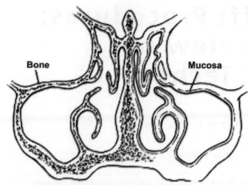

Fig. 1. Coronal view of the ostiomeatal complex. The uncinate process lies in a sagittal plane. The maxillary sinus ostium drains into the infundibulum. (*From* Flint PW, Haughey BH, Lund V, et al. Cummings otolaryngology head and neck surgery review. 5th edition. St Louis (MO): Mosby; 2011; with permission.)

affect a treatment plan, and failure to identify them preoperatively may result in perioperative complications, as discussed later.

Of physiologic importance is that the membrane cilia guide mucous discharge and debris toward the ostium so that in normal-functioning sinuses drainage is constantly maintained. Some conditions may predispose certain patients to chronic sinusitis. Allergic rhinitis causes inflammation of the mucosa at the ostium, leading to local swelling and subsequent blockage of the outflowing mucous discharge, resulting in painful sinus pressure as well as infection of the stagnant fluid. Dysfunctional sinus cilia may also lead to accumulation of mucus and debris, resulting in infection due to the inability of the sinus to clear normal discharge and associated debris.[5]

INDICATIONS AND CONTRAINDICATIONS FOR SINUS RECONSTRUCTION

The primary indication for sinus graft surgery is the planned implant reconstruction of the edentulous posterior maxilla afflicted with postextraction alveolar bone loss and sinus pneumatization, resulting in bone too atrophic for said implant placement (**Table 1**). Sinus graft surgery is indicated for single-tooth and multiple-teeth reconstruction as well as reconstruction of the completely edentulous posterior maxilla.

PREOPERATIVE EVALUATION

A comprehensive history and physical examination should be performed before initiating surgical treatment. Pertinent positives in the history such as recent upper respiratory infection, chronic sinus disease, chronic sinus/facial pain, otitis media, history of nasal/sinus surgery, history of prior attempts at maxillary reconstruction, and history of smoking are important to note. Research has shown that the complication rate for sinus lift grafts performed on smokers is similar to the complication rate for the general population. However, there is evidence that smokers with implants placed in sinus-grafted bone have an increased failure rate when compared with nonsmokers.[6,7] A preoperative computed tomography (CT) scan is recommended to assess the existing bone volume, rule out preexisting sinus disease, and evaluate for the presence of bony septae.[8]

Table 1
Indications for sinus lift surgery

Condition	Treatment
Edentulous maxilla with severely atrophic maxilla and pneumatized sinus	Open sinus lift via lateral maxilla sinus antrostomy; delayed implant placement
Edentulous maxilla with some remaining alveolar bone (0–4 mm)	Open sinus lift via lateral maxilla sinus antrostomy; delayed implant placement
Edentulous maxilla with some remaining alveolar bone (5–10 mm)	Open sinus lift via lateral maxilla sinus antrostomy; immediate implant placement
Single-tooth edentulous space with 5–7 mm alveolar bone remaining	Open sinus lift via lateral maxilla sinus antrostomy; immediate implant placement
Single-tooth edentulous space with >8 mm bone remaining	Open sinus lift via lateral maxilla sinus antrostomy or closed (crestal approach) osteotome technique; immediate implant placement

INFORMED CONSENT

As with all surgical procedures, an informed consent discussion must take place before initiation of the procedure. The discussion must include the usual elements of the informed consent process including the risks, benefits, and alternatives to the procedure as well as the risks of the alternatives to the procedure. Typically the risks of maxillary sinus grafting include (but are not limited to) pain, bleeding from the incision site, infection (acute and/or chronic), swelling, graft failure, need for future surgery, hypesthesia, paresthesia, and/or dysesthesia in the distribution of the second branch of cranial nerve V (which includes the lateral nose, lower eyelid, cheek, upper lip, upper teeth and gums), and that this sensation change may be permanent although usually it resolves within 6 months. Smokers should be counseled that although the graft procedure may be successful, they place themselves at higher risk for implant failure with continued smoking. The benefit of the procedure is the ability to eventually reconstruct the edentulous maxilla. Although this benefit is obvious, it must be clearly stated as part of this discussion so that the patient is clear about the indication for the surgery. The most common alternatives to the procedure include a shorter implant, a 3-unit bridge, or a partial denture. Zygomaticus implants and angled implants may also be alternatives. The risks of the alternatives should be discussed as well. In addition, it is important to stress that this surgery is completely elective and that after considering the possible alternatives, the decision to proceed is the patient's alone. It is also imperative to emphasize that the expected timeframe from this procedure to dental restoration can commonly exceed 1 year, as well as the costs associated with all additional procedures. Patient education videos are available, which provide a multimedia overview of the informed consent process and thus can help solidify difficult concepts. Using other visual aids such as models and radiographs also helps.

SURGICAL TECHNIQUES

There are currently two techniques widely used for maxillary sinus augmentation, the lateral window technique and sinus intrusion osteotomy technique. These methods have been shown to be two of the most stable techniques for vertical augmentation in the oral cavity. When performing these techniques several types of bone graft material can be used including autogenous bone, allograft, xenograft, and alloplastic materials. The graft material chosen must provide adequate viable bone to stabilize the implant initially and encourage osseointegration.[9] Autogenous bone is considered the ideal graft for the sinus lift technique. Although other graft materials can provide adequate bone levels initially, recent studies have shown that autogenous bone grafts have adequate height of alveolar ridge 5 to 10 years after initial placement.[10] Often demineralized freeze-dried bone can be added to autogenous bone to increase the volume of bone placed into the maxillary sinus. Studies have shown that the addition of demineralized freeze-dried bone to autogenous bone slightly lowers the bone level obtained. This lowering was statistically significant, but minimal clinical difference existed due to the implants being still covered with bone.[9]

Autogenous bone grafts are the only graft materials that contain endosteal osteoblasts, giving them osteogenic properties and the ability to directly form bone. In addition to providing osteoblasts for direct bone formation, a corticocancellous graft will provide bone morphogenic proteins (BMPs) and growth factors that will induce bone formation.[11] Many different sites can be used to obtain bone grafts, including the anterior iliac crest, calvarium, proximal tibia, and maxillofacial regions. Most of these techniques are outside the scope of this article, and their individual techniques are not discussed here.

Several sites can be used to harvest bone intraorally. These sites can come from the maxillary tuberosity, the symphysis, the ramus, posterior maxilla, and mandibular third molar site. The maxillary tuberosity offers a small amount of bone (1–2 mL) but should be considered because it is in the same surgical field as the lateral approach to the maxillary sinus.[12] To obtain the graft a crestal incision is made in the posterior maxilla to the area of the hamular notch, with vertical releasing incisions as needed. If the lateral window approach is to be used to access the maxillary sinus, the incision is extended posteriorly to allow access to the tuberosity. A full-thickness mucoperiosteal flap is raised to expose the posterior maxilla. A rongeur can then be used to harvest the bone. When performing this technique care must be taken to avoid the maxillary sinus, pterygoid plates, molar teeth, and the greater palatine canal (**Fig. 2**). The symphysis donor site offers the greatest volume of intraoral bone.[13] To access this region a vestibular incision is made from canine to canine. The incision should be placed at least 3 mm from the mucogingival junction. The periosteum is elevated and the osteotomy is performed 10 mm inferior to the apex of the incisor teeth.

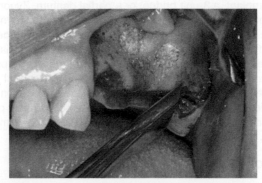

Fig. 2. Bone harvesting. (*From* Fonseca RJ, Marciani RD, Turvey TA. Oral and maxillofacial surgery. 2nd edition. Philadelphia: Saunders; 2008. p. 409; with permission.)

A trephine with a collecting device placed within the suction line can be used to harvest the bone.[9] If needed, the cortical plate can be removed and the marrow harvested (**Fig. 3**). Care must be taken to avoid the mental nerve, and the patient should be informed of the increased chance of V3 paresthesia from this procedure. Similar to this procedure, a scraping device with a collection container attached to the suction can be used to obtain bone from the posterior maxilla and mandibular third molar sites.

The lateral window technique was first demonstrated by Tatum[14] by using a modified Caldwell-Luc approach. The surgical technique consists of osteotomies to form a bony window and either the removal or medial rotation of this window without perforating the sinus membrane. Before starting, local anesthetic with epinephrine is administered by performing a posterior superior alveolar nerve block, anterior superior alveolar nerve block, and palatal infiltration. Local anesthesia can be used with intravenous sedation or general anesthesia if indicated. Conventionally, prophylactic antibiotics and steroids are administered before starting the procedure. The surgeon should use his or her discretion when using perioperative steroids and antibiotics. There is no solid evidence to suggest whether the surgeon should use these medications preoperatively, therefore one should weigh the benefits and risks before administering these medications. Before making the incision it is recommended to have the patient rinse and expectorate with 0.12% chlorhexidine rinse. A crestal incision is made from the maxillary tuberosity to a point just anterior to the anterior border of the sinus. Vertical releasing incisions are then made in the anterior and posterior aspect to the depth of the vestibule. The incisions must allow adequate exposure of the sinus and should not be placed in the area of the sinus window. A full-thickness mucoperiosteal flap is then elevated, exposing the lateral wall of the maxilla (**Fig. 4**). At this point the 4 linear osteotomies are performed with a #6 or #8 round bur. The first to be done is the inferior horizontal osteotomy, which is made as close as possible to the floor of the sinus and no more than 2 to 3 mm above the floor. The osteotomy runs from the area of the first or second molar posteriorly to the anterior extent of the maxillary sinus (**Fig. 5**). When performing the osteotomies one must take care to do so with a light touch and a brushing stroke so not to tear the Schneiderian membrane. When bicuspid teeth are present, care must be taken not to damage them and one should limit the osteotomy 4 mm from the distal aspect of the tooth. The superior horizontal osteotomy is performed next at the level of the planned augmentation height. The superior and inferior osteotomies are connected with the anterior and posterior vertical osteotomies. The vertical osteotomies are

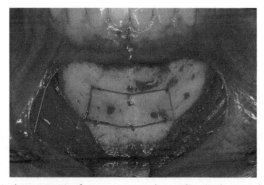

Fig. 3. The unicortical osteotomies form a rectangular outline in the symphysis. (*From* Fonseca RJ, Marciani RD, Turvey TA. Oral and maxillofacial surgery. 2nd edition. Philadelphia: Saunders; 2008. p. 410; with permission.)

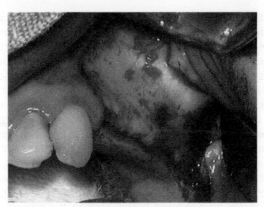

Fig. 4. Incision and mucoperiosteal flap reflection. (*From* Fonseca RJ, Marciani RD, Turvey TA. Oral and maxillofacial Surgery. 2nd edition. Philadelphia: Saunders; 2008. p. 459; with permission.)

made parallel to the lateral nasal wall and the anterior border of the maxillary tuberosity (or the maxillary buttress), respectively (**Fig. 6**). Once the window is created and the membrane exposed, the bone that is adherent is either removed or rotated in medially. If the bony window is rotated inward it then becomes the new floor of the maxillary sinus.

The Schneiderian membrane is then elevated by starting at the edges and then gradually increasing the amount of membrane elevation. If elevation is too excessive in one area, perforation may occur. The elevation can be performed using broad-based freers or curettes. The membrane can and should be elevated higher than the superior osteotomy. It is important to do this to prevent excessive pressure on

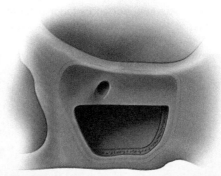

Fig. 5. Diagram demonstrating the ideal location of sinus window preparation of the lateral maxillary wall. The inferior ostectomy should be approximately 1 mm superior to or level with the floor of the sinus. The posterior ostectomy should be at the corner of the maxillary buttress. The anterior ostectomy should be adjacent to and parallel with the lateral wall of the nose, and the superior ostectomy should be at the height of the intended graft. (*From* Block MS. Color atlas of dental implant surgery. 2nd edition. Philadelphia: Saunders; 2007. p. 129; with permission.)

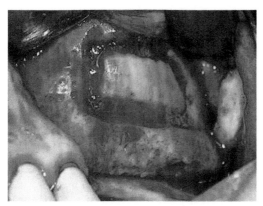

Fig. 6. Complete quadrilateral osteotomy. (*From* Fonseca RJ, Marciani RD, Turvey TA. Oral and maxillofacial surgery. 2nd edition. Philadelphia: Saunders; 2008. p. 460; with permission.)

the bone graft material (**Fig. 7**). Perforation of the sinus membrane is a possibility, and may occur (**Fig. 8**). Small perforations can be left untreated, but if a large perforation occurs the clinician should either abort the procedure or use a collagen membrane to patch the membrane. If the procedure is aborted, it should not be reattempted for an additional 4 to 6 months. Once the membrane is elevated, the bone graft material is placed under the membrane in an anterior and inferior direction. The graft should contact the medial wall of the maxillary sinus. The graft is placed in the cavity loosely and should not be overpacked. The surgeon should add an additional 20% of bone graft to compensate for loss of graft volume (**Fig. 9**). After the bone is placed in the sinus, the mucoperiosteal flap is repositioned and sutured. Implants can be placed 6 months after the sinus lift procedure is performed. If there is adequate alveolar bone to stabilize the implants, the implant sites are prepared and the implants are placed before the bone graft, with the bone graft material being packed around the implants (**Fig. 10**). It is recommended to place the patient on postoperative antibiotics and decongestants for 2 weeks. Patients should also be placed on sinus precautions, should not blow their nose, and should cough or sneeze with their mouth open.

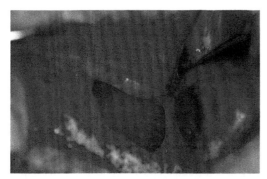

Fig. 7. Membrane is carefully elevated and reflected medially into the sinus. (*From* Block MS. Color atlas of dental implant surgery. 2nd edition. Philadelphia: Saunders; 2007. p. 134; with permission.)

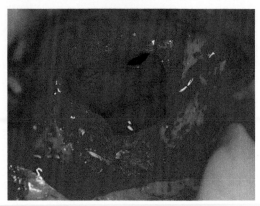

Fig. 8. Crestal incision is combined with anterior and posterior vertical release incisions to allow for exposure of lateral wall of the maxilla. Lateral wall of the sinus is rotated medially with membrane reflection. A small perforation is present. (*From* Block MS. Color atlas of dental implant surgery. 2nd edition. Philadelphia: Saunders; 2007. p. 145; with permission.)

Piezoelectric technology is an ultrasonic device that is used to make the osteotomies. This system has been shown to help avoid perforating the sinus membrane. The piezoelectric surgery systems have been designed to use a specific power that is higher than traditional ultrasonic instruments. This higher power allows the osteotomies to be made even in thicker, more compact cortical bone. The real advantage of this system is that it does not cut soft tissue and helps to reduce the chance of perforating the membrane. The surgical instrument can even be used to assist in the elevation of the sinus membrane. This instrument is helpful with robust areas of bone and thin membranes. The piezoelectric surgery systems come with many different inserts, from osteotomes, to diamond-cutting inserts, to inserts to help elevate the sinus membrane. Once the window is made the lifting of the membrane is accomplished by separating the endosteum from bone, and a hydropneumatic pressure of the physiologic saline solution is subjected to the piezoelectric cavitation (**Fig. 11**).[15] A study by Vercellotti and colleagues[16] was performed on 15 patients, creating 21 bony window

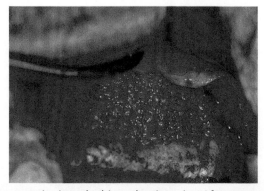

Fig. 9. Bone graft composite is packed into the sinus site. After approximately 6 months, implants are placed; after an additional 6 months, the final restoration is completed. (*From* Block MS. Color atlas of dental implant surgery. 2nd edition. Philadelphia: Saunders; 2007. p. 135; with permission.)

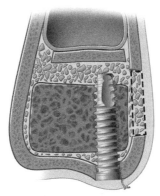

Fig. 10. Diagram showing the lateral wall of the maxilla rotated medially into the sinus, which is optional. Bone graft material is placed into the sinus, either in particulate material or block form, to support the implant. Ideally, the block grafts should engage the superior surface of the implant. (*From* Block MS. Color atlas of dental implant surgery. 2nd edition. Philadelphia: Saunders; 2007. p. 130; with permission.)

osteotomies with a Mectron Piezosurgery System (Mectron Medical Technology, Mectron SPA, Carasco, Italy). The inserts were used with a vibration between 60 and 210 μm with a power exceeding 5 W. All osteotomies are made under irrigation provided by a pump in the surgical system. After reflection of the flap the piezoelectric scalpel is used to make the bony window. The membrane elevator tip is then used beginning at the apical position, then moving to the mesial and distal aspects. Then attention is drawn to the floor of the sinus, a common place to find adhesions, where the membrane is elevated and the risk of perforation reduced. All sinus augmentations in this study were performed with autogenous bone grafts and platelet-rich plasma. Of the 21 cases, only 1 resulted in perforation of the membrane and there was a 95% success rate.

The sinus intrusion osteotomy is indicated when at least 5 to 6 mm of alveolar bone is present. This approach has been shown to add 4 to 8 mm of bone height, but is best indicated when minimal bone height is needed and there is sufficient bone for

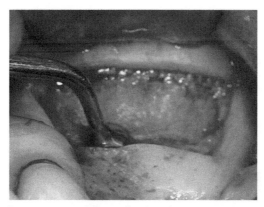

Fig. 11. Incision and mucoperiosteal flap reflection. (*From* Fonseca RJ, Marciani RD, Turvey TA. Oral and maxillofacial surgery, vol. 1. 2nd edition. Philadelphia: Saunders; 2008. p. 462; with permission.)

stabilization of an implant.[17] This technique was developed in 1994 by Summers,[18] and consisted of a crestal incision, preparation of the bone, and elevation of the sinus by several millimeters. When performing this technique one will not only compact bone apically and elevate the sinus but also compact bone laterally by using osteotomes of progressively increasing diameter (**Fig. 12**). Summers performed this procedure in 46 patients, placing 143 implants, and showed a 96% success rate 5 years postoperatively. When performing this procedure a crestal incision is made and the implant drills are used to create an osteotomy, leaving 1 mm of bone between the site and the sinus membrane. After preparing the site with the implant drills, sequential osteotomes are used to the depth of desired implant length; this compacts bone lateral and apical, and elevates the sinus membrane. Once at the desired length and diameter, bone graft material is placed in the apical portion of the prepared site (**Fig. 13**). The implant is placed next to the desired length, and care is taken to ensure that the implant is stable. A coverscrew is placed and primary closure is achieved. After 4 to 6 months of healing the implant can be uncovered and the healing abutment placed. Komarnyckys and London[19] performed this procedure in 16 patients and placed 43 implants, showing a 95.3% success rate. This study had a follow-up that ranged from 9 to 47 months and showed a mean bone gain of 3.25 mm.

An alternative to bone graft material is bone morphogenic protein (BMP), which is becoming more and more popular. BMPs are transforming growth factors that contain bone-inductive properties.[20] There are two recombinant human proteins that are currently available: rhBMP-2 and rhBMP-7. This material is used in place of bone graft material for spinal fusion, treatment of bone defects, fracture repair, and reconstruction of the maxillofacial region. Advantages of using this material include no harvest-site morbidity, enhanced soft-tissue healing, ease of use, and possible use in patients who are not autogenous graft candidates.[9] BMP comes in the form of a powder that is reconstituted with sterile water and applied to a carrier at the time of the surgery. The carrier material is resorbed over time, and its purpose is to maintain the rhBMP at the treatment site and to act as a temporary scaffold for osteogenesis. The most commonly used carrier for maxillary sinus augmentation is the collagen carrier. This carrier is adequate for maxillary sinus augmentation, but does not have any mechanical strength and must be used in an area that has borders in all dimensions.[9] The following discussion describes the use of BMP-2 on a collagen sponge. When using

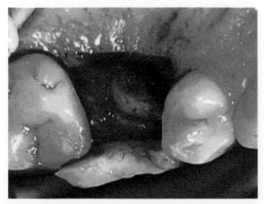

Fig. 12. Trephined bone core partially intruded into sinus cavity. (*From* Fonseca RJ, Marciani RD, Turvey TA. Oral and maxillofacial surgery. 2nd edition. Philadelphia: Saunders; 2008. p. 465; with permission.)

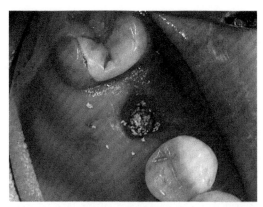

Fig. 13. Graft placed through implant receptor site into sinus cavity. (*From* Fonseca RJ, Marciani RD, Turvey TA. Oral and maxillofacial surgery. 2nd edition. Philadelphia: Saunders; 2008. p. 468; with permission.)

BMP-2 for maxillary sinus augmentation the lateral window method is preferred, and there are very few data to show success through the sinus intrusion osteotomy. Local anesthetic is administered, an incision is made, full-thickness mucoperiosteal flap is raised, bony osteotomies are made, and sinus membrane is elevated as previously described. If a membrane perforation is encountered it is not necessary to repair this when using BMP, but it may be done if the surgeon prefers to.

The BMP comes packaged as a lyophilized powder and is reconstituted into the sterile water as per the manufacturer's recommendations. The reconstituted BMP is then placed in a sterile syringe and applied to the collagen sponge (**Fig. 14**). When placing the liquid on the sponge, drops are applied equally along the sponge and allowed to sit for at least 15 minutes. This period of time allows the BMP to adhere to the collagen sponge. The sponge can then be cut into 15-mm strips and placed into the sinus between the bony floor and membrane (**Fig. 15**). Primary closure is then achieved with chromic gut sutures. Antibiotics are given for 1 week and the

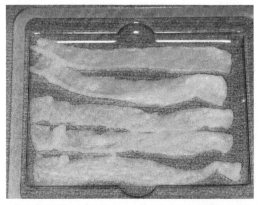

Fig. 14. BMP is placed onto collagen sponge and the sponge is cut into five or six strips. (*From* Block MS. Color atlas of dental implant surgery. Philadelphia: Saunders; 2007. p. 147; with permission.)

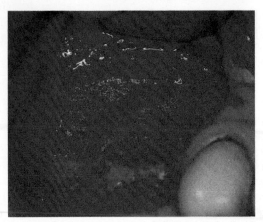

Fig. 15. BMP impregnated collagen membrane is placed into the sinus with no membranes used to cover the sinus graft site. (*From* Block MS. Color atlas of dental implant surgery. Philadelphia: Saunders; 2007. p. 147; with permission.)

patient is placed on sinus precautions. One should advise the patient that significant swelling is likely to occur. After 4 months a postoperative panoramic radiograph can be obtained showing bone formation, and implants can be placed 6 months after the procedure. One of the earliest studies showing the successful use of rhBMP-2 was done by Boyne and colleagues,[21] in which 12 patients had rhBMP-2 placed into their maxillary sinus. The mean height of bone was 8.51 mm. The most significant postoperative side effects were facial edema, erythema, pain, and rhinitis. In another study rhBMP-2 was compared with anterior iliac crest grafts in 30 rabbits.[22] Implants were placed in the augmented sinuses 12 weeks later and allowed to integrate for 3 months. The mean vertical bone gain was greatest in the rhBMP-2 group, and showed that the bone between both groups was of similar quality. Recombinant BMP is contraindicated in patients with hypersensitivity to the protein, carrier, or any other components of the formulation. It should not be used in patients with an active malignancy or being treated for a malignancy, in areas of existing or resected tumors, in skeletally immature patients, in pregnant women, or in areas of active infection. BMP is an excellent alternative for patients who do not wish to undergo a separate procedure to obtain bone graft material, and should be considered.

POSTOPERATIVE INSTRUCTIONS AND MANAGEMENT

The patient should be provided with a printed set of postoperative instructions as well as an oral review of the instructions with the surgeon. Typically the patient is cautioned against consuming anything hard or rough that may damage the sutures and lead to wound dehiscence. Sinus precautions are advised as well, and include avoiding anything that can cause sudden pressure changes in the sinus such as nose blowing and sneezing. The patient should be instructed to sneeze only with an open mouth so that pressure can be directed away from the sinus. There are several things that the patient should be told to expect after surgery. Soreness is, of course, normal and expected for several days after surgery. It is normal for some patients to experience some bleeding from the surgical incision for up to 24 hours after surgery. This bleeding will appear to be worse than it is, due to the blood mixing with saliva. The blood should be swallowed (not expectorated), and if bothersome is controllable with direct wet gauze pressure. If after 2 applications of gauze of 1 hour each the bleeding persists or if the volume is of concern, the patient should inform the surgeon. Swelling and occasional skin bruising is not uncommon after sinus lift surgery.

MANAGEMENT OF COMPLICATIONS

The most common surgical complication of the maxillary sinus lift is perforation of the Schneiderian membrane (**Table 2**). In a recent prospective observational uncontrolled study, 70 patients underwent 81 sinus lifts and were followed through to loading of a total of 212 implants. Forty-four percent of the sinuses were perforated intraoperatively but were repaired, and the procedure was completed without other complications. Two percent of the sinuses suffered perforations so severe that the procedure was aborted. Thirty-three percent of the perforations occurred in sinuses that had septae noted on preoperative radiographs, and of those sinuses with septae 52% suffered perforations. Two of the 36 perforations were so severe that the surgeon aborted the procedure. Common modalities for dealing with sinus perforation include doing nothing if the perforation is less than 2 mm in diameter and placement of a slowly resorbing collagen membrane if larger than 2 mm. Postoperative complications in the study included graft extrusion into the sinus cavity in one patient presenting as an acute sinusitis after implant placement. After surgical and medical treatment, the infection resolved and the implants went on to be restored. Late complications included persistent peri-implantitis and a peri-impant cyst. Of importance is that although membrane perforations were associated with postoperative complications such as swelling, pain, and local infection, there is no association between intraoperative perforations and long-term implant survival. Overall, this study demonstrated a 95.5% 7-year survival rate for implants placed in the grafted sinuses. Also of note is that of the 9 implants that failed, 5 were placed in patients who were heavy smokers. Chronic infections leading to severe sinusitis and possible graft exposure, extrusion, and/or failure are rare events. Management typically involves treatment based on the presenting symptoms, and can range from antibiotics to surgical debridement drainage to a Caldwell-Luc procedure.[23–25]

Table 2
Common sinus lift surgery complications

Complication	Treatment
Graft exposure	Gentle daily normal saline irrigation, allow for creeping epithelialization
No graft present after maturation phase	Assess for possible etiology and retreat
Paresthesia CN V2 distribution immediately postop	Medrol dose pack if no contraindication
Facial swelling 2–3 days post surgery	No treatment, normal postop
Severe facial ecchymosis appearing 1–3 days postop	No treatment, normal postop
Facial pain and swelling, 1 week postop	Clinical examination, CT scan, consider antibiotics
Swelling, acute onset	Possible air-emphysema; antibiotics, reinforce nasal precautions

SUMMARY

The maxillary sinus lift has, over the last 30 years, been established as an accepted standard for treatment of the edentulous maxilla. Alternatives such as short implants, although shown to be effective in the short term, lack long-term studies to support routine use. While there are some relative contraindications for the procedure, there are almost no absolute contraindications. With preparation, education, and experience, the maxillary sinus augmentation/elevation graft is a procedure that greatly benefits the patient, with a predictable outcome.

REFERENCES

1. Boyne PJ, James RA. Grafting of the maxillary sinus floor with autogenous marrow and bone. J Oral Surg 1980;38(8):613–6.
2. Gosau M, Rink D, Driemel O, et al. Maxillary sinus anatomy: a cadaveric study with clinical implications. Anat Rec (Hoboken) 2009;292(3):352–4.
3. Yanagisawa E, Yanagisawa K. Endoscopic view of the infraorbital nerve. Ear Nose Throat J 1999;78(4):226–8.
4. Park YB, Jeon HS, Shim JS, et al. Analysis of the anatomy of the maxillary sinus septum using 3-dimensional computed tomography. J Oral Maxillofac Surg 2011; 69(4):1070–8.
5. Gudis DA, Cohen NA. Cilia dysfunction. Otolaryngol Clin North Am 2010;43(3): 461–72, vii.
6. Kan JY, Rungcharassaeng K, Lozada JL, et al. Effects of smoking on implant success in grafted maxillary sinuses. J Prosthet Dent 1999;82(3):307–11.
7. Levin L, Herzberg R, Dolev E, et al. Smoking and complications of onlay bone grafts and sinus lift operations. Int J Oral Maxillofac Implants 2004;19(3): 369–73.
8. Cote MT, Segelnick SL, Rastogi A, et al. New York State ear, nose, and throat specialists' views on pre-sinus lift referral. J Periodontol 2011;82(2):227–33.
9. Block MS. Color atlas of dental implant surgery. St Louis (MO): Saunders/Elsevier; 2007.
10. Block MS, Kent JN, Kallukaran FU, et al. Bone maintenance 5 to 10 years after sinus grafting. J Oral Maxillofac Surg 1998;56:706.
11. Goldberg VM, Stevenson S. The biology of bone grafts. Semin Arthroplasty 1993; 4:58–63.
12. Misch CE. Maxillary sinus augmentation for endosteal implants: organized alternative treatment plans. Int J Oral Implantol 1987;4:49–58.
13. Misch C. Autogenous bone grafting for dental implants. St Louis (MO): Saunders; 2009.
14. Tatum H Jr. Maxillary and sinus implant reconstructions. Dent Clin North Am 1986; 30:207.
15. Raja SV. Managament of the posterior maxilla sinus lift: review of techniques. J Oral Maxillofac Surg 2009;67:1730–4.
16. Vercellotti T, De Paoli S, Nevins M. The piezoelectric bony window osteotomy and sinus membrane elevation: introduction of a new technique for simplification of sinus augmentation procedures. Int J Periodontics Restorative Dent 2001; 21:561.
17. Smiler D, Soltan M, Ghostine MS. Contemporary sinus-lift subantral surgery and graft. St Louis (MO): Saunders; 2009.
18. Summers RB. A new concept in maxillary implant surgery: the osteotome technique. Compend Contin Educ Dent 1994;15:152.

19. Komarnyckys OG, London RM. Osteotome single-stage dental implant placement with and without sinus elevation: a clinical report. Int J Oral Maxillofac Implants 1998;13:219.
20. Reddi AH. Role of morphogenetic proteins in skeletal tissue engineering and regeneration. Nat Biotechnol 1998;16:247.
21. Boyne PJ, Marx RE, Nevins M, et al. A feasibility study evaluating rhBMP-2/absorbable collagen sponge for maxillary sinus floor augmentation. Int J Periodontics Restorative Dent 1997;17(1):11.
22. Wada K, Niimi A, Watanabe K, et al. Maxillary sinus floor augmentation in rabbits: a comparative histologic histomorphogenetic study between rhBMP-2 and autogenous bone. Int J Periodontics Restorative Dent 2001;21:253.
23. Schwartz-Arad D, Herzberg R, Dolev E. The prevalence of surgical complications of the sinus graft procedure and their impact on implant survival. J Periodontol 2004;75(4):511-6.
24. Becker ST, Terheyden H, Steinriede A, et al. Prospective observation of 41 perforations of the Schneiderian membrane during sinus floor elevation. Clin Oral Implants Res 2008;19(12):1285-9.
25. Vandeweghe S, De Ferrerre R, Tschakaloff A, et al. A wide-body implant as an alternative for sinus lift or bone grafting. J Oral Maxillofac Surg 2011;69(6):e67-74.

Review of Antibiotics and Indications for Prophylaxis

Adam Weiss, DDS[a],*, Harry Dym, DDS[b]

KEYWORDS

- Antibiotic prophylaxis • Joint replacement
- Methicillin-resistant *Staphylococcus aureus* • Endocarditis
- American Heart Association guidelines • Heart valves
- Bacteremia

Antibiotic prophylaxis as an attempt to prevent infective endocarditis (IE) is an extremely important, controversial, and evolving topic that is important for dental professionals to address. IE is an uncommon, but life-threatening infection of the inner lining of the heart (endocardium). This infection is characterized by the presence of vegetations composed of platelets, fibrin, microorganisms, and inflammatory cells. The pathogenesis of IE involves a complex sequence or confluence of events. Endothelial damage caused by turbulent blood flow normally seen in congenital or acquired heart disease causes platelets and fibrin deposition leading to formation of nonbacterial thrombotic endocarditis (NBTE). In this environment, an incidence of bacteremia could result in bacterial adherence to NBTE, bacterial proliferation within the NBTE, and formation of vegetations, the typical lesions of IE. This infection usually happens when bacteria or other germs from another part of the body, such as the mouth, spread through the bloodstream and attach to damaged areas in the heart. IE most commonly occurs in conjunction with invasive dental, gastrointestinal (GI), or genitourinary (GU) tract procedures. Certain underlying cardiac conditions may predispose an individual to developing endocarditis, such as artificial heart valves. If left untreated, endocarditis can damage or destroy heart valves and can lead to life-threatening complications. Often patients with IE have substantial morbidity and mortality despite technological and medical advancements.

[a] Division of Oral and Maxillofacial Surgery, The Brooklyn Hospital Center, 121 DeKalb Avenue, Brooklyn, NY 11201, USA
[b] Department of Dentistry/Oral and Maxillofacial Surgery, The Brooklyn Hospital Center, 121 DeKalb Avenue, Brooklyn, NY 11201, USA
* Corresponding author.
E-mail address: aweissdds@gmail.com

Dent Clin N Am 56 (2012) 235–244
doi:10.1016/j.cden.2011.07.003
0011-8532/12/$ – see front matter © 2012 Elsevier Inc. All rights reserved.

WHY WERE THE PREVIOUS GUIDELINES CHANGED?

The most recent guidelines on IE prophylaxis were published by the American Heart Association (AHA) in 1997.[1] This separated cardiac conditions into high-, moderate-and low-risk (negligible risk) categories, with prophylaxis not advised for the low-risk group. A detailed list of dental, respiratory, GI and GU, tract procedures for which prophylaxis was and was not recommended was included. The decision to revise the old IE prophylaxis guidelines and issue a revised document was made for a variety of reasons. It was found that the basis for recommendations for IE prophylaxis was not well-established, and the quality of evidence was limited to a few case–control studies or was based on expert opinion, clinical experience, and descriptive studies, which used surrogate measures of risk.[2] There were no definitive published data that accurately determined the absolute risk of IE resulting from a dental procedure. One study reported that 10% to 20% of patients with IE caused by oral flora had a prior dental procedure (within 30 or 180 days of onset).[3] Also, the number of cases of IE that could be prevented by antibiotic prophylaxis, even if 100% effective, is very small.[2] Most endocarditis cases caused by oral microflora are the result of bacteremia caused by routine daily activities (eg, tooth brushing and flossing). As a result, the current AHA guidelines shift the emphasis away from antibiotic prophylaxis for dental procedures and toward improved access to dental care and oral health for patients, especially those with underlying cardiac risk factors. Many authorities and advisory bodies have questioned the efficacy of antimicrobial prophylaxis to prevent endocarditis in patients who undergo a dental, GI, or GU tract procedure and have pushed for alterations to the 1997 AHA guidelines. Following along these lines, the British Society for Antimicrobial Chemotherapy recently issued new guidelines for endocarditis prophylaxis that recommended prophylaxis before dental procedures only for patients who have a history of previous endocarditis or who have had cardiac valve replacement or surgically constructed pulmonary shunts or conduits.[4]

2007 UPDATED ANTIBIOTIC PROPHYLAXIS GUIDELINES

In 2007, the AHA released its newly revised guidelines for the prevention of IE. As shown in **Box 1**, the new guidelines[2] include a much more restrictive list of cardiac conditions for which antibiotic prophylaxis is recommended. In contrast to the 1997 guidelines, the AHA now recommends antibiotic prophylaxis only for those whose underlying cardiac conditions are associated with the highest risk of adverse outcome should they contract IE. Such conditions include prosthetic heart valves, previous history of IE, unrepaired cyanotic congenital heart disease (CHD), completely repaired congenital heart defect with prosthetic material or device during the first 6 months after the procedure, repaired CHD with residual defects at the site or adjacent to the site of a prosthetic patch or device, and cardiac transplantation recipients who develop valvulopathy.[2] The committee members believed that prophylaxis for dental procedures in patients with underlying cardiac conditions associated with the highest risk of adverse outcome was reasonable even though its effectiveness is unknown. In contrast to mentioning specific dental procedures that would require prophylaxis as in the old guidelines, the new guidelines suggest that antibiotic prophylaxis is reasonable for all dental procedures that involve manipulation of gingival tissues or the periapical region of teeth or perforation of oral mucosa only for patients with underlying cardiac conditions associated with the highest risk of adverse outcome from IE.[2] However, certain procedures do not require antibiotic prophylaxis, including the routine anesthetic injections through noninfected tissue, the taking of dental radiographs, the placement of removable prosthodontic or orthodontic appliances, and the adjustment

---

Box 1
Cardiac conditions associated with the highest risk of adverse outcome from endocardities for which prophylaxis with dental procedures is reasonable

1. Prosthetic cardiac valve or prosthetic material used for cardiac valve repair

2. Previous infective endocarditis

3. Congenital heart disease (CHD)[a]

    a. Unrepaired cyanotic CHD, including palliative shunts and conduits

    b. Completely repaired congenital heart defect with prosthetic material or device, whether placed by surgery or by catheter intervention, during the first 6 months after the procedure[b]

    c. Repaired CHD with residual defects at the site or adjacent to the site of a prosthetic patch or prosthetic device (which inhibit endothelialization)

4. Cardiac transplantation recipients who develop cardiac valvulopathy

[a] Except for the conditions listed, antibiotic prophylaxis is no longer recommended for any other form of CHD.
[b] Prophylaxis is reasonable, because endothelialization of prosthetic material occurs within 6 months after the procedure.
From Wilson W, Taubert KA, Gewitz M, et al. Prevention of infective endocarditis: guidelines from the American Heart Association: a guideline from the American Heart Association Rheumatic Fever, Endocarditis and Kawasaki Disease Committee, Council on Cardiovascular Disease in the Young, and the Council on Clinical Cardiology, Council on Cardiovascular Surgery and Anesthesia, and the Quality of Care and Outcomes Research Interdisciplinary Working Group. J Am Dent Assoc 2007;138:739–45.

---

of orthodontic appliances **Fig. 1**[2] represents a diagram that dentists can follow when determining whether to suggest antibiotic prophylaxis for their patients before dental treatment.

Antibiotics Used for Prophylaxis

The antibiotics suggested for prophylaxis are shown in **Table 1**. Antibiotics should be given 30 to 60 minutes before starting the indicated procedure. According to the AHA, if the drug is inadvertently omitted before the procedure, it may be administrated up to 2 hours after the procedure with some protective benefit.

Amoxicillin is the preferred option for oral prophylaxis, because it is well-absorbed in the GI tract and provides high and sustained serum concentrations. Ampicillin and amoxicillin are aminopenicillins that have identical coverage as penicillin against the same non–β-lactamase containing gram-positive pathogens. This group has additional coverage against non–β-lactamase producing strains of *Haemophilus influenzae*, *Escherichia coli*, *Proteus mirabilis*, *Salmonella*, and *Shigella* but lacks coverage against *Pseudomonas aeruginosa*. Aminopenicillins have an increased incidence of drug hypersensitivity reactions with rashes as compared with other penicillins.[5]

Cephalosporins are another category of antibiotics that are included as options in the prophylactic regimen. These antibiotics are β-lactam agents that cover a broad spectrum of organisms and are easy to administer with low toxicity issues. They can often be used in place of penicillins when patients have a history of mild rashes associated with penicillin use. However, cephalosporins should not be used in patients who describe anaphylaxis, angioedema, urticaria, or asthma when using

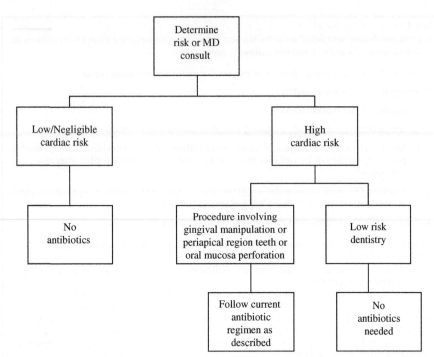

Fig. 1. Preprocedural plan for patients with a history of increased risk of infective endocarditis.

penicillin.[6] Cefazolin the most commonly used intravenous first-generation cephalosporin available and is recommended for patients who those patients who are allergic to penicillin. It has similar activity against most gram-positive cocci including *Staphylococcus aureus*, group A β-hemolytic *Streptococcus* (*Streptococcus pyogenes*), and penicillin-susceptible *Streptococcus pneumonia.* Cephalexin is also a first-generation oral cephalosporin. This agent has high oral bioavailability and is most effective against *Streptococcus pyogenes*. Ceftriaxone is a third-generation cephalosporin that covers many important infections because of its broad coverage, high potency, low toxicity issues, and favorable pharmacokinetics, such as high levels in the cerebrospinal fluid. However, this agent has less activity against gram-positive pathogens compared with the first-generation cephalosporins.[4]

Clarithromycin and azithromycin are bacteriostatic commonly used macrolide antibiotics. Macrolide antibiotics are used to treat infections caused by gram-positive bacteria, *Streptococcus pneumoniae*, and *Haemophilus influenzae* infections such as respiratory tract and soft-tissue infections. The antimicrobial spectrum of macrolides is slightly wider than that of penicillin, and, therefore, macrolides remain a common alternative for patients with a penicillin allergy. Concerns with macrolide antibiotics include GI distress, drug–drug interactions, and QT prolongation.[7]

Clindamycin can also be used for IE prophylaxis before an invasive dental procedure. It is a semisynthetic derivative of lincomycin, a natural antibiotic produced by the actinobacterium *Streptomyces lincolnensis*.[5] It is bacteriostatic by inhibiting protein synthesis. Clindamycin is an excellent agent for the treatment of infections of the oral cavity. It is effective against most pneumococci and streptococci and most penicillin-resistant staphylococci including some methicillin-resistant *Staphylococcus aureus* (MRSA) isolates. *Clostridium difficile* pseudomembranous colitis is

Table 1
Regimens for a dental procedure

Situation	Agent	Regimen: Single Dose 30–60 Minutes Before Procedure	
		Adults	Children
Oral	Amoxicillin	2 g	50 mg/kg
Unable to take oral medicates	Ampicillin or cefazolin or ceftriaxone	2 g IM[a] or IV[b] 1 g IM or IV	50 mg/kg IM or IV 50 mg/kg IM or IV
Allergic to penicillins or ampicillin oral	Cephalexin[c,d] or Clindamycin or Azithromycin or clarithromycin	2 g 600 mg 500 mg	50 mg/kg 20 mg/kg 12 mg/kg
Allergic to penicillins or ampicillin and unable to take oral medication	Cefazolin or ceftriaxonel[d] or clindamycin	1 g IM or IV 600 mg IM or IV	50 mg/kg IM or IV 20 mg/kg IM or IV

[a] IM: Intramuscular.
[b] IV Intravenous.
[c] Or other first- or second-generation oral cephalosporin to equivalent adult or podiatric.
[d] cephalosporin should not be used in a person with a history of anaphylaxis angioedema or urticaria with penicillins or ampicillin.
From Wilson W, Taubert KA, Gewitz M, et al. Prevention of infective endocarditis: guidelines from the American Heart Association: a guideline from the American Heart Association Rheumatic Fever, Endocarditis and Kawasaki Disease Committee, Council on Cardiovascular Disease in the Young, and the Council on Clinical Cardiology, Council on Cardiovascular Surgery and Anesthesia, and the Quality of Care and Outcomes Research Interdisciplinary Working Group. J Am Dent Assoc 2007;138:739–45.

a complication that may occur after all antibacterial agents but has been linked most often with clindamycin. Treatment includes discontinuation of the antibiotic and treatment with oral metronidazole, vancomycin, or nitazoxanide.[5]

Antibiotic Prophylaxis for Full Joint Replacement

Antibiotic prophylaxis for those individuals who have undergone full joint replacement has also been a controversial topic in the past years. Joint guidelines were published in 2003[8] by the American Dental Association (ADA) and the American Academy of Orthopedic Surgeons (AAOS) regarding antibiotic prophylaxis for dental patients with total joint replacements. The 2003 ADA/AAOS guidelines contained the following statement: "The risk/benefit and cost/effectiveness ratios fail to justify the administration of routine antibiotic prophylaxis" for individuals with joint replacements.[8] However, these guidelines also suggest that patients at greater risk because of specific medical conditions should be considered for prophylaxis. These include patients whose prostheses are less than 2 years old or those who have high-risk conditions such as inflammatory arthropathies (rheumatoid arthritis, systemic lupus erythematosus), drug-induced or radiation-induced immunosuppression, previous joint infection, malnourishment, hemophilia, human immunodeficiency virus infection, insulin-dependent diabetes, or malignancy.[8]

In February 2009, without a joint effort with organized dentistry or nonorthopedic physician specialties, the AAOS published what it called an "Information Statement"[9] entitled "Antibiotic Prophylaxis for Bacteremia in Patients With Joint Replacements." It states that it "was developed as an educational tool based on the opinions of the authors. Readers are encouraged to consider the information presented and reach their own conclusions."[9] This new 2009 AAOS statement suggests a different position: "Given the potential adverse outcomes and cost of treating an infected joint replacement, the AAOS recommends that clinicians consider antibiotic prophylaxis for all total joint replacement patients before any invasive procedure that may cause bacteremia."[9] In a position paper from the American Academy of Oral Medicine (AAOM), it was suggested that the statement issued by the AAOS was made with little or no scientific data to suggest a link between late prosthetic joint infections and organisms specific to the mouth.[9,10]

Currently, the ADA and the AAOS are working together to develop evidence-based, clinical practice guidelines for antibiotic prophylaxis for dental patients with total joint replacement. The new guidelines, expected to be complete by the end of 2011, will go through a meticulous evidence-based approach by the AAOS, ADA, and others who participate in the work group put together by the AAOS Guidelines and Technology Oversight Committee.[11]

Antibiotic Prophylaxis for Nonvavular Cardiovascular Devices

The AHA does not recommend secondary antibiotic prophylaxis for patients with non-valvular cardiovascular devices who are undergoing dental, respiratory, GI, or genito-urinary procedures.[12] In most cases of infections of these devices, staphylococci, and not viridans streptococci (found in oral cavity), are the responsible bacteria. As a result, this finding does not support an oral origin for the infecting organisms.[12] Even when viridans streptococci are found in a rare instance, the bacteria are much more likely to result from the cumulative exposure to multiple daily physiologic bacteremias.

Based on this scientific statement, dental patients with nonvalvular cardiovascular devices (prosthetic valves, pacemakers, defibrillators, ventriculoatrial shunts, closure devices, patches, stents, vascular grafts, dacron grafts or patches, vena caval filters, vascular closure devices, total artificial hearts, and L ventricular assist devices) do not require antibiotic prophylaxis for dental treatment. An exception involves patients with nonvalvular cardiovascular devices that undergo incision and drainage for infection at other sites or to replace an infected device.[12] So, patients with any of these devices who undergo incision and drainage for a dental abscess or those having teeth extracted or undergoing surgical procedures in areas of acute infection should receive antibiotic prophylaxis.

Renal dialysis shunts

Some authors in the dental literature have supported antibiotic prophylaxis on the basis of a proposed risk of shunt infection,[13] and others have done so because of concern for prevention of IE, given the higher incidence of native heart valve disease in this patient population. In the past, most publications concerning antibiotic prophylaxis either did not mention peritoneal dialysis (PD) catheters or recommended against prophylaxis.[14] Guidelines for PD were updated in 2005 with a greater emphasis on prevention of infection.[15] These guidelines suggest that "invasive procedures may infrequently cause peritonitis in PD patients," and suggest that "a single dose of amoxicillin (2 g) 2 hours before extensive dental procedures," but point out that "there are no studies to support this approach." The literature continues to show a wide range of opinions on prophylaxis because of the lack of scientific evidence. Patients undergoing hemodialysis are at increased risk for bacterial endocarditis and endarteritis (at the site of the arteriovenous fistula, graft, or shunt that is constructed to insert the large-gauge needle for connecting to the dialysis machine). However, staphylococci are the usual causative agents for most of these infections. Bacteria found in the oral cavity have been implicated rarely. In those few cases caused by oral bacteria, the source was much more likely to come from physiologic bacteremias rather than from the brief bacteremias associated with invasive dental procedures. The AHA does not recommend antibiotic prophylaxis for patients undergoing hemodialysis when they are receiving invasive dental procedures.[16]

Immunosuppression secondary to cancer and cancer chemotherapy
The dental professional must also decide whether to offer antibiotic prophylaxis to those patients who are immunosuppressed secondary to cancer and cancer chemotherapy. Baddour and colleagues. state that "patients with low granulocyte counts should only be treated on an emergency basis,"[12] and another source states that dental bacteremia can result in "overwhelming septicemia ... and the spread and severity of the infection can potentially be rapid and life-threatening."[14] The National Cancer Institute Web site suggests that patients with indwelling venous access lines and neutrophil counts between 1000 and 2000 mm^3 receive the AHA-recommended regimen for antibiotics, with consideration given to a more aggressive antibiotic therapy in the presence of infection.[17]

Insulin-dependent diabetes
There is also controversy over whether of offer prophylaxis to insulin-dependent diabetics. Some articles and opinion papers suggest that patients with unstable, insulin-dependent diabetes should receive coverage with prophylactic antibiotics for invasive dental procedures.[18] Others, however, suggest prophylaxis only in the presence of an acute oral infection.

Vascular Grafts

The clinician must also decide whether to recommend antibiotic prophylaxis to those patients who have had vascular grafts placed. Some texts and narrative review papers recommend that patients be warned about the possibility of graft infection resulting from a bacteremia, and stress the importance of antibiotic prophylaxis.[19] In a survey of infection disease specialists, 35% indicated that they either always or usually recommended prophylaxis for patients with vascular grafts.[20] In contrast, other authors have suggested that there is no indication for antibiotic prophylaxis.

Organ Transplants

For organ transplant patients, antibiotic prophylaxis has been suggested for dental treatment because of the patient's life-long use of immunosuppressive drugs to avoid organ rejection. However, there are limited data to support doing this. The new AHA IE prevention guidelines state that there is lack of evidence to support prophylaxis in heart transplant patients; however, the AHA did recommend it for those patients who developed cardiac valvulopathy. Antibiotic prophylaxis for invasive dental procedures offers no benefit when the transplant is functioning well, rejection does not occur, and there is no evidence of obvious signs of immunosuppression.[21]

As a general guideline, antibiotic prophylaxis for invasive dental procedures should be considered for patients with a suppressed immune response, regardless of the cause that is, neutropenia (<1000/mm^3) or a low CD4 count (<200/mm^3).[22] The clinician and the patient's physician should decide together whether antibiotic prophylaxis is required to prevent systemic infection from invasive dental procedures.

Antibiotic Resistance

When deciding to advise patients to take antibiotic prophylaxis, the clinician should keep in mind that the widespread use of antibiotic therapy promotes the emergence of resistant microorganisms most likely to cause endocarditis, such as viridans group streptococci and enterococci. The frequency of multidrug-resistant viridans group streptococci and enterococci has increased dramatically during the past 20 years. This increased resistance has reduced the efficacy and number of antibiotics available for the treatment of IE. Antibiotic resistance has also contributed to the rise of methicillin-resistant MRSA.

MRSA refers to Staphylococcus aureus that is resistant to all currently available β-lactam antimicrobial agents, including antistaphylococcal penicillins (methicillin, oxacillin, nafcillin) and cephalosporins.[23] There has been a rise in both health care-associated and community outbreaks of MRSA infections. Health care-associated MRSA infections most commonly present as surgical site infections, pneumonia, or bloodstream infections, and they require treatment with systemic antimicrobial agents. In the community, outbreaks of MRSA infections have been reported in settings in which people are crowded, have frequent skin-to-skin contact, and have cuts or abrasions on their skin, lack adequate hygiene practices, and share personal items. About 77% of community-associated MRSA infections are localized in the skin in the form of pustules, boils, or abscesses.[24] In 2005, revised MRSA infection control guidelines for hospitals from the Joint Working Party of the British Society for Antimicrobial Chemotherapy, Hospital Infection Society and Infection Control Nurses Association included the rational use of antibiotics and an antibiotic policy among the basic infection control measures.[24] A limited use of glycopeptides, cephalosporins, and fluoroquinolones was strongly recommended.[25] Additionally, Tacconelli and colleagues.[26] performed a meta-analysis using data of 24,230 patients that demonstrated that subjects who had been exposed to antibiotic therapy had an almost twofold chance of acquiring MRSA as opposed to nonexposed subjects. They concluded that a controlled use of antibiotics may be the key adjustable factor for the primary prevention of MRSA colonization.[26]

DISCUSSION

In conclusion, antibiotic prophylaxis to prevent IE has been a controversial issue through the years, with a variety of changes made to recommendations provided to treating physicians and dentists. As recommended by the ADA, the dentist must always use his or her best judgment when applying any guideline. However, it is important for the dentist to keep in mind that the guidelines may be cited in any malpractice litigation as evidence of the standard of care. For those patients who received antibiotic prophylaxis in the past and no longer require antibiotic prophylaxis according to the updated guidelines, the dentist should explain to the patient that discontinuing antibiotic prophylaxis according to the current guidelines does not mean that the clinical characteristics that increase their risks of developing endocarditis have been changed. It is important to emphasize that these patients continue to be at an increased risk of developing endocarditis. Good dental hygiene is particularly important in this patient population. Also, these patients need to be educated regarding the signs and symptoms of endocarditis so that they seek prompt medical treatment at the early stage of the disease. Early diagnosis with prompt treatment with effective antimicrobial therapy is the best way to lower the mortality and morbidity of endocarditis. In terms of antibiotic prophylaxis for joint replacement, the dentist must decide to follow the 2003 or the 2009 informational statement provided by the AAOS. The dentist may consult the patient's orthopedist and come to a joint decision. If there is a disagreement, the information may be presented to the patient in order for the patient to make an informed decision. When prescribing antibiotics, the clinician must realize that the overprescription of antibiotics has led to resistance to antibiotic regimens and the rise of antibiotic-resistant strains of bacteria, such as MRSA.

REFERENCES

1. Dajani AS, Taubert KA, Wilson W, et al. Prevention of bacterial endocarditis: recommendations by the American Heart Association. JAMA 1997;277(22):1794–801.
2. Wilson W, Taubert KA, Gewitz M, et al, American Heart Association Rheumatic Fever, Endocarditis Kawasaki Disease Committee, Council on Cardiovascular Disease in the Young; Council on Clinical Cardiology; Council on Cardiovascular Surgery and Anesthesia; Quality of Care and Outcomes Research Interdisciplinary Working Group; American Dental Association. Prevention of infective endocarditis: guidelines from the American Heart Association: a guideline from the American Heart Association Rheumatic Fever, Endocarditis and Kawasaki Disease Committee, Council on Cardiovascular Disease in the Young, and the Council on Clinical Cardiology, Council on Cardiovascular Surgery and Anesthesia, and the Quality of Care and Outcomes Research Interdisciplinary Working Group. J Am Dent Assoc 2007;138:739–45.
3. van der Meer JT, Thompson J, Valkenburg HA, et al. Epidemiology of bacterial endocarditis in The Netherlands, part II: antecedent procedures and use of prophylaxis. Arch Intern Med 1992;152(9):1869–73.
4. Gould FK, Elliott TS, Foweraker J, et al. Guidelines for the prevention of endocarditis: report of the Working Party of the British Society for Antimicrobial Chemotherapy. J Antimicrob Chemother 2006;57:1035–42.
5. Levi M, Eusterman V. Oral infections and antibiotic therapy. Otolaryngol Clin North Am 2011;44:57–78.
6. Pichichero ME. A review of evidence supporting the American Academy of Pediatrics recommendation for prescribing cephalosporin antibiotics for penicillin allergic patients. Pediatrics 2005;115:1048–57.
7. Fairbanks DN. Pocket guide to antimicrobial therapy in otolaryngology-head and neck surgery. 13th edition. Alexandria (VA): American Academy of Otolaryngology-Head and Neck Surgery Foundation, Incorporated; 2007. p. 10–11.
8. American Dental Association; American Academy of Orthopaedic Surgeons. Antibiotic prophylaxis for dental patients with total joint replacements. JADA 2003;134(7):895–9.
9. American Academy of Orthopaedic Surgeons and American Association of Orthopaedic Surgeons information statement: antibiotic prophylaxis for bacteremia in patients with joint replacements. February 2009. Revised June 2010. Available at: http://www6.aaos.org/news/PDFopen/PDFopen.cfm?page_url=http://www.aaos.org/about/papers/advadvis/1033.asp. Accessed February 2, 2011.
10. Little J, Jacobson J, Lockhart P. The dental treatment of patients with joint replacements: a position paper from the American Academy of Oral Medicine. J Am Dent Assoc 2010;141:667–71.
11. Goldie M. New evidence on bacteraemia. Int J Dent Hygiene 2010;8:317–8.
12. Baddour LM, Bettmann MA, Bolger AF, et al. Nonvalvular cardiovascular device-related infections. Circulation 2003;108:2015–31.
13. Seymour RA, Whitworth JM. Antibiotic prophylaxis for endocarditis, prosthetic joints, and surgery. Dent Clin North Am 2002;46(4):635–51.
14. Tong DC, Rothwell BR. Antibiotic prophylaxis in dentistry: a review and practice recommendations. JADA 2000;131(3):366–74.
15. Piraino B, Bailie GR, Bernardini J, et al. Peritoneal dialysis-related infections recommendations: 2005 update. Perit Dial Int 2005;25(2):107–31.
16. Pallasch TJ, Slots J. Antibiotic prophylaxis and the medically compromised patient. Periodontol 2000 1996;10:107–38.

17. National Cancer Institute, US National Institutes of Health. Oral complications of chemotherapy and head/neck radiation (PDQ). Available at: www.cancer. gov/cancertopics/pdq/supportivecare/oralcomplications/HealthProfessional. Accessed February 17, 2007.
18. Hallmon WW, Mealey BL. Implications of diabetes mellitus and periodontal disease. Diabetes Educ 1992;18(4):310–5.
19. Rutherford RB, editor. Vascular surgery. 5th edition. Philadelphia: Saunders; 2000.
20. Lockhart PB, Brennan MT, Fox PC, et al. Decision-making on the use of antimicrobial prophylaxis for dental procedures: a survey of infectious disease consultants and review. Clin Infect Dis 2002;34(12):1621–6.
21. Little JW, Falace DA, Miller CS, et al. Dental management of the medically compromised patient. 6th edition. St Louis (MO): Mosby; 2002. 501–525.
22. McKenna SJ. Immunocompromised host and infection. In: Topazian RG, Goldberg MH, Hupp JR, editors. Oral and maxillofacial infections. 4th edition. Philadelphia: Elsevier; 2002. p. 456–68.
23. Klevens R, Gorwitz R, Collins A. Methicillin-resistant *Staphylococcus aureus*: a primer for dentists. J Am Dent Assoc 2008;139:1328–37.
24. Fridkin SK, Hageman JC, Morrison M, et al. Methicillin-resistant *Staphylococcus aureus* disease in three communities. (published correction appears in N Engl J Med 2005;352(22):2362). N Engl J Med 2005;352(14):1436–44.
25. Gemmell CG, Edwards DI, Fraise AP, et al. Guidelines for the prophylaxis and treatment of methicillin-resistant *Staphylococcus aureus* (MRSA) infections in the UK. J Antimicrob Chemother 2006;57:589–608.
26. Tacconelli E, Angelis G, Cataldo M, et al. Does antibiotic exposure increase the risk of methicillin-resistant *Staphylococcus aureus* (MRSA) isolation? A systematic review and meta-analysis. J Antimicrob Chemother 2008;61:26–38.

Exodontia: Tips and Techniques for Better Outcomes

Harry Dym, DDS[a],*, Adam Weiss, DDS[b]

KEYWORDS

- Powered periotome • Piezosurgery • Immediate implants
- Bone grafting • Physics forceps

Exodontia is a procedure that all dentists are taught to perform in dental school and used by most general clinicians in their practice. With the growth of implant dentistry because of its high success rate and predictability, more questionable teeth that in the past may have been salvaged through extreme endodontic or periodontic procedures are now extracted for implant placement. A good skill set in basic and complex exodontia is therefore essential for well-trained general dentists who wish to be clinically involved in this facet of their practice.

This article reviews and highlights exodontia tips as well as new techniques to make simple and complex exodontia (**Box 1**) more predictable and efficient with improved patient outcomes. Included in this article is a discussion of a powered periotome that has been developed to aid in the atraumatic extraction of teeth. This instrument is particularly useful for immediate or delayed implant placement. Another new device, the piezosurgery, is also being increasingly used for outpatient oral surgery procedures, including complex exodontia. The precise and effortless nature of piezosurgery has been used in the removal of difficult broken down teeth and in bone grafting. A brief discussion on the physics forceps, a new type of exodontia forceps, which uses class 1 lever mechanics to extract teeth without having to use excessive force or squeezing motion, is also included in this article on basic and complex exodontia.

PRINCIPLE OF SIMPLE EXTRACTION

In the process of a simple extraction, surgeons must exercise a great deal of finesse and a certain degree of controlled force to be able to deliver a simple tooth extraction.

[a] Department of Dentistry/Oral and Maxillofacial Surgery, The Brooklyn Hospital Center, 121 DeKalb Avenue, Brooklyn, NY 11201, USA
[b] Division of Oral and Maxillofacial Surgery, The Brooklyn Hospital Center, 121 DeKalb Avenue, Brooklyn, NY 11201, USA
* Corresponding author.
E-mail address: hdymdds@yahoo.com

Dent Clin N Am 56 (2012) 245–266
doi:10.1016/j.cden.2011.07.002
0011-8532/12/$ – see front matter © 2012 Elsevier Inc. All rights reserved.

> **Box 1**
> **Exodontia: basic and complex**
>
> *Definition*
>
> 1. Basic exodontia: simple luxation techniques, bone expansion, and forceps delivery
> 2. Complex exodontia: techniques used to remove teeth other than by simple luxation and forceps delivery

If surgeons find themselves in a situation in which they have to exercise a significant degree of force to be able to deliver a certain tooth, they must stop and reassess the situation before resuming.

A simple extraction process involves minor alveolar bone expansion, separation of the periodontal ligament (PDL), and simple coronal forceps delivery of the tooth. Successful extractions also depend on the surgeon's thorough and detailed understanding of the anatomy of the teeth involved, the root form, angulation, attachment of the teeth to the periodontal apparatus, and the bony structure underneath.[1]

Experience will enhance the surgeon's tactile sense. As the tooth is being removed, the surgeon will be able to appreciate the lateral forces applied on the tooth's roots and their effect on the alveolar bone. This recognition leads to avoidance of any excessive forces that would produce root and alveolar bone fractures.

The patient needs to be positioned in the dental chair to allow for the surgeon's optimal control and visibility. When extractions are being performed in the lower arch, it is preferable that the patient's mandible is positioned in a parallel line with the floor. Then the patient's height should be adjusted up and down to allow for the mandible to be positioned at the same level at the surgeon's elbow so that when the surgeon is performing the extraction, the forearm is parallel with the floor as well. When extracting a maxillary tooth, the patient's maxillary occlusal plane should fall at almost 60° angle with the floor.

The surgeon's position, relative to the patient's position, varies as well, depending on which tooth is being extracted, and is also dependant on the surgeon's dominant hand (**Fig. 1**).[1]

Using the appropriate specialized instrumentation facilitates the procedure and makes it more predictable. Typically, the surgeon starts by separating the superior portion of the PDL and then subluxating with an elevator. Choosing the right forceps is important to be able to grasp the cervical portion of the tooth and position it as apically as possible to try to shift the center of rotation toward the root. This positioning allows the most effective central bone expansion movement and prevention of the fracture of roots or crown at the same time. Sharp elevators and forceps are always more desirable to use because they engage the tooth in a more firm and predictable manner and prevent slippage and/or lack of efficient delivery of force.

Pursuant to the separation of the PDL, one must find an appropriate purchase point for the elevator. The clinician must try to position the elevator between the bony socket wall and the tooth itself and direct the elevator in an apical direction trying to subluxate the root and push it coronally. Most of the time, an effective elevation prevents injury to the adjacent teeth, maintains the integrity of the alveolar bony structure, and makes the forceps delivery extremely simple. During the introduction of the elevator, the surgeon's free hand should, if possible, always hold the alveolar process with the thumb on one side and the forefinger on the other side and try to sense and direct the degree and direction of force being applied to the alveolar process of the tooth (**Fig. 2**).[1]

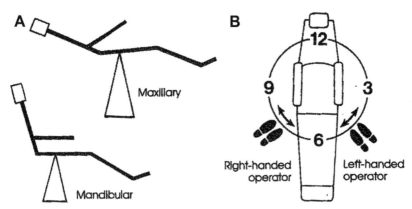

Fig. 1. Chair position for dental extractions. (*A*) Controlled force is delivered most effectively when a low upright chair position is used for the extraction of mandibular teeth. A higher more reclined chair position is used for extraction of maxillary teeth. (*B*) Most extraction instruments are designed to be used from the right (or left) front chair location. (*From* Pederson GW. Uncomplicated extraction. In: Oral surgery. Philadelphia: WB Saunders; 1998.)

When extracting one of the maxillary anterior lateral and central incisors and/or mandibular premolars, the predominant extraction force is mainly rotational with the use of a universal maxillary forceps No. 150 for the maxillary teeth and Asch forceps for the lower teeth (**Fig. 3**).[1]

The maxillary canines and the lower anterior teeth, however, seem to have flatter roots and require more lateral buccal and lingual forces application in the process of the extraction first. The maxillary premolars could have roots that are thin. A maxillary universal forceps is typically used for these teeth to be extracted. The forceps is positioned to grasp the crown portion of the tooth and seated as apically as possible. Lateral force in a buccal fashion is applied first and then in palatal aspect with extreme care to prevent fracturing those thin roots. Careful repetition of the same movement is done until the tooth is subluxated. The alveolar bone is expanded, and the tooth can then be delivered coronally (**Fig. 4**).[1]

A very similar technique is used for maxillary molars as well. Great attention must be paid not to cause excessive force, which could fracture the buccal plate. A variety of other maxillary forceps have been designed to allow for the breaks of the extraction forceps to enter in between the 2 buccal roots, such as in a maxillary cowhorn (**Fig. 5**).[1]

Extraction of lower molars could be the most difficult extraction in the mouth because of the density of the posterior mandible, the root form of lower molars, and proximity to vital anatomic structures. A lower universal forceps No. 151 is best used. A variety of cowhorn forceps are used to allow for the beaks to seat into the furca with very gentle digital pressure. Once the cowhorn beaks are seated into the furca, gentle approximation of handles of the forceps takes place. That process luxates the tooth coronally, and then simple delivery of the tooth follows. One must still pay great attention to prevent causing any damage to the soft tissue surrounding the extracted tooth (**Fig. 6**).[1]

Bone loss after tooth extraction without replacement is a well-documented phenomenon. A skilled surgeon should avoid any traumatic extraction leading to

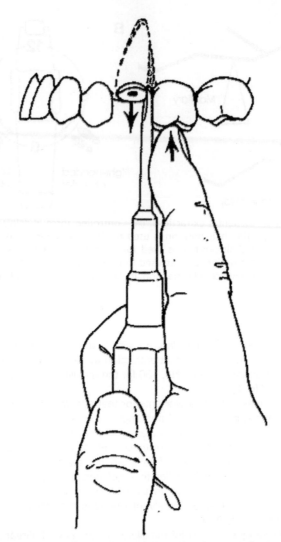

Fig. 2. Use of straight elevator for tooth extractions. The elevator is forcing the root upward and outward as its blade is being forced apically into the socket. As the surgeon's experience increases, such forces can be used to direct the tooth's delivery. Note that the index finger is extended and can be used to control the forces required to remove the root. (*Modified from* Peterson LJ, editor. Contemporary oral and maxillofacial surgery. 3rd edition. St Louis (MO): Mosby; 1998; with permission.)

further bone remodeling and ultimately more bone resorption. Should the surgeon expect a traumatic extraction with possible excessive bone removal, then the patient must be counseled for the need of socket preservation and extensive augmentation procedures by the various grafting techniques currently available.

COMPLICATED EXODONTIA

Complicated exodontia involves techniques to remove teeth other than by simple luxation of the tooth and forceps delivery. As all dentists are aware, not all extractions

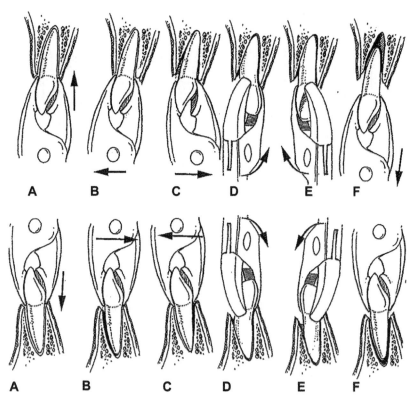

Fig. 3. Use of extraction forceps. (*Upper panel*) Rotation is performed with a No. 1 forceps or a No. 150 (maxillary universal) forceps. The forceps is seated against the tooth (*A*) and then forced apically. Continued apical pressure is applied, and buccal luxation begins (*B*), followed by palatal luxation. Once some mobility is noted, the conical root of the anterior maxillary teeth allows rotational forces to be used. The tooth is rotated distally (*C*) and then mesially (*D*). The process is repeated until the tooth can be delivered from its socket (*E, F*). This technique can be used for the maxillary lateral incisor and the canine. However, the canine often requires greater force and effort to remove it from its socket. (*Lower panel*) The ideal forceps for the removal of mandibular premolar is the English/Asch forceps or the No. 151 (mandibular universal) forceps. All the anterior mandibular teeth can be extracted similarly with this technique. The forceps are placed and seated apically (*A*), and then light luxation is used to push the tooth buccally (*B*), followed closely by lingual movements (*C*). Rotational movements can be used because the roots are frequently single or conical in nature (*D–F*). Care must be taken when evaluating these teeth radiographically because they are in close proximity to the mental foramen. The foramen's location should be determined to prevent possible compression of the nerve.

can be done by simply grasping the tooth with forceps and expanding the alveolar bone to deliver the tooth. Conditions such as advanced caries, abnormal root morphology, or difficult anatomic locations can make the extraction of a tooth complicated and necessitate a surgical extraction using specialized techniques.

Experience has taught that any planned simple extraction can develop complications that will lead to a surgical extraction, and the oral surgeon must therefore be

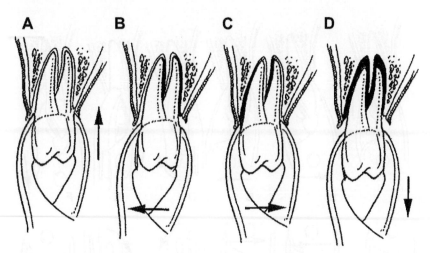

Fig. 4. Extraction of maxillary premolars. The maxillary premolar has 2 thin and slender roots. These roots can be easily fractured if proper technique is not used. A No. 1 or No. 150 forceps is used for this extraction. Initially, the forceps is seated and pushed apically (*A*). Then the tooth is luxated buccally to begin alveolar expansion (*B*), and then it is pushed palatally (*C*). This is repeated in a deliberate manner. Occasionally, figurements can be used until the tooth is removed from its socket (*D*).

prepared to routinely convert to using specialized techniques that are discussed in this section. Although complicated surgical exodontia often emanate from attempts at simple forceps extraction, it is best when surgical extractions are planned. In most cases, proper diagnosis and careful surgical planning before initiation of the procedure save time, decrease morbidity, and increase efficiency.

INDICATIONS

Common indications for surgical extractions are listed in **Box 2**.
    Surgical extraction usually involves 3 or more of the following steps:

1. Elevation of a mucoperiosteal flap
2. Ostectomy
3. Sectioning of the tooth
4. Luxation and removal of the roots
5. Removal of radicular pathologic condition when present
6. Debridement of the surgical field and the removal of sharp bony edges
7. Wound closure.

As is mandatory for simple extractions, good-quality radiographs to visualize decay, root morphology, intrabony pathologic conditions, and approximation to critical anatomic structures are even more critical for surgical extractions. In general, the panoramic radiograph is the preferred imaging modality for complex exodontia because it shows the entire teeth-bearing areas, the full extent of any intrabony pathologic conditions that may be present, along with their relationship to vital anatomic structures. When periapical radiographs are used, they should be of good quality and show the entire tooth along with close anatomic structures. For some unerupted

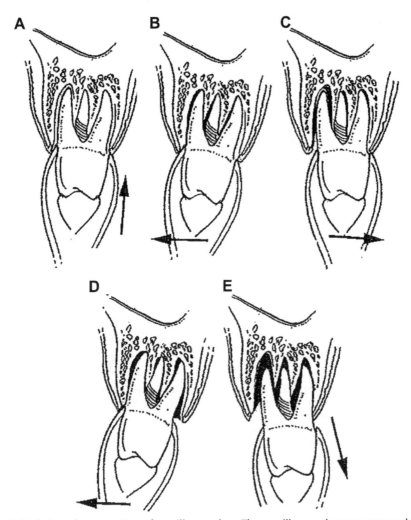

Fig. 5. Technique for extraction of maxillary molars. The maxillary molars are commonly in close proximity to the maxillary sinuses, and careful radiographic interpretation can prevent possible antral involvement. These teeth are removed with a No. 150 (maxillary universal), No. 210s, No. 53, or No. 88 forceps. Their 3-rooted nature can make a relatively simple look-ing extraction more complex owing to root dilacerations or diligence. The initial step is to seat the forceps and apply apical force. (*A*) The next step is to apply slow and deliberate forces in the buccal and palatal directions, allowing for initial expansion of the alveolus. (*B*) Because the maxillary bone is less compact, large initial forces can result in buccal plate fractures and occasionally tuberosity fractures. Larger forces and movements follow in a buccal and lingual direction, allowing for increased expansion of the bone (*C, D*). The tooth is then carefully delivered out of the mouth buccally. (*E*) If the gingival begins to tear, stop the extraction so that the likely buccal plate fracture causing it can be dissected free of the gingival.

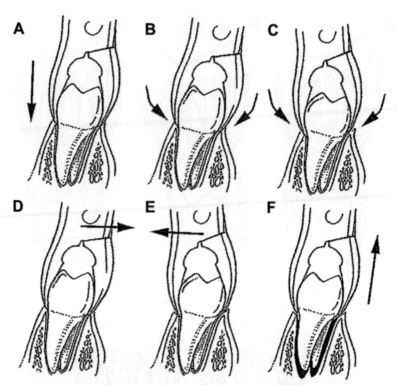

Fig. 6. Technique for extraction of mandibular molars. Mandibular molars are often the most difficult teeth to remove owing to various factors, and they can have the most complications because of anatomic considerations. They are best removed with No. 151 (universal) or No. 23 (cowhorn) forceps. Once the forceps is seated (*A*), heavy apical pressure is applied. If a cowhorn forceps is being used, the tips of the beaks should be wedged into the furca of the tooth by squeezing the handles of the instrument and gently rocking the beaks into position (*B, C*). Once the beaks are tightly seated around the crown, heavy luxation of the tooth occurs in a buccal and lingual direction (*D, E*). When the tooth is adequately mobile, a wiggling motion can be used to extract it from the socket (*F*). The figure-of-eight technique is also used at this point, and, all the while, apical pressure is applied.

teeth, panoramic radiograph or the sole periapical radiograph will not provide complete or accurate information as to tooth position, and localizing radiographs are needed to properly determine their position.

FLAP DESIGN

In surgical exodontia, a full-thickness mucoperiosteal flap is the type of flap used to facilitate the removal of the desired tooth or root fragment. Reasons for reflecting the flap are to

1. Allow for complete visualization of the operative field
2. Prevent unnecessary trauma to the adjacent soft tissue when removing bone or teeth
3. Provide an adequate working area that allows for the full removal of intrabony pathologic conditions when present.

Box 2
Indications for surgical extractions

Accidental fracture of the crown during simple extraction that leaves the root buried in the socket

Retained roots

Severely carious teeth that will fracture with forceps extraction

Endodontically treated teeth

Teeth with internal resorption

Teeth with divergent roots

Teeth with dilacerated or greatly curved roots

Ectopic teeth in positions where forceps cannot be used

Teeth that are positioned close to vital anatomic structures

Unerupted teeth other than third molars

Hypercementosis

Ankylosed teeth

Mandibular third molar in the proximal segment of a fracture of the mandibular angle region

Multirooted teeth located in areas of the jaw where bone preservation is critical for implant placement.

Tooth that will be used for autotransplant

Careful consideration must be given to the position of the incisions and to the type and shape of the flap. The following are guidelines for flap design for surgical extractions:

- Incisions should be placed over bone not planned for removal.
- The incision should be long enough to allow for a flap that will give clear and adequate hard tissue visualization and permit easy retraction without tearing.
- The base of the flap should be wider than the reflected free margin to ensure proper blood supply to the reflected soft tissue.
- Incisions should not be placed over vital structures (mental foramen and lingual nerve).

The soft tissue flap configuration can be of 3 basic designs: the envelope flap, triangle flap, and trapezoidal flap.

The most common flap used in exodontia is possibly the envelope flap. The incision is made with a No. 15 blade around the necks of the teeth within the dental sulcus, including the interdental papillae. The length of the incision usually involves 3 to 4 teeth, but the length should be that which provides adequate access to the area of intervention without the need for excessive retraction. Elevation of the flap is started at the sulcular incision, where a sharp periosteal elevator is used to firmly lift the free gingival margins and the incised dental papillae. The periosteum along the supraperiosteal structures is gently elevated from the bone (**Fig. 7**).[1] Procedures that involve more than one tooth or in which the level of surgery is located beyond the apices of the tooth require vertical releasing incisions to improve the access. The horizontal circumdental incision is made first; then the vertical arm or arms are added in a manner that allows a sufficient quantity of the papilla to remain intact (**Fig. 8**).[1]

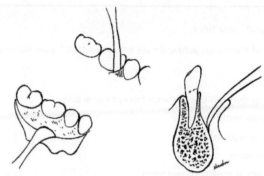

Fig. 7. Creation of an envelope flap. The envelope flap made with a periosteal elevator. (*From* Costich ER, White RP. Fundamentals of oral surgery. Philadelphia: WB Saunders; 1971; with permission.)

This intact papilla serves as an anchoring point for sutures and has the least wound contraction on closure. The releasing incision should never be placed on the facial aspect of the tooth in the midsulcular area because this frequently results in periodontal defect.

When additional working access is necessary, the sulcular incision can be lengthened or a second vertical incision tapered in the opposite direction may be added to convert the triangular flap into a trapezoidal flap (**Fig. 9**).[1]

BONE REMOVAL

Sometimes it is necessary to remove alveolar bone from the crown of the tooth or form the retained root to facilitate its removal. This removal is most often done with a dental bur in a high-speed handpiece under constant irrigation. In some instances, a rongeur may be used. Alveolar bone removal must be as conservative as possible, removing

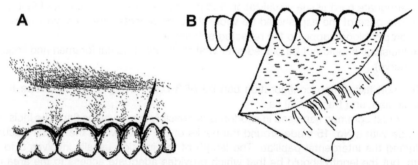

Fig. 8. Flaps with releasing incisions. (*A*) A sulcular incision with a vertical release. The vertical release is done in the alveolar mucosa and is tapered to provide a wide base for the flap that will be elevated from the bone. The vertical incision joins the sulcular incision in such a way as to save the interdental papilla. The fixed papilla provides a stable point onto which the repositioned flap may be anchored. (*B*) A mucoperiosteal flap with an anteriorly based releasing incision. The base of the flap is kept larger than the apex to ensure an adequate blood supply. (*From* Dym H, Ogle OE. Atlas of minor and oral surgery. Philadelphia: WB Saunders; 2001, with permission [*A*]; and Costich ER, White RP. Fundamentals of oral surgery. Philadelphia: WB Saunders; 1971, with permission [*B*].)

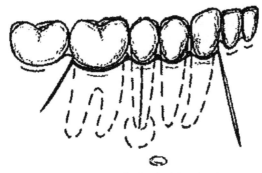

Fig. 9. Flaps with releasing incisions. A sulcular incision in the posterior mandible with vertical releases anteriorly and posteriorly. The vertical release anteriorly should be at the canine or lateral incisor area to prevent injury to the mental nerve. (*From* Dym H, Ogle OE. Atlas of minor and oral surgery. Philadelphia: WB Saunders; 2001; with permission.)

only the amount of bone required to achieve access that is needed to remove the tooth or roots. The amount of bone removed depends on the physical state of the crown or root and the level at which the fracture of the root occurred. The osteotomy should expose enough root structure to permit elevation without crumbling. In general, buccal bone removal should be done to expose 20% to 40% of the remaining root length. Bone can also be removed within the socket to allow the introduction of a narrow elevator (**Fig. 10**).[1]

SECTIONING OF TEETH AND REMOVAL

Any teeth that radiographically demonstrate abnormal root morphology, which would impede its removal, or a tooth that requires excessive force to elevate or luxate should be surgically sectioned so as to provide a mechanical advantage. Sectioning the tooth

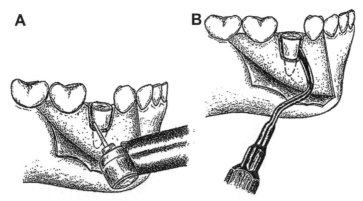

Fig. 10. Removal of dental root tips. (*A*) Teeth often fracture during extraction, leaving root fragments in alveolar bone. Adequate access must first be established by wither an envelope or 3-cornered triangle flap. Buccal plate is removed with a bur to expose root fragment. Space should be made to allow introduction of narrow elevator. (*B*) Root is removed with elevator wedged between root and alveolar bone. Controlled luxation is performed to prevent root displacement and soft tissue injury. (*From* Dym H, Ogle OE. Atlas of minor and oral surgery. Philadelphia: WB Saunders; 2001; with permission.)

into multiple segments allows the surgeon to remove tooth fragments as several single-rooted teeth, improve leveraging, and minimize trauma to adjacent bone.

When a multirooted tooth fractures at the cementoenamel junction and leaves the roots joined, it should be sectioned and then removed with either forceps or elevators. There are several roots tip forceps available for this purpose. Sectioning of the mandibular molar tooth in a buccolingual direction allows easy removal in most instances (**Fig. 11**).[1]

Sometimes it may be necessary to remove bone around the roots as previously mentioned. In cases in which the interradicular bone is present, this removal may be eliminated to facilitate root removal with east-west, crane pick, or other types of elevators (**Fig. 12**).[1]

Purchase points directed toward the root apex can also be placed with the drill to improve the leveraging during elevation. A mandibular tooth with widely divergent roots can be sectioned and extracted like 2 individual premolars (**Fig. 13**).[1]

In some cases, a modification of the open surgical procedure should be performed, when attempting to remove small remaining root tips, in order to preserve the buccal cortical crestal bone. In cases in which an endosseous implant is planned or in bicuspid extractions for planned orthodontia, a "window" technique is used. In this procedure, a small window is drilled and opened in the buccal plate adjacent to the root fragment and a fine instrument is then inserted into the window and the root pushed out through the socket (**Figs. 14** and **15**).[2]

Like mandibular multirooted teeth, maxillary molars and first premolars can also be sectioned into individual roots to allow easier removal. Depending on the root morphology of the maxillary molars, their roots may be partitioned in a T or Y configuration using a rotary instrument (**Fig. 16**). The buccal roots should be removed first. Great care should be taken to avoid pushing the roots into the maxillary sinus. The risk is highest with maxillary second premolar, first molar, and second molar teeth.

Compression of the buccal and lingual plates should be minimal and should be avoided in orthodontic extractions and potential implant sites. Aggressive removal of the interseptal or interradicular bone leads to greater postoperative bone resorption and should also be avoided.

At the termination of the procedure, the extraction socket and the space under the soft tissue flap should be generously irrigated to remove bone dust and tooth particles that may be present. Leaving bone dust and clotted blood below the flap could result in an infection. The surgeon should keep in mind that the elevation of a flap and bone cutting will be additional surgical traumas that result in additional swelling and possibly

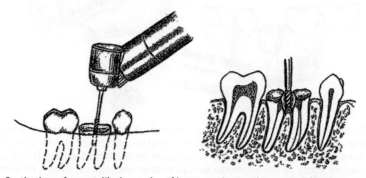

Fig. 11. Sectioning of a mandibular molar. If lower molar tooth proves difficult to extract, it is sectioned through the furcation area, resulting in 2 single-rooted teeth. (*From* Dym H, Ogle OE. Atlas of minor and oral surgery. Philadelphia: WB Saunders; 2001; with permission.)

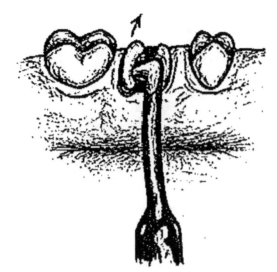

Fig. 12. Use of east-west elevator to remove root tips. After one root of molar roots has been removed, the Cryer elevator (east-west) is placed into empty mesial socket and turned with sharp point, engaging interseptal bone and root to elevate remaining distal root. (*From* Dym H, Ogle OE. Atlas of minor and oral surgery. Philadelphia: WB Saunders; 2001; with permission.)

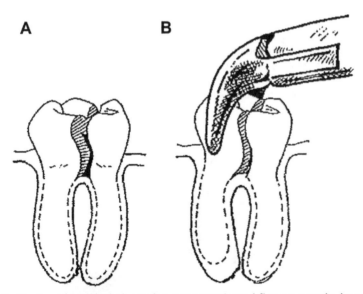

Fig. 13. Sectioning of a mandibular molar. A mucoperiosteal flap exposes the buccal aspect of the molar tooth requiring sectioning. The tooth is sectioned from the buccal to lingual though the furcation (*A*). This allows removal of the tooth with simple elevation and luxation (*B*). (*From* Archer WH, editor. Oral and maxillofacial surgery, vol. 1. 5th edition. Philadelphia: WB Saunders; 1975; with permission.)

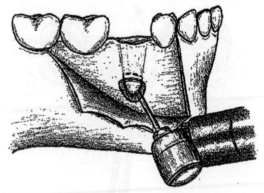

Fig. 14. Creation of bony window to remove root tip. In an attempt to maintain buccal plate and alveolar bone, a bony window can be opened at the apical root area with a bur. (*From* Dym H, Ogle OE. Atlas of minor and oral surgery. Philadelphia: WB Saunders; 2001; with permission.)

an increase in postoperative pain and should make the patient aware of these consequences. A summary of techniques to aid in safe and effective exodontia is provided in the following boxes. Following all exodontia procedures, whether it be simple or complex, the patient should be given both verbal and written postoperative instructions along with doctor/office emergency contact numbers (**Boxes 3–5**).

PERIOTOME

A periotome is a surgical instrument that can be used to sever the PDL of the tooth before extraction, with the surrounding tissue subjected to less trauma, and, in many cases, allows for immediate placement of an implant. To use a periotome, the blade of the instrument is placed down into the sulcus, severing the PDL. The blade is then lifted out of the sulcus and the process repeated, moving circumferentially around the tooth. This procedure severs the PDL except for where it connects at

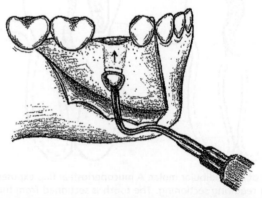

Fig. 15. Extraction root tip through bony window. An angled root tip elevator is used to drive root apically through window in bone, helping to preserve buccal plate. (*From* Dym H, Ogle OE. Atlas of minor and oral surgery. Philadelphia: WB Saunders; 2001; with permission.)

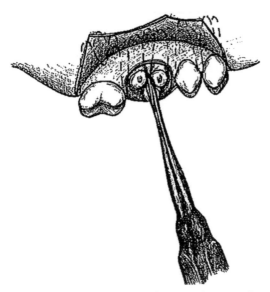

Fig. 16. Separation and removal of maxillary molar root tips. Buccal roots are then separated and delivered with a straight elevator. (*From* Dym H, Ogle OE. Atlas of minor and oral surgery. Philadelphia: WB Saunders; 2001; with permission.)

the most apical part of the tooth. Afterward, a periosteal elevator and extraction forceps are used in the usual atraumatic manner.

POWERED PERIOTOME

The traditional means of extracting teeth often involving creation of a mucoperiosteal flap, elevation, and luxation with forceps often results in fracture or deformation of the

---

Box 3
Postextraction patient instructions

Instructions following extractions

1. Avoid vigorous exercise

2. No smoking for 3 days

3. No rinsing or spitting for 24 hours

4. No drinking with straws

5. No alcohol beverages while on narcotic medications

6. Rest for remainder of day

7. Elevate head for 24 hours

8. Take medications as instructed

9. Soft foods and liquids for 24 hours

10. Keep gauze in place for 2 hours on leaving office

11. Ice packs to face 20 minutes on and 20 minutes off for 1 day

12. Call emergency number if any problems occur

Box 4
Exodontia: tips and strategies

- Office must be well equipped for any exodontia, simple or complex. Never assume that any tooth will be easily delivered.

- Always use specialized surgical handpiece when performing surgical exodontia (avoid air emphysema).

- Have backup handpiece available.

- Always look to preserve alveolar bone when performing exodontia. Assume all patients may come to request implant reconstruction at a later date.

- Have hemostatic material available in case of severe oozing or bleeding.

- Be prepared to leave behind root fragment (4 mm or less) if removal will lead to significant trauma or potential damage to patient.

- Have patient bite on mouth prop to help avoid temporomandibular joint pain.

- Always perform vigorous irrigation of surgical site following surgical extraction.

- Never fully begin any exodontia without recent diagnostic radiograph.

- Discuss postexodontia home care instructions. Give written instructions and include emergency contact/number.

- Know when to refer to oral and maxillofacial surgeon. It is best to not begin a procedure you are not sure if you will finish.

dentoalveolar complex.[2] This trauma could lead to ridge defects, making the placement of implants very difficult or even impossible in some cases. Also, elevation of the mucoperiosteum may compromise the periosteal blood supply to the alveolus, leading to loss of marginal alveolar bone even in relatively atraumatic extractions. In addition, if the teeth adjacent to the tooth to be extracted have extensive restorations or crown coverage, the powered periotome eliminates the need to elevate against and possibly damage these restorations.

A powered periotome (Powertome 100S, Westport Medical Inc., Salem, OR, USA), as shown in **Fig. 17**, has been developed that allows for the precise extraction of a tooth while producing minimal or no alveolar bone loss. This atraumatic means of dental extraction preserves bone and gingival architecture and gives the clinician the option of placing future or even immediate implants. The powered periotome functions by using the mechanisms of wedging and severing to aid in tooth extraction.[3] As shown in **Fig. 18**, these instruments are made of very thin metal blades that are gently wedged down the PDL space in a circumferential manner. This device severs Sharpey fibers, which function to secure the tooth within the alveolar socket. After most of the Sharpey fibers have been severed from the root surface, gentle rotational movement with minimal lateral pressure facilitates tooth removal.

A powered periotome is an electric unit that contains a handpiece with a periotome that is activated by a foot control. This device allows precise control over the quantity of force that the periotome tip exerts and the distance it travels into the PDL space. This instrument has a microprocessor-run actuator that eliminates uncertainty while extracting a tooth. As shown in **Fig. 17**, this device comes with a controller box that can be adjusted to 10 different power settings. In addition, the use of the Powertome 100S system frequently allows flapless removal of teeth, decreasing postoperative pain and discomfort while maintaining the periosteal blood supply to the alveolus.[4] The automated powered periotome system also reduces concern for fracture of

Box 5	
Basic instruments for complex exodontia	
Technique	Instruments
Cheek retraction and visualization of the surgical area incision	Mouth mirror, wide retractor (Seldin No. 23, Minnesota) Scalpel handle with No. 15 blade
Flap development and reflection	No. 9 periosteal elevator, Woodson, Molt
Flap retraction	Wide retractor (Seldin No. 23, Minnesota)
Bone removal	Handpieces: high-speed surgical handpiece (no air into the surgical field), 2-speed straight handpiece (using the higher speed), surgical straight handpiece (used by many oral surgeons)
	Burs: crosscut tapered fissure (702, 558); nontapered crosscut fissure; round (high-speed burs should be of surgical length) and straight elevators, such as the 301 and 34 or 34S and Cryer East-West elevators
Luxation and sectioning	
Tooth removal	Forceps such as No. 150 and No. 151
Suture cutting, distal wedge excision, severing fibrotic tissue	Surgical scissors, such as Dean
Tying sutures, traction on follicle removing loose pieces of tooth	Needle holder, such as Mayo-Hegar 6
Suturing material	4-0 or 3-0 silk or chromic gut suture with 3/8 circle reverse cutting needle
Curetting follicle or infection	Surgical spoon curette
Suctioning	Surgical suction tip, preferably tapered, plastic, or metal
Irrigation	Device: (1) through the handpiece, (2) with 3-way syringe (irrigation medium from a reservoir), (3) 15–30 mL irrigation syringe with a blunt irrigation needle, (4) bulb syringe, or (5) plastic-modeled irrigation syringe
	Medium: sterile saline or sterile water

lingual bone or buccal plate during difficult extractions. The use of a standard periotome is a much more tedious process and can actually cause unneeded discomfort for the patient, especially if a mallet is also needed to separate the tooth from bone.

When using the powered periotome, the authors have found that starting interproximally seems to work most efficiently because of the thickness of the interproximal bone. It is important to keep the blade parallel along the long axis of the tooth being removed. The blade should follow the tooth anatomy circumferentially in an apical direction in 2- to 3-mm increments. When extracting a multirooted tooth, the authors have found it most efficient to section the tooth and treat each sectioned root as a single-rooted tooth.[5] This instrument has a very small learning curve and has been used by both general practice and oral surgery residents for tooth extractions. Photographs from a clinical case taken in the authors' clinic are shown in this article (**Figs. 19** and **20**).

Clinical use by the authors has shown that this product works efficiently to deliver an intact extraction socket with excellent patient acceptance while at the same time adding little to no additional time as compared with other surgical extraction techniques.[6] This device and technique used is also very easy and intuitive with a very rapid learning

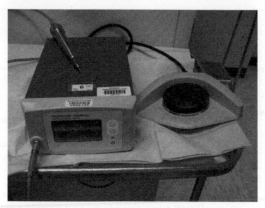

Fig. 17. Powered periotome.

curve, so even the beginner can become very comfortable with the technique almost immediately.

Regardless of whether an implant is placed immediately postextraction or if the socket is grafted in preparation for future implant placement, the preservation of alveolar bone allows for more aesthetic and functional implant restorations. Millimeters do count when it comes to implants.

PIEZOSURGERY

Piezosurgery was introduced in 1988 and has been improved upon since then. Piezosurgery is an innovative bone surgery technique that produces a modulated ultrasonic frequency of 24 to 29 kHz and a microvibration amplitude between 60 and 200 mm/s.[7] The amplitude of the vibrations created allows a very clean and precise surgical cut. Piezosurgery is very effective in the creation of osteotomies because it works selectively, without harming soft tissues such as nerves and blood vessels even with accidental contact with the cutting tip.[8] This is a tremendous advantage over the use of burs and surgical saws that have the potential to cause destruction to soft tissue. When compared with oscillating microsaws, the oscillation of the piezosurgery scalpel tip is very small, which performs more precise and safe ostetomies.[9] Traditional burs and microsaws do not distinguish hard and soft tissue.[10] Piezosurgery also gives the

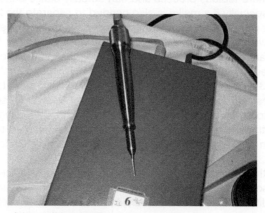

Fig. 18. Powered periotome instrument.

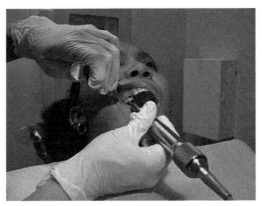

Fig. 19. Intraoperative clinical case.

operator a clearer field of vision by producing a very restricted bloody region. In addition, as shown in **Fig. 21**, the surgical control of the device is effortless compared with rotational burs or oscillating saws because there is no need for an additional force to oppose rotation or oscillation of the instrument.[11]

In a recent study by Sortino and colleagues,[7] rotary and piezoelectric techniques were compared in terms of postoperative outcome. The average time of surgery was 25.83% higher with the piezoelectric technique in comparison with the rotary technique. Despite the longer time of the procedure, the investigators also noted that the piezoelectric osteotomy reduced the postoperative facial swelling and trismus.

The ability of piezosurgery to allow precise and selective cuts makes this a useful technique when performing surgery close to the inferior alveolar neurovascular bundle and/or the roots of adjacent teeth. The removal of the body of the mandible lateral cortical bone with piezoelectric instrumentation allows adequate access to the surgical area, terrific visibility, minimal bone loss, precise cutting ability, and protection of the inferior alveolar nerve (IAN) by sparing the soft tissue when osteotomy was performed blind.[12] Because the bone cutting ability is so precise with minimal bone loss, investigators using this technique have found it easy to readapt the bone windows to their former location and fixate them.[11]

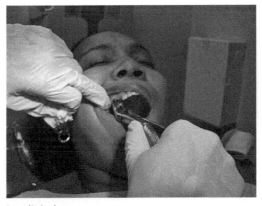

Fig. 20. Intraoperative clinical case.

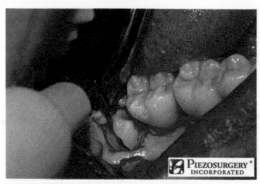

Fig. 21. Piezosurgery used to extract affected wisdom tooth.

In contrast, manual and/or mechanical instruments used in the close proximity of delicate structures (vascular, nervous tissue) do not allow for control of the cutting depth and can damage these structures by accidental contact.[7] This new bone lid technique described uses the piezosurgery device to cut and elevate a precisely defined bone lid on the lateral cortex of the mandible to provide access to the teeth needing extraction or even a lesion that needs to be excised. The bone window is then elevated with the help of a curved osteotome. The tooth or lesion can then be seen and subsequently removed atraumatically by either sectioning with piezosurgery or circular piezo-osteotomy. After the visual confirmation of an undamaged IAN and adjacent tissues, the bone lid was placed back into its original position and fixated with absorbable miniplates.

USE OF PHYSICS FORCEPS FOR TOOTH EXTRACTION

The physics forceps[13] uses first-class level mechanics to atraumatically extract a tooth from its socket. As seen on **Fig. 22**, one handle of the device is connected to a "bumper," which acts as a fulcrum during the extraction. This bumper is usually placed on the facial aspect of the dental alveolus, typically at the mucogingival junction. It is critical that the bumper side of the forceps always be seated higher than the beak side before beginning the extraction.

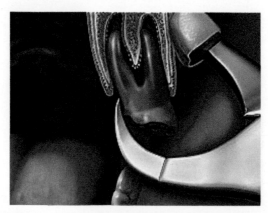

Fig. 22. Physics forceps.

The beak of the extractor is positioned most often on the lingual or palatal root of the tooth and into the gingival sulcus.[14]

Unlike conventional forceps, only one point of contact is made on the tooth being extracted. Together the beak and bumper design acts as a simple first-class lever. A squeezing motion should not be used with these forceps. By contrast, the handles are actually rotated as one unit using a steady yet gentle rotational force with wrist movement only. Once the tooth is loosened, it may be removed with traditional instruments such as a conventional forceps or rongeur. With this technique, no prior elevator use is required before attempting the extraction and no mucosal flap need be used. The dentist requires some practice before achieving complete mastery in the use of the physics forceps because the technique is significantly different from what is used for conventional forceps extractions; however, once comfortable, the clinician will marvel at the ease and the little force required to remove even difficult teeth.

SUMMARY

General dentists are incorporating oral surgical procedures into their everyday practice, including complex exodontia, more than ever before. Simply removing the entire tooth is no longer the only goal of exodontia; in the present environment of implant dentistry, the ultimate goal is preservation of alveolar bone following all teeth removal. This goal obviously implies an increased awareness of new surgical techniques and devices that may be used to render this aspect of dentistry more predictable, less traumatic for the patient, and less anxiety-producing for the treating dentist. A variety of new instruments and techniques are enabling surgeons to provide patients services in a shorter period with higher accuracy. The powered periotome functions by aiding the surgeon in atraumatically extracting teeth, which allows for either immediate or delayed implant placement into a preserved socket. Piezosurgery is also being used as many surgeons are taking advantage of its precise and effortless nature. This type of surgery provides the patient with safe and accurate procedure because soft tissue remains unharmed. Also, the physics forceps has been invented, which allows its operator to remove teeth without the use of excessive force or pulling motion. No matter what technique is used, the dentist must approach all office exodontia procedures prepared and confident, having both the necessary clinical skill, appropriate surgical equipment, and knowledge base to make exodontia procedures efficient and less traumatic for both the patient and the clinician.

REFERENCES

1. Saker M, Ogle OE, Dym H. Complex exodontia and surgical management of impacted teeth. In: Fonseca R, editor. Oral and maxillofacial surgery, vol. 1. 2nd edition. Philadelphia: Elsevier; 2009.
2. Dym H, Ogle O. Atlas of minor oral surgery. Philadelphia: W.B. Saunders Company; 2001.
3. White J, Holtzclaw D, Toscano N. Powertome assisted atraumatic tooth extraction. J Implant Adv Clin Dent 2009;1:6.
4. Levitt D. Atraumatic extraction and root retrieval using the periotome: a precursor to immediate placement of dental implants. Dent Today 2001;20(11):53–7.
5. Misch CE, Perez H. Atraumatic extractions: a biologic rationale. Dent Today 2008; 27(8):100–1.
6. Kang J, Dym H, Stern A. Use of the powertome periotome to preserve alveolar bone during tooth extraction—a preliminary study. Oral Surg Oral Med Oral Pathol Oral Radiol Endod 2009;108:4.

7. Sortino F, Pedulla E, Masoli V. The piezoelectric and rotatory osteotomy technique in impacted third molar surgery: comparison of postoperative recovery. J Oral Maxillofac Surg 2008;66:2444–8.

8. Kotrikova B, Wirtz R, Krempien R, et al. Piezosurgery—a new safe technique in cranial osteoplasty? Int J Oral Maxillofac Surg 2006;35:461–5.

9. Stubinger S, Kuttenberger J, Filippi A, et al. Intraoral piezosurgery: preliminary results of a new technique. J Oral Maxillofac Surg 2005;63:1283–7.

10. Grenga V, Bovi M. Piezoelectric surgery for exposure of palatally impacted canines. J Clin Orthod 2004;38:446–8.

11. Eggers G, Klein J, Blank J, et al. Piezosurgery: an ultrasound device for cutting bone and its use and limitations in maxillofacial surgery. Br J Oral Maxillofac Surg 2004;42:451–3.

12. Degerliyurt K, Akar V, Denizci S, et al. Bone lid technique with piezosurgery to preserve inferior alveolar nerve. Oral Surg Oral Med Oral Pathol Oral Radiol Endod 2009;108:e1–5.

13. Golden RM, inventor; GoldenMisch Inc, assignee. Dental plier design with offsetting jaw and pad elements for assisting in removing upper and lower teeth utilizing the dental plier design. US patent 6,910,890. June 28, 2005.

14. Misch C, Perez H. Atraumatic extractions: a biomechanical route. Dent Today 2008;27:8.

Surgical Management of Cosmetic Mucogingival Defects

Harry Dym, DDS, Jonathan M. Tagliareni, DDS*

KEYWORDS

- Cosmetic mucogingival defects • Free gingival autograft
- Subepithelial connective tissue graft • Pedicle grafts

Mucogingival conditions are deviations from the normal anatomic relationship between the gingival margin and the mucogingival junction. The term mucogingival surgery was introduced in the literature by Friedman in 1957 and was defined as surgical procedures for the correction of the relationship between the gingiva and the oral mucous membrane regarding problems associated with attached gingiva, shallow vestibules, and frenum attachments that interfere with the marginal gingiva.

Mucogingival surgery is defined as plastic surgical procedures designed to correct defects in the morphology, position, and/or amount of gingiva surrounding the teeth. In 1993, Miller proposed using the term periodontal plastic surgery. Miller thought the name was more appropriate with mucogingival surgery moving beyond the traditional treatment of problems associated with the gingiva and recession-type defects, including the correction of ridge form and soft tissue esthetics. Periodontal plastic surgery is now defined as surgical procedures performed to prevent or correct anatomic, developmental, traumatic, or plaque disease–induced defects of the gingiva, alveolar mucosa, or bone.[1]

Common mucogingival conditions are recession, absence, or reduction of keratinized tissue, and probing depths extending beyond the mucogingival junction. Tooth position, frenum insertions, and vestibular depth are anatomic variations that can complicate the management of these conditions.

Mucogingival conditions may be detected during a comprehensive or problem-focused periodontal examination (**Box 1**). The problem-focused examination should also include appropriate screening techniques to evaluate for periodontal or other oral diseases.

Surgical procedures should be performed in a plaque-free and inflammation-free environment, enabling firm tissue management. When the tissue is inflamed and

Department of Dentistry/Oral & Maxillofacial Surgery, The Brooklyn Hospital, 121 DeKalb Avenue, Box 187, Brooklyn, NY 11201, USA
* Corresponding author.
E-mail address: JTagliarenidds@gmail.com

Dent Clin N Am 56 (2012) 267–279
doi:10.1016/j.cden.2011.09.007
0011-8532/12/$ – see front matter © 2012 Elsevier Inc. All rights reserved.

Box 1
Problem-focused examination for mucogingival conditions

1. Comprehensive medical history should be taken to identify predisposing conditions that may affect treatment or patient management
2. Comprehensive dental history
3. General periodontal examination including probing depths and visual examination
4. Identifying deficiencies of keratinized tissue, abnormal frenulum insertions, and other tissue abnormalities
5. Causal factors affecting the results of therapy
6. Variations in ridge configuration

edematous, precise incision lines and flap reflection cannot be achieved. The patient's teeth must undergo careful and thorough scaling, root planing, and meticulous plaque control before any surgical procedure (**Box 2**).

The goals of mucogingival therapy are to help maintain good health with good function and esthetics in the dentition or its replacements, and may include restoring anatomic form and function. Furthermore, the long-term goal is to reduce the risk of progressive recession. Reducing progressive recession and cosmetic defects can be accomplished with a variety of procedures including root coverage, gingival augmentation, pocket reduction, and ridge reconstruction, as well as control of causal factors (**Box 3**).

Surgical techniques used to augment cosmetic mucogingival defects include the free gingival autograft, the subepithelial connective tissue graft, rotational flaps, lateral sliding flaps, coronally repositioned flaps, and the use of acellular dermal matrix grafts (**Box 4**).

FREE GINGIVAL AUTOGRAFT

The free gingival autograft was first described by Bjorn[2] in 1963, and Sullivan and Atkins in 1968. Initially, the autograft was used to increase the amount of attached gingiva and extend the vestibule.[2] A versatile surgical technique, the free gingival autograft is simple and highly predictable when used to increase the amount of attached gingiva (**Box 5**).

Box 2
Criteria for predictable success when repairing cosmetic mucogingival defects

1. Calculus-free and plaque-free environment
2. Anatomy of recipients and donor site
3. Donor tissue availability
4. Adequate blood supply
5. Graft stability
6. Esthetic demands

Box 3
The desired outcomes of periodontal therapy for patients with mucogingival conditions

1. Correction of the mucogingival condition

2. Cessation of further recession

3. Tissues free of clinical signs of inflammation

4. Return to function in health and comfort

5. Satisfactory esthetics

TECHNIQUE
Recipient Site Preparation

Using a no. 15 blade, a horizontal incision is made below the gingival recession. Adjacent to the affected teeth, 2 vertical releasing incisions are created extending beyond the mucogingival junction. A partial-thickness flap is elevated, leaving the periosteum intact. It is critical to dissect as close to the periosteum as possible, removing all movable soft tissue, including the epithelium, connective tissue, and muscle fibers. The superficial flap can now be excised. Some investigators advocate the placement of the graft on denuded bone, reporting less shrinkage and a firmer, less mobile graft.[3,4] In this technique, the surgeon removes the periosteum, as well as the other structures mentioned previously, such as the epithelium, connective tissue, and muscle fibers, to expose the alveolar bone. The incisions go down to the bone, incising through the periosteum. Using a periosteal elevator, a full-thickness flap is elevated. Using a round bur, it is important to decorticate the alveolar plate and prepare the graft placement on the denuded bone. Revascularization of the graft is accelerated through the formation of capillary outgrowths (**Fig. 1**).

GRAFT HARVESTING

The graft area should be outlined, extending from the palatal root of the first molar and the distal line angle of the canine. Keratinized tissue can be harvested from any area including an edentulous ridge, attached gingiva, or tuberosities. Knowledge of surgical anatomy is important when harvesting keratinized tissue from the palate. The neurovascular bundle enters the palate through the greater and lesser palatine foramina, apical to the third molars, and then travels across the palate and into the incisive foramen.

Box 4
Elements of surgical management of cosmetic mucogingival defects

1. Free gingival autografts

2. Subepithelial connective tissue grafts

3. Pedicled rotational flaps

4. Lateral sliding flaps

5. Coronally repositioned flaps

6. Acellular dermal matrix grafts

> **Box 5**
> **Uses of free gingival autograft**
>
> 1. Increasing the amount of keratinized tissue
> 2. Increasing the vestibular depth
> 3. Increasing the volume of gingival tissues in edentulous spaces
> 4. Covering roots in areas of gingival recession

Reiser and colleagues[5] in 1996 reported that the neurovascular bundle could be located 7 to 17 mm from the cementoenamel junction (CEJ) of the maxillary premolars and molars.

In the average palatal vault, the distance from the CEJ to the neurovascular bundle is 12 mm. That distance is shortened to 7 mm in shallow palatal vaults and lengthened to 17 mm in high palatal vaults.[5] Using a periodontal probe, the measurements of the palate should be recorded and the graft outline traced with the scalpel. The thickness of the graft should be close to 1.5 mm. The dissection is done with a no. 15 blade kept parallel to the epithelial outer side of the graft. The harvested graft should immediately be sutured onto the recipient site with the connective tissue facing down against the periosteum of the recipient site.

Single interrupted sutures are placed to secure the graft mesially and distally. A mesiodistal horizontal suture is added to wrap the lower half of the graft. Immobilization of the graft is critical, and reduction of dead space between the recipient site and the graft minimizes the size of the blood clot, resulting in better adaptation and revascularization. To check for mobility of the graft, the cheek or lip may be pulled once the graft is sutured. If the graft moves, then the suturing is inadequate. A periodontal dressing may be applied to the graft site. The donor site heals by secondary intention. To assist in patient comfort, surgicel or gelfoam may be applied to the donor site.

Graft healing is initially based on plasmic circulation. The graft is dependant on diffusion from its host bed, occurring most efficiently through the fibrin clot.[6] The graft then reestablishes vascularization, with capillary proliferation beginning on postoperative day 1. By day 2 and 3, capillaries have extended and penetrated the free graft.[6] Davis

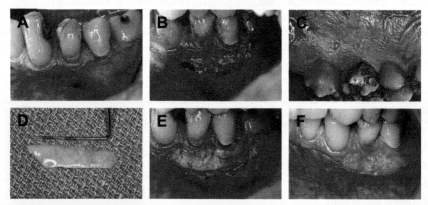

Fig. 1. Free gingival graft. (*A*) Before treatment; minimal keratinized gingiva. (*B*) Recipient site prepared for free gingival graft. (*C*) Palate will be donor site. (*D*) Free graft. (*E*) Graft transferred to recipient site. (*F*) At 6 months, showing widened zone of attached gingiva. (*Courtesy of* Dr Perry Klokkevold, Los Angeles, CA.)

and Traut[7] discuss blood supply to the graft appearing at day 8. By the end of day 10, an organic connective tissue union between the host bed and graft can be seen. This union is responsible for secondary contraction, and may shrink as much as 33%.[8] Possible complications may include bleeding from the donor site, swelling, bruising, and graft mobility.

SUBEPITHELIAL CONNECTIVE TISSUE GRAFT

Langer and Langer[9] first described the advantages of the subepithelial connective tissue graft in 1985. The subepithelial connective tissue graft benefits from double vascularization, combining the use of a partial-thickness flap with the placement of a connective tissue graft.[9] In addition, the connective tissue carries a genetic component for the overlying epithelium to be keratinized.[10] Only connective tissue from a keratinized mucosa can be used for this graft.[11] A highly predictable and esthetic graft, the subepithelial connective tissue graft is the gold standard for root coverage. Comparing root coverage using a connective tissue graft versus a free gingival graft, Jahnke and colleagues[12] reported success rates 5 times greater for the subepithelial graft in achieving 100% root coverage (**Box 6**).

TECHNIQUE

The recipient site needs to be prepared, which includes scaling and root planing along with elimination of concavities and convexities of the root surface. Miller[13] advocates the use of saturated citric acid applied with a cotton pellet to the root surface for a time of 5 minutes. The acid etch removes the smear layer, which could act as a barrier to the connective tissue attachment from the root surface.[14] Using a no. 15 blade and keeping the blade parallel to the long axis of the tooth, an envelope flap is made from the CEJ to CEJ of each adjacent tooth to the gingival recession. Dissecting sharply creates a pouch, moving apically beyond the mucogingival line. Adequate dissection is critical to mobilize the buccal flap, advancing it coronally to the CEJ of the affected surface.

The subepithelial graft should be harvested from the palate using 2 parallel incisions and 2 vertical releasing incisions. Surgical anatomy is critical: the graft should be anterior to the palatal root of the first molar and within 12 mm of the CEJ.[9] The trap door is elevated and the connective tissue graft is retrieved. The palatal flap should be sutured immediately after the graft is harvested. Primary closure is indicated using a horizontal mattress suture. The connective tissue is then placed in the subepithelial space beneath the flap. The coronal portion of the graft lies adjacent to the CEJ. The graft is sutured to the papilla using a resorbable interrupted suture. The buccal flap is then advanced, pulling over the graft, and secured. To optimize vascular supply, maximal buccal coverage is indicated. Mild pressure with wet gauze minimizes the dead space between the graft and flap. A periodontal dressing may be placed on the graft site (**Fig. 2**).

Box 6
Indications for subepithelial connective tissue graft

Root coverage

Gingival coverage of exposed implant or collar

Increase in width of attached gingiva

Ridge augmentation

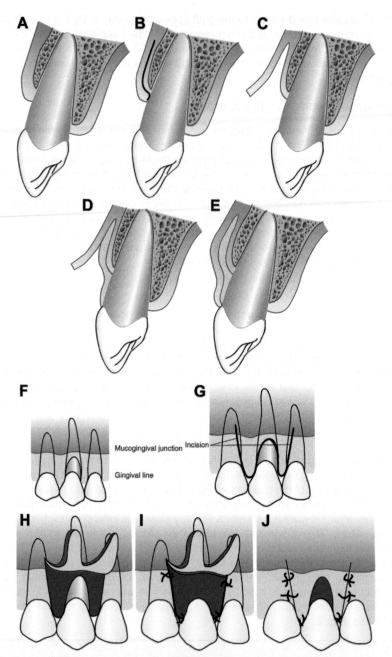

Fig. 2. Subepithelial connective tissue graft for root coverage. (*A–E*) Sagittal views. (*A*) Preoperative view of facial recession on maxillary central incisor. (*B*) Split-thickness incision for recipient site. (*C*) Split-thickness flap reflected. (*D*) Connective tissue placed over denuded root surface. Note that apical portion of the donor tissue is placed between the split flap. (*E*) Recipient flap is closed. Subepithelial connective tissue graft for root coverage. (*F*) Gingival recession. (*G*) Vertical incisions to prepare recipient site. (*H*) Split-thickness flap reflected. (*I*) Connective tissue sutured over denuded root surface. (*J*) Split-thickness flap sutured over donor connective tissue.

PEDICLE GRAFTS: ROTATIONAL FLAPS

Isolated gingival defects can be repaired using various pedicle flaps, including the rotational flap and the coronal advancement flap. In 1956, Grupe and Warren[15] described the use of sliding flaps as a method to repair gingival defects, rotating a full-thickness flap from an adjacent tooth to cover the recession. In addition, Cohen and Ross described a technique in which the interproximal papillae were used to correct defects in areas not suitable for a lateral sliding flap. Having the presence of its own blood supply, the pedicle flap is able to nourish the graft and facilitate re establishment of vascular anastamoses at the recipient site during the healing phase (**Box 7**).[16]

LATERAL SLIDING FLAPS
Technique

Local anesthesia is administered to the patient, and the area of recession is root planed and prepared for the flap. Using a no. 15 blade, the tissue adjacent to the defect is trimmed free of sulcular epithelium. A partial-thickness flap twice as wide as the defect is elevated and reflected beyond the mucogingival junction. To avoid any tension that could compromise the vasculature, releasing incisions are made at the base of the flap. The periosteum is left intact and heals by secondary intention. The flap is repositioned laterally, covering the defect and secured using a single interrupted suture. Gentle pressure with wet gauze and application of the periodontal dressing reduces the risk of hematoma formation, encouraging fibrinous adhesion. When successful attachment occurs on the exposed root, the attachment can be a combination of connective tissue attachment or long junctional attachment (**Figs. 3 and 4**).[17]

PEDICLE GRAFTS: CORONALLY ADVANCED FLAPS

Pedicle grafts are defined as surgical flaps sustained by a blood-carrying stem from the donor site during transfer. Tarnow[18] discussed the grafting of mild shallow gingival recessions using a 1-stage, sutureless coronally repositioning flap. In addition, Allen and Miller[19] reported the use of a 1-stage coronally repositioned flap to correct marginal recessions measuring 2.4 mm to 4.0 mm. These pedicle flaps are used to cover gingival recession affecting natural teeth. This technique requires the patient to have an adequate width of keratinized gingiva, absence of excessive protrusive labial ridge contours, and thick gingiva.[20]

Technique

Sutureless coronally repositioned flap
Adequate root planing of the area of recession is always indicated. Using a no. 15 blade, a semilunar incision is made following the curvature of the free gingival margin and extending into the papilla, staying 2 mm from the papilla tip on either side. It is

Box 7
Indications for pedicle flaps to correct cosmetic mucogingival defects
Single or multiple adjacent gingival recessions that have adequate donor tissue laterally
Inadequate amount of attached gingiva
Recession next to an edentulous area

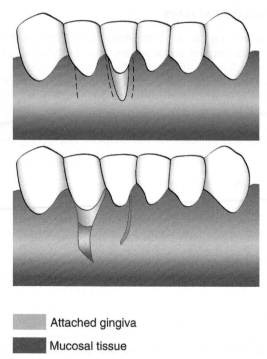

■ Attached gingiva
■ Mucosal tissue

Fig. 3. Laterally displaced flap for coverage of denuded root. (*Top*) Incisions removing the gingival margin around the exposed root and outlining the flap. (*Bottom*) After the gingiva around the exposed root is removed, the flap is separated, transferred, and sutured.

necessary to avoid extending the incision through and releasing the papilla tips. A split-thickness flap is created by making a sulcular incision, which connects apically to the semilunar incision. With the papilla intact, the flap is loosened and coronally repositioned, covering the recession. Wet gauze and mild pressure is applied to the

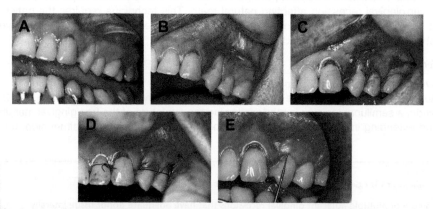

Fig. 4. Laterally displaced flap. (*A*) Preoperative view, maxillary bicuspid. (*B*) Recipient site is prepared by exposing the connective tissue around the recession. (*C*) Incisions are made at the donor site in preparation of moving the tissue laterally. (*D*) Pedicle flap is sutured in position. (*E*) Postoperative result at 1 year. (*Courtesy of* Dr E.B. Kenney, Los Angeles, CA.)

Box 8
Advantages of the semilunar coronally positioned flap

1. No tension on the flap after repositioning

2. No shortening of the vestibule

3. No reflection of the papillae, thereby avoiding esthetic compromise

4. No suturing

---

flap, and periodontal dressing is placed. The advantages of this technique include a passively lying flap on the recession, the vestibular depth stays the same, papillae stay intact, there is no esthetic compromise, and no suturing is required (**Box 8** and **Fig. 5**).[18]

One-stage coronally repositioned flap

The following requirements are critical when evaluating long-term success using coronally positioned flaps: shallow cervical depths on proximal surfaces, normal intraproximal bone heights, tissue height within 1 mm of the CEJ of adjacent teeth, reduction in root prominence, and adequate release of flap to prevent retraction during healing (**Box 9**).

Technique

The area of recession requires root preparation and conditioning with citric acid at pH 1 (40%). A chisel or bur is used to reduce prominent concavities or convexities to the grafting site. Using a no. 15 blade, a sulcular incision is created around the facial or buccal surface of the affected tooth site. Mesial and distal vertical releasing incisions are made at the line angles of the adjacent teeth. A partial-thickness pedicle flap is elevated, leaving the periosteum intact. Sharp dissection beyond the mucogingival junction creates a flap that is mobile enough to be repositioned coronally. Using a new no. 15 blade, the papilla adjacent to the recession are deepithelialized and sutured 0.5 to 1.0 mm coronally to the CEJ. A single interrupted suturing technique

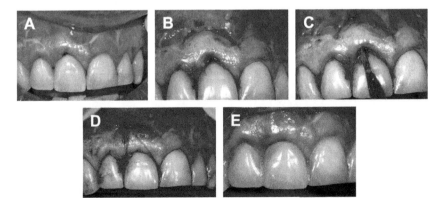

Fig. 5. (A–E) Semilunar coronally positioned flap. (A) Slight recession in facial of the upper left canine. (B) After thorough scaling and root planing of the area, a semilunar incision is made and the tissue separated from the underlying bone. The flap collapses, covering the recession. (C) Appearance after 7 weeks. Note coverage of the previous root denudation. (Courtesy of Dr J.J. Elbaz, Beverly Hills, CA.)

> **Box 9**
> **Prerequisites for coronally positioned flap**
>
> Shallow marginal recession
>
> Minimum keratinized tissue width (3 mm)
>
> Thick periodontal bio type

> **Box 10**
> **Indications for acellular dermal matrix grafts**
>
> Soft tissue augmentation
>
> Multiple adjacent gingival recessions
>
> Patient reluctant for second site morbidity
>
> Correction of gingival amalgam tattoos

is adequate to stabilize the papilla and vertical releases. Periodontal dressing is placed and postoperative instructions are given to the patient. This procedure is indicated when root sensitivity and/or cosmetic concerns relative to recession become therapeutic issues.

ALLODERM: ACELLULAR DERMAL MATRIX GRAFT

When patients are reluctant to have a second surgical site, allograft materials should be considered. Originally intended for burn wounds, Wainwright discussed the use of a cellular dermal matrix allograft. The acellular dermal matrix is a freeze-dried, cell-free

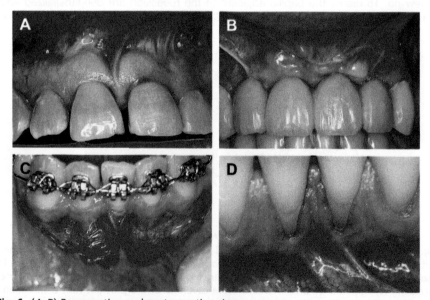

Fig. 6. (*A–D*) Preoperative and postoperative view.

dermal matrix consisting of a structurally integrated basement membrane complex and extracellular matrix.[21] Studies show mean defect coverage ranging from 66% to 99%, with a mean for all studies of 86%. Predictability data indicate that 90% or greater defect coverage was achieved 74% of the time (**Box 10**).

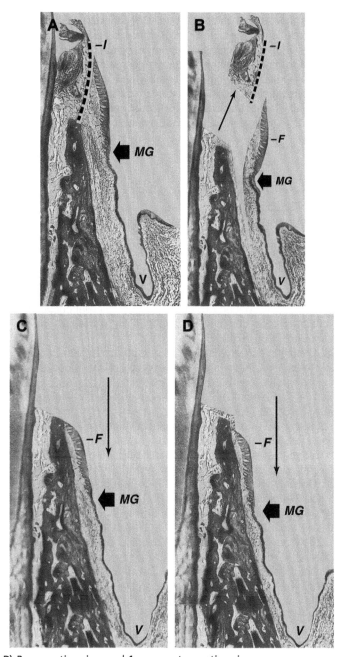

Fig. 7. (*A–D*) Preoperative view and 1 year postoperative view.

Technique

Adequate local anesthesia is administered to the patient using standard technique. The area of recession needs to be prepared by scaling and root planing. Using a no. 15 blade, a partial-thickness flap is created. Careful and methodical sharp dissection ensures the prevention of perforating the buccal flap. Using sterile saline baths for 10 to 15 minutes, the AlloDerm is rehydrated and inserted against the connective tissue side of the recipient bed. Deepithelialization of the papilla with a fresh no. 15 blade is required, and the graft is stabilized with resorbable sutures at the level of the CEJ. The buccal flap is then advanced and sutured over the Allo-Derm. It is critical to cover as much of the dermal matrix as possible. One-hundred percent coverage is ideal, ensuring graft stability and increasing the long-term prognosis. The graft is revascularized in a week and remodels for the next 3 to 4 months. The graft eventually takes the characteristics of the underlying and surrounding tissues. It takes 2 to 3 years for the final results of the graft to be appreciated (**Figs. 6** and **7**).

REFERENCES

1. American Academy of Periodontology (AAP). Consensus report: mucogingival therapy. Ann Periodontol 1996;1:702–6.
2. Bjorn H. Free transplantation of gingival propria. Sven Tandlak Tidskr 1963;22: 684–5.
3. James WC, McFall WT. Placement of free gingival grafts on denuded alveolar bone. J Periodontol 1978;49:283–90.
4. Dordick B, Coslet JG, Seibert JS. Clinical evaluation of free autogenous gingival grafts placed on alveolar bone. J Periodontol 1976;41:559–67.
5. Reiser GM, Bruno JF, Mahan PE, et al. The subepithelial connective tissue graft palatal donor site: anatomic considerations for surgeons. Int J Periodontics Restorative Dent 1996;16:131–7.
6. Foman S. Cosmetic surgery. Philadelphia: Lippincott; 1960.
7. Davis JS, Traut HF. Origin and development of the blood supply of whole-thickness skin grafts. Ann Surg 1925;82:871–9.
8. Egli U, Vollmer W, Rateitschak KH. Follow-up studies of free gingival grafts. J Clin Periodontol 1975;2:98–104.
9. Langer B, Langer L. Subepithelial connective tissue graft technique for root coverage. J Periodontol 1985;56:715–20.
10. Edel A. Clinical evaluation of free connective tissue grafts used to increase the width of keratinized gingiva. J Clin Periodontol 1974;1:185–96.
11. Bruno JF. Connective tissue graft technique assuring wide root coverage. Int J Periodontics Restorative Dent 1994;14:127–37.
12. Jahnke PV, Sandifer JB, Gher ME, et al. Thick free gingival and connective tissue autografts for root coverage. J Periodontol 1993;64:315–22.
13. Miller PD. Root coverage using the free soft tissue autograft following citric acid application. III. A successful and predictable procedure in areas of deep wide recession. Int J Periodontics Restorative Dent 1985;5(2):15–37.
14. Isik AG, Tarim B, Hafez AA, et al. A comparative scanning electron microscopic study on the characteristics of demineralized dentin root surface using different tetracycline HCl concentrations and application times. J Periodontol 2000;71: 219–25.
15. Grupe HE, Warren RF. Repair of gingival defects by a sliding flap operation. J Periodontol 1956;27:92–5.

16. Wood DL, Hoag FM, Donnenfeld OW, et al. Alveolar crest resorption following full and partial thickness flaps. J Periodontol 1972;43:141–4.

17. Wilderman MN, Wentz FM. Repair of a dentogingival defect with a pedicle flap. J Periodontol 1965;35:218–31.

18. Tarnow DP. Semilunar coronally repositioned flap. J Clin Periodontol 1986;13: 182–5.

19. Allen EP, Miller PD. Coronal positioning of existing gingiva: short term results in the treatment of shallow marginal tissue recession. J Periodontol 1989;60:316–9.

20. Block MS. Color atlas of dental implant surgery. 2nd edition. Philadelphia (PA): Saunders; 2007.

21. Wei PC, Laurell L, Geivelis M, et al. Acellular dermal matrix allografts to achieve increased attached gingiva. Part 1. A clinical study. J Periodontol 2000;71(8): 1297–305.

Suturing Principles for the Dentoalveolar Surgeon

M. Todd Brandt, DDS, MD[a],*, W. Scott Jenkins, DMD, MD[b]

KEYWORDS

• Sutures • Suturing • Dentoalveolar • Oral surgery

Successful dentoalveolar surgery begins with a detailed presurgical assessment, consideration of potential postoperative sequelae, proper selection of surgical instrumentation and materials, and sound surgical technique using those instruments and materials. One of the most important aspects for general practitioners who routinely perform dentoalveolar surgery to master is adequate closure of the surgical wound. Dentists who begin to perform more extensive dentoalveolar surgery often encounter surgical cases in which the removal of the tooth, excision of a mass or lesion, or placement of a graft or implant is less technically demanding than the wound closure. Inadequate or improper wound closure can lead to inadequate or delayed healing, or worse, including surgical failure. Thus, proper healing requires proper positioning of the soft tissues closest to their original position in a stable fashion, with the least amount of tension. Closure in this fashion decreases fibrous scarring, decreases the risk for infection, provides enhanced cosmesis, and facilitates hemostasis. The variety of suture material available is expansive and many companies manufacture sutures with seemingly unlimited sizes, needle designs, and materials. Dentists have traditionally selected sutures based on materials that were available during training. However, a decision made in this manner may overlook the distinct physical properties of a given suture or its effect on the surrounding tissues. This article focuses on the physical properties of suture materials and their tissue reactivity, and reviews various suturing techniques used in contemporary dentoalveolar surgery.

SUTURE MATERIAL

A suture is a strand of material used to ligate vessels and reapproximate lacerated or incised tissue. Evidence of suture use dates back to 50,000 BC.[1] Materials historically

---

The authors have nothing to disclose.
a Blue Ridge Oral and Maxillofacial Surgery, 54 South Medical Park Drive, Fishersville, VA 22939, USA
b Jenkins and Morrow, PLLC, 216 Fountain Court, 110, Lexington, KY 40509, USA
* Corresponding author.
E-mail address: mtbrandtoms@gmail.com

used have included linen, horsehair, flax, silkworm gut, kangaroo tendon, umbilical tape, ligament, cotton, iron wire, bark fibers, stainless steel, gold, and silver.[1–3] Synthetic fibers, such as nylon and polyester, first appeared in the 1940s.[2] Polyglycolic acid (Dexon) and polyglactin 910 (Vicryl) were developed in the early 1970s and polydioxanone (PDS) was introduced in the 1980s.[2] Suture materials are classified by performance, size, and physical configuration. Suture performance is categorized as either absorbable or nonabsorbable. The United States Pharmacopeia (USP) and the European Pharmacopeia (EP) govern the size or diameter of sutures and needles and prescribe the maximum and minimum standards and the diameter tolerances to which each manufacturer must adhere.[4] Physical configuration describes whether the suture is a monofilament or in braided, multifilament form.[1,3,5] The various suture characteristics all contribute to tissue reactivity, breaking strength, tensile strength, breaking strength retention, knot security, extensibility, memory, and absorbability (**Tables 1–3**).[1,2,5–15] A thorough knowledge of these properties is essential for the selection and proper use of the most appropriate suture for a specific clinical use.

Ideally, suture material should persist and retain adequate tensile strength after surgery, until healing has reached a stage at which wound separation is unlikely to occur.[1,2,5–15] The chosen suture material should have adequate and easy handling qualities and excellent knot security.[1,2,5–15] The material should not impede healing or elicit an inflammatory response or toxic effect.[3,5,10–16] Ideal sutures should also be affordable, available, easily sterilized, and nonconducive to bacterial growth.[2] Dentists should also be able to predict the absorption or encapsulation of the suture in the tissue.[1,2,8] No single ideal suture material exists, so dentists must choose a suture material that has most of the aforementioned qualities.

PHYSICAL PROPERTIES

The physical properties of sutures must be reviewed before discussing individual suture characteristics.

Tissue Reactivity

Sutures are foreign bodies that elicit an inflammatory response. Tissue reaction can be slight, minimal, or severe.[1,2,8–16] Specific perisutural cellular and enzymatic changes vary with each suture material.[16]

Breaking Strength

Breaking strength is the maximum force applied to a suture at the point of breaking or disruption.[16]

Tensile Strength

Tensile strength is the ratio of maximum load a suture can withstand without breaking while being stretched (breaking strength) to the original cross-sectional area of the given material.[5,7] The suture first deforms and then returns to the original size or shape when a stress less than the tensile strength is applied and then removed.[5,7] Tensile strength is measured in units of force per unit area.[5,7]

Breaking Strength Retention

Breaking strength retention is a measure of the tensile strength retained by a suture in vivo over time,[5,7] and is typically measured as a percent loss of the tensile strength calculated from peri-implantation tensile strength.[5,7]

Knot Security

Knot security is a force defined as the force applied to a loop (knot) suture at the point of knot slippage or disruption.[5,7,8]

Extensibility

During closure of a wound, sutures inevitably stretch during knot tying. This stretch in a suture varies for each material; as surgeons become familiar with a suture material's extensibility, their knot-tying ability improves, with less breakage of that suture material.[5,8]

Memory

Most materials used in dentoalveolar surgery have memory, that is, the tendency to not lay flat but to return to an original shape set by the material's manufacturing process or packaging.[5] This must be remembered during wound closure and knot tying.

Absorbable Sutures

The USP defines an absorbable suture as a "flexible strand prepared from collagen derived from health mammals, or from a synthetic polymer. It is capable of being absorbed by living mammalian tissue, but may be treated to modify its resistance to absorption. It may be impregnated or treated with a suitable coating, softening, or antimicrobial agent. It may be colored by a color additive approved by the Food and Drug Administration (FDA)."[4]

Nonabsorbable Sutures

The USP defines a nonabsorbable suture as a "flexible strand of material that is suitably resistant to the action of living mammalian tissue. It may be impregnated or treated with a suitable coating, softening, or antimicrobial agent. It may be colored by a color additive approved by the Food and Drug Administration (FDA)."[4]

Monofilament Sutures

Monofilament sutures are a single strand or filament.

Multifilament Sutures

Multifilament sutures are made of several braided or twisted strands or filaments.[1,3,5]

BIOLOGIC RESPONSE TO SUTURE MATERIALS

Regardless of their physical composition, all sutures implanted in the human body act as foreign bodies.[1-3,5,6,9-16] Intraoral placement of sutures produces a different inflammatory response than that witnessed elsewhere in the body.[16] Confounding factors in the oral cavity include humidity and an indigenous flora, which increases the likelihood for bacterial migration along the suture, resulting in infection.[14,16] Natural absorbable sutures are generally digested by enzymatic and macrophage activity.[14,15] This produces a greater degree of tissue reaction in the breakdown of synthetic absorbable sutures, which occur by hydrolysis.[3,16] Water gradually penetrates the synthetic suture, causing a breakdown in the polymer chain.[3,16]

Some generalities exist regarding suture tissue reactivity.[1] Multifilament sutures elicit a greater inflammatory response than monofilament sutures.[2] Polypropylene and steel elicit the least inflammatory response, whereas nylon, polyester, cotton, and silk all cause an increased tissue response.[1,2] Histologic analysis shows discrete

Table 1
Characteristics of absorbable suture material

Suture	Types	Raw Material	Tensile Strength	Absorption Rate	Tissue Reaction	Contraindications	Frequent Uses
Surgical gut	Plain	Collagen derived from healthy beef and sheep	Individual patient characteristics can affect rate of tensile strength	Absorbed by proteolytic enzymatic digestive process	Moderate reaction	Being absorbable, should not be used where extended approximation of tissues under stress is required; should not be used in patients with known sensitivities or allergies to collagen or chromium	General soft tissue approximation and/or ligation
Surgical gut	Chronic	Collagen derived from healthy beef and sheep	Individual patient characteristics can affect rate of tensile strength	Absorbed by proteolytic enzymatic digestive process	Moderate reaction	Being absorbable, should not be used where extended approximation of tissues under stress is required; should not be used in patients with known sensitivities or allergies to collagen or chromium	General soft tissue approximation and/or ligation

Polyglactin 910 Vicryl (Ethicon)	Braided monofilament	Copolymer of lactide and glycolide coated with polyglactin 370 and calcium stearate	~75% remains at 2 wk; ~ 50% remains at 3 wk	Complete between 56 and 90 d Absorbed by hydrolysis	Minimal acute inflammatory reaction	Being absorbable, should not be used where extended approximation of tissue is required	General soft tissue approximation and/or ligation
Polyglycolic acid Dexon (USS/DG)	Braided (coated)	Polyglycolic acid polycaprolate coating system (copolymer of glycolide and ε-caprolactone)	~65% remains at 2 wk; ~ 35% remains at 3 wk	Essentially complete between 60 and 90 d, absorbed by hydrolysis	Minimal acute inflammatory reaction	Being absorbable, should not be used where extended approximation of tissue is required	General soft tissue approximation and/or ligation

Table 2
Characteristics of absorbable suture material

Suture	Types	Raw Material	Tensile Strength	Absorption Rate	Tissue Reaction	Contraindications	Frequent Uses
Poliglecaprone 25 Monocryl (Ethicon)	Monofilament	Copolymer of glycolide and ε-caprolactone	~50%–60% (violet 60%–70%) remains at 1 wk; ~20%–30% (violet 30%–40%) remains at 2 wk; lost within 3 wk (violet 4 wk)	Complete at 91–119 d; absorbed by hydrolysis	Minimal acute inflammatory reaction	Being absorbable, should not be used where extended approximation of tissue under stress is required; undyed not indicated for use in fascia	General soft tissue approximation and/or ligation; not for use in cardiovascular or neurologic tissues, microsurgery, or ophthalmic surgery
Polydioxanone PDS II (Ethicon)	Monofilament	Polyester polymer	~70% remains at 2 wk; ~50% remains at 4 wk; ~25% remains at 6 wk	Minimal until ~90th day Complete between 18 and 30 mo Absorbed by slow hydrolysis	Slight reaction	Being absorbable, should not be used where prolonged approximation of tissues under stress is required; should not be used with prosthetic heart valves or synthetic grafts	All types of soft tissue approximation, including pediatric cardiovascular and ophthalmic procedures; not for use in adult cardiovascular tissue, microsurgery, and neural tissue
Polyglyconate Maxon (USS/DG)	Monofilament	Polyglyconate	~75% remains at 2 wk; ~65% remains at 3 wk; ~25% remains at 6 wk	Essentially complete by 6 mo Absorbed by slow hydrolysis	Slight reaction	Being absorbable, should not be used where prolonged approximation of tissues under stress is required; should not be used with prosthetic heart valves or synthetic grafts	All types of soft tissue approximation; not for use in adult cardiovascular tissue, microsurgery, and neural tissue

Table 3
Characteristics of nonabsorbable suture material

Suture	Types	Raw Material	Tensile Strength	Absorption Rate	Tissue Reaction	Contraindications	Frequent Uses
Silk suture	Braided	Organic protein called fibroin	Progressive degradation of fiber may result in gradual loss of tensile strength over time	Gradual encapsulation by fibrous connective tissue	Acute inflammatory reaction	Should not be used in patients with known sensitivities or allergies to silk	General soft tissue approximation and/or ligation, including cardiovascular, ophthalmic, and neurologic procedures
Nylon suture Ethilon (Ethicon) Dermalon (USS/DG)	Monofilament	Long-chain aliphatic polymers nylon 6 or nylon 6,6	Progressive hydrolysis may result in a gradual loss of tensile strength over time	Gradual encapsulation by fibrous connective tissue	Minimal inflammatory reaction	Should not be used where permanent retention of tensile strength is required	Same
Polyester fiber suture ersiline (Ethicon) Dacron (USS/DG)	Braided monofilament	Poly (ethylene terephthalate)	No significant change known to occur in vivo	Gradual encapsulation by fibrous connective tissue	Minimal inflammatory reaction	None known	Same
Polypropylene suture Prolene (Ethicon) Surgiline (USS/DG)	Monofilament	Isotactic crystalline stereoisomer of polypropylene	Not subject to degradation or weakening by action of tissue enzymes	Nonabsorbable	Minimal inflammatory reaction	None known	

temporal phases of tissue reactivity around sutures.[16] Selvig and colleagues[16] found distinct concentric perisutural zones after histologic processing and analysis. An acute-phase response of neutrophil infiltration was observed up to 3 days, mainly reflecting the initial surgical trauma in suture placement. This response was comparable in all suture materials tested.[16] The neutrophilic infiltration is soon replaced by chronic cellular infiltrates, including monocytes, plasma cells, and lymphocytes.[13] These stages of tissue reactivity remove cellular debris and suture material.[13] Peak tissue reaction occurs between the second and seventh days.[16] Theoretically, in favorable healing conditions, this acute phase should be replaced by the formation of granulation tissue in the absence of inflammatory cells.[16] Progressive inflammatory reactions caused by sutures may persist for as long as 7 to 14 days.[16]

Bacterial migration along the suture track has been documented.[2,3,16] Although braided suture has been reported to promote bacterial retention and growth because of its physical composition, Selvig and colleagues[16] found bacteria plaque migration extending more than 100 μm into suture channels at 14 days regardless of the suture material tested, except for gut, which had rapidly dissipated by this time. Sutures that remain in intraoral wounds, such as silk, cause epithelial tracks, thereby increasing the propensity for bacterial migration.[16] In general, sutures should be removed no later than 7 to 10 days.[16] The loss of tensile strength and rate of absorption are separate and distinct phenomena.[3] Sutures may rapidly lose adequate tensile strength, but be absorbed slowly, or vice versa. Fever, infection, or protein-deficient states may accelerate the absorption process and cause an increase in loss of tensile strength.[2,7] Moist or fluid-filled tissue such as the oral cavity, or soaking sutures in saline for extended periods, may also accelerate the absorption process.[2,3,7]

SUTURE SELECTION

When selecting a suture material, consideration must be given to the duration the suture must remain and the relationship the suture has with adjacent tissue. The smallest suture that couples the least immunogenicity with the highest tensile strength is preferable.[5] This article examines suture performance by degree of absorbability.

Nonabsorbable sutures resist enzymatic activity and hydrolysis. One of the most widely used nonabsorbable sutures is silk. This raw fiber is harvested while the silkworm larvae are spinning the cocoons. This material is processed into a braided fiber, sterilized, and used in a variety of surgical settings. Although it is classified as a nonabsorbable suture, histologic analysis of silk in vivo after 2 years revealed no evidence of remaining suture.[5] Synthetic absorbable sutures include nylon, polypropylene, and polyester. These sutures are chemically synthesized polymers that vary in their physical properties and chemical structure, and are manufactured as monofilament or braided strands. Nylon is a polyamide polymer that may either be monofilament or braided and can be dyed in a variety of colors.[5] Polyester sutures are polyethylene terephthalate braided multifilament strands that produce little inflammatory response but tend to create more tissue tearing.[5] Polypropylene-based sutures have low immunogenicity compared with most other nonabsorbable sutures with high breaking strength.

As with nonabsorbable sutures, absorbable sutures are classified as either monofilament or multifilament. The natural form of absorbable sutures is surgical gut that may be further subdivided as plain or chromic. Gut suture is rendered from bovine or sheep submucosal intestinal layer and processed to the desired size. Once processed, the gut suture is either packaged as plain gut or is treated to lengthen the absorption time. In vivo, gut is digested by proteolytic enzymes in macrophage activity. This absorption can be prolonged if the suture is treated with acromion salt solution. Thus, in infected wounds, dentists may choose to use chromic gut suture for wound closure because of the delayed absorption.

Synthetic absorbable sutures were designed to bypass problems encountered with gut suture immunogenicity and unpredictability in absorption. Historically, the synthetic absorbable sutures include polyglycolic acid (Dexon), polyglactin 910 (Vicryl), and polydioxanone (PDS). Polyglycolic acid (Dexon) was the first synthetic absorbable suture with handling characteristics similar to silk, but has greater tensile strength than gut.[2] It is produced in a braided multifilament form. Polyglactin 910 (Vicryl) is a copolymer of lactic and polyglycolic acid that has a 50% tensile strength for 3 weeks and then resorbs within 90 days. It is produced in a braided multifilament form. Poliglecaprone 25 (Monocryl) is composed of glycoside and ε-caprolactone. It offers high initial tensile strength and absorbs by 119 days. Another synthetic material suture is PDS, a polydioxanone polymer that forms a monofilament suture with enhanced flexibility and significantly greater tensile strength than both polyglycolic acid and polyglactin 910.[2] Absorbable synthetic suture can also be obtained in a coated form that inhibits bacterial colonization of the suture. Ethicon Vicryl Plus coated antibacterial suture contains Irgacare MP, a pure form of triclosan, which is a broad-spectrum antibacterial agent that creates a zone of inhibition, preventing bacterial colonization by the pathogens that most often cause surgical site infections.

NEEDLE SELECTION

The purpose of the needle is to transport the chosen suture material through the soft tissues with the least amount of traumatic injury. A balance must be maintained between needle rigidity and flexibility. Too rigid a needle may fracture when met with resistance, whereas one that is too flexible may not accurately travel to the designated exit point.[5] The material of choice in contemporary needle design is a corrosion-resistant stainless steel alloy. The needle itself has 3 designated regions: the eye, the body, and the point. The entire complex begins as a sharp point and expands in diameter to the eye. The eye of the needle harbors the interface of the suture material. There are 3 types of needle eyes: closed, split (French), and swaged. The closed and split types are less desirable because the junction of the needle and the suture is often enlarged, increasing the risk of tissue trauma, and must be threaded, which is time consuming. The needle of choice today is a swaged eyeless needle, in which the junction of the needle and suture is uniform and permanent. The body of the needle is manufactured in a variety of sizes, shapes, and curvatures. Needles may be round, flat, triangular, oval, or tapered. The needles most frequently used in dentoalveolar surgery are curved needles that range in shape from 1/4 to 5/8 of a circle (**Fig. 1**). The appropriate needle must be based on the dimensions of the wound to be closed. The point of the needle is the initial contact point of the needle with the tissue. Three basic needle points exist: tapered, blunt, or cutting. In dentoalveolar surgery, cutting needles are preferred because of the thickness, resilience, and resistance of the gingiva and oral mucosa. The 2 basic cutting needles used in dentoalveolar surgery are conventional (cutting) and reverse cutting needles (**Fig. 2**). Each has 3 cutting edges with 2 edges opposing each other. The conventional has a third edge facing upwards (toward the inside of the circle), whereas, in the reverse cutting needle, it faces down.

Suture materials have their own classification system for needle size and shape. When selecting the desired suture and needle combination, close attention must be paid to each manufacturer's supply-order charts for the proper needle selection.

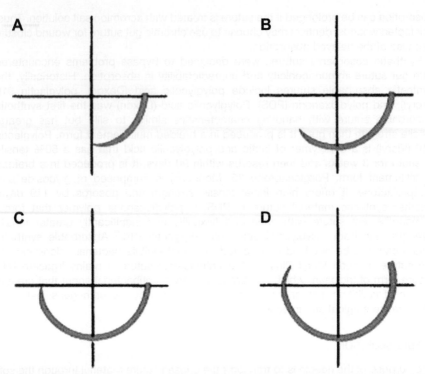

Fig. 1. Degree of needle curvature: (A) 1/4 circle, (B) 3/8 circle, (C) 1/2 circle, (D) 3/4 circle. (*From* Peterson LJ, editor. Contemporary oral and maxillofacial surgery. 3rd edition: Mosby Year Book; 1998. p. 54; with permission.)

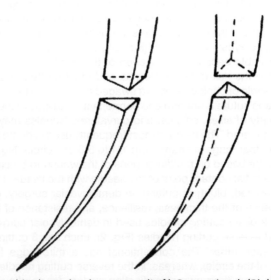

Fig. 2. Needles used in dentoalveolar surgery. (*Left*) Conventional. (*Right*) Reverse cutting, regular cutting. (*From* Peterson LJ, editor. Contemporary oral and maxillofacial surgery. 3rd edition: Mosby Year Book; 1998. p. 54; with permission.)

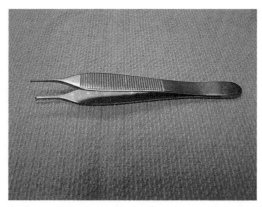

Fig. 3. Common tissue forceps, single-toothed Adson, 7.6 cm (3 inches).

INSTRUMENTATION

Intraoral suturing requires 2 main instruments: the needle driver and the suture scissors. Tissue forceps may occasionally be used to ensure proper needle entrance through tissue by ensuring stability of the soft tissue flap. These tissue forceps are manufactured in various sizes, with and without teeth. The most common tissue forceps used is a single-toothed 7.6-cm (3-inch) Adson forceps (**Fig. 3**). The needle driver most commonly used is the 15.2-cm (6-inch) version of the Hegar-Mayo type (**Fig. 4**).[17] Needle drivers are also manufactured with a variety of sizes and beaks, with or without teeth. A needle driver is most effective when using proper hand position. The needle driver is held in the palm with the fourth (ring) finger and the thumb within the rings of the instrument. The second finger is placed along the lower straight arm for stabilization, and the third ring finger is laid passively outside the ring of the fourth finger (**Fig. 5**). The beaks of the needle driver should be perpendicular to the needle and held one-third of the distance from the origin of the suture (**Fig. 6**). The weakest part of the needle is located at the junction of the needle body in the portion where the suture is affixed to the needle. If the beaks of the needle driver are placed too close to the swaged end, bending or breakage of the needle may occur on insertion in the tissue. A bend in the needle may not be visible to the clinician, but

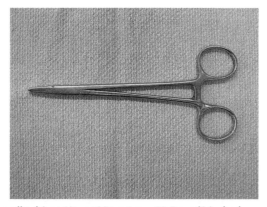

Fig. 4. Common needle driver, Hegar-Mayo type, 15.2 cm (6 inches).

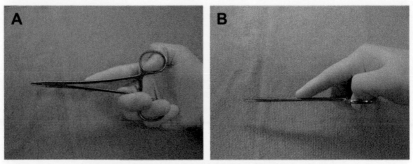

Fig. 5. (*A, B*) Proper hand positioning of ringed instruments.

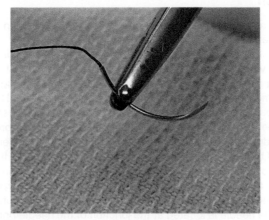

Fig. 6. Proper relationship between needle and needle driver.

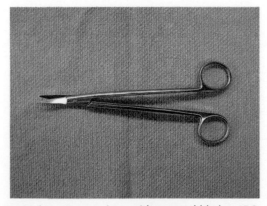

Fig. 7. Common suture scissor, Deans scissor with serrated blades, 17.8 cm (7 inches).

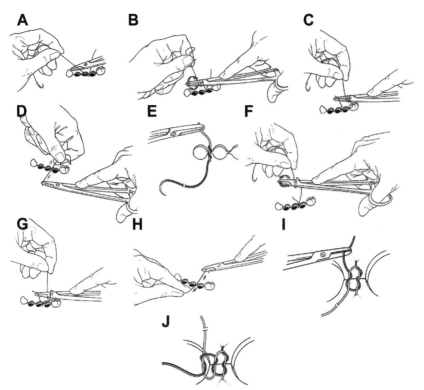

Fig. 8. Most intraoral sutures are tied with instrument tie. (*A*) Suture is pulled through tissue until short tail of suture (approximately 1.3–5 cm long) remains. Needle holder is held horizontally by right hand in preparation for knot-tying procedure. (*B*) Left hand then wraps long end of suture around needle holder twice in clockwise direction to make 2 loops of suture around needle holder. (*C*) Surgeon then opens needle holder and grasps short end of suture near its end. (*D*) Ends of suture are then pulled to tighten knot. Needle holder should not pull until knot is nearly tied, to avoid lengthening that portion of suture. (*E*) End of first step of surgeon's knot. Note that double wrap has resulted in double overhand knot, which increases friction in knot and keeps wound edges together until second portion of knot is tied. (*F*) Needle holder is then released from short end of suture and held in same position as when knot-tying procedure began. Left hand then makes single wrap in counterclockwise direction. (*G*) Needle holder then grasps short end of suture at its end. (*H*) This portion of knot is completed by pulling this loop firmly down against previous portion of knot. (*I*) This completes surgeon's knot. Double loop of first pass holds tissue together until second portion of square knot can be tied. (*J*) Most surgeons add a third throw to their instrument tie. Needle holder is repositioned in original position, and 1 wrap is placed around needle holder in original clockwise direction. Short end of suture is grasped and tightened down firmly to form second square knot. Final throw of 3 knots is tightened firmly. (*From* Peterson LJ, editor. Contemporary oral and maxillofacial surgery, 3rd edition: Mosby Year Book; 1998. p. 188–9; with permission.)

nonetheless can cause sufficient metal fatigue to result in unexpected needle breakage. Holding the needle too close to the sharp tip limits the length of needle available to pass through tissue. The most common suture scissor is the Dean scissor, an instrument that is 17.8 cm (7 inches) long and has offset serrated blades (**Fig. 7**).[17] It should be held in the same fashion as the needle driver. It is most efficient when cutting the suture perpendicular to its blades. The Dean scissor is also a general-purpose scissor that may be used in trimming or removing tissue.

SUTURE TECHNIQUES

There is a multitude of suturing techniques available to the dentist. The technique selected depends on the breadth and length of the wound, the closure tension required, and the distance to which wound edges must move. Techniques are broadly categorized as interrupted and continuous: interrupted techniques include simple interrupted, horizontal/vertical mattress, and sling; continuous suturing is divided into running, locking, and continuous sling. Choosing between an interrupted and continuous technique requires striking a balance between the ease and rapidity of the continuous techniques and the additional stability and control of wound edges offered by interrupted techniques.

Simple Interrupted

This is the most universal technique in practice today and may be used for small wounds, or evenly spaced or continuous to close larger wounds. Placement requires entrance of the suture through both wound margins, with the surgeons knot for stability. Placed correctly, the suture should slightly evert the wound edges (**Fig. 8**).[18]

Vertical Mattress

This technique is primarily used extraorally and may be used when everted wound edges are desired. By its nature, this technique provides wound support at 2 levels: deep and superficial (**Figs. 9A and 10**). These 2 levels of closure provide great resistance to wound separation. When fibrous scarring and tissue contraction occur during healing, the everted wound edges created by this technique enhance the appearance of the final scar. It can be difficult to place a vertical mattress suture in intraoral tissues because the limited degree of tissue elasticity often prevents placement of the deep portion of the mattress across the wound edges. Furthermore, there is less wound contracture that occurs during healing because of the thinness of submucosal tissue, so creating everted wound edges is not essential for formation of a cosmetic scar.

Horizontal Mattress

This technique is ideal for closure of soft tissue wounds across small bony defects because it everts the mucosal margins and provides a broader area of support (see **Figs. 9B and 10**). Considerable wound tension can be created using the horizontal

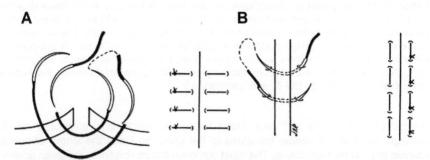

Fig. 9. (A) Vertical mattress suture. (B) Horizontal mattress suture. (*From* Pedersen GW. Oral surgery. Philadelphia: WB Saunders; 1988. p. 55; with permission.)

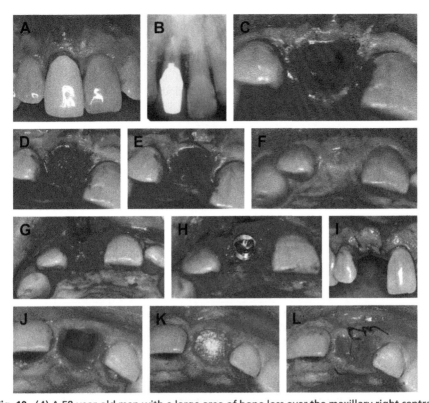

Fig. 10. (*A*) A 58-year-old man with a large area of bone loss over the maxillary right central incisor. The tooth was mobile and had a draining fissure present over the labial surface of the tooth at the level of the apex of the tooth. (*B*) Periapical radiograph showing significant bone loss to approximately 3 mm from the apex of the tooth. This large restoration had been stable for 14 years before the current problem. The patient was placed on antibiotics and prescribed a mouth rinse to decrease the bacteria flora and was appointed for surgery. (*C*) The tooth was extracted easily after incisions were made around the neck of the tooth. After the tooth was removed, there was a large area of bone loss, extending 9 mm from the gingival margin. Even with the 9-mm pocket that was present on the labial aspect of the tooth, the gingiva form matched the level on the adjacent tooth. (*D*) A graft of human mineralized bone was placed into the defect and compacted to recreate root form anatomy and the labial aspect of the socket. (*E*) A piece of collagen was placed and retained by a horizontal mattress suture. (*F*) The area approximately 4 months after graft placement, indicating sufficient form of the gingiva and root prominence. (*G*) After a crestal incision and small reflection in the sulci of the adjacent teeth, sufficient bone was found for placement of a 4-mm diameter implant. (*H*) The implant was placed approximately 3 mm apical to the adjacent gingival margin. After the implant was placed, bone harvested from the drills was placed over the labial aspect to further augment the site. (*I*) The site was closed with 2 vertical mattress sutures everting the interdental papilla and to advance the flaps coronally. (*J*) A central incisor was extracted with loss of a significant amount of labial bone. There was vertical palatal bone present but no labial bone superior to the nasal floor. (*K*) Bovine mineralized bone was compacted into the site to recreate the root prominence and to fill the space that was previously occupied by the root of the tooth. (*L*) A collagen material (Collaplug) was placed over the bovine graft and was retained in position with 2 horizontal mattress silk sutures. (*From* Block MS, Jackson WC. Techniques for grafting the extraction site in preparation for dental implant placement. Atlas of oral and maxillofacial surgery. vol. 14. Elsevier; 2006. p. 2; with permission.)

mattress technique; the mattress spreads the forces along the horizontal band of tissue instead of focusing at a single point, thus decreasing the chance for the suture to pull through and lacerate tissue during wound approximation and knot tying. The horizontal mattress technique is frequently used during closure of an oroantral opening, where tension-free, watertight wound closure is required to prevent exchange of air, saliva, and mucus between the sinus and oral cavity.

Figure-eight

This technique can be used effectively to close the tissue of an extraction site. Although not frequently used to gain primary closure, it can provide a barrier to dislodgment of a clot after tooth extraction and may help stabilize materials placed into an extraction socket, such as Gelfoam, bone grafting materials, collagen plugs, or other packing materials (**Figs. 11** and **12**).

Sling Ligation

This technique is ideally used in surgery where a flap is elevated only on one side of the alveolus. This technique allows repositioning of the flap without entering the opposing intact soft tissue (**Figs. 13** and **14**).

Anchor Suture

This technique is indicated for closure of mucosa in edentulous areas either mesial or distal to a tooth. This technique offers tight closure of the buccal and lingual soft tissues and causes increased adaptation to the adjacent tooth (**Fig. 15**).

Continuous Sutures

This technique is commonly used in dentoalveolar surgery when longer wounds result. Dentists often use this technique following multiple or full-mouth tooth extractions that leave a wound that spans the entire alveolus. This method offers quicker closure because few knots are placed over the entire length of the wound. A major disadvantage in this type of suturing is that, if one knot fails, the closure is compromised. This simple technique has a potential to obliquely apply pressure along the length of the wound, whereas the locked technique has a lesser potential (**Figs. 16** and **17**).[18]

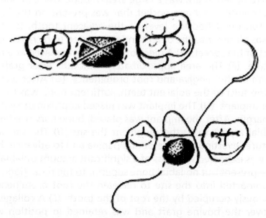

Fig. 11. Figure-of-eight suture techniques. (*From* Kwon PH, Laskin DM. Clinician's manual of oral and maxillofacial surgery. 2nd edition: Quintessence Publishing; 1997. p. 249; with permission.)

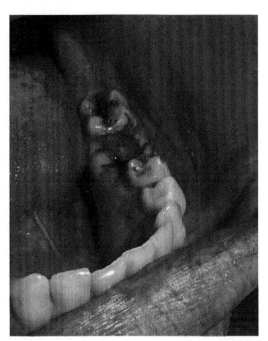

Fig. 12. Socket bone grafting technique showing containment of the particulate bone graft material with a collagen plug and figure-of-eight suture. (*From* Roden RD. Principles of bone grafting. Oral Maxillofacial Surg Clin N Am 2010;22(3):299; with permission.)

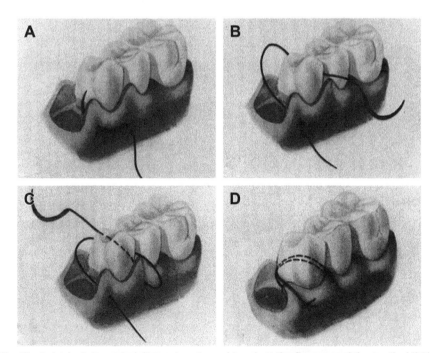

Fig. 13. A single, interrupted sling suture is used to adapt the flap around the tooth. (*A*) The needle engages the outer surface of the flap, and (*B*) encircles the tooth. (*C*) The outer surface of the same flap of the adjacent interdental area is engaged, and (*D*) the suture is returned to the initial site and the knot tied. (*From* Carranza FA. Glickman's clinical periodontology. 7th edition. Philadelphia: WB Saunders; 1990. p. 803; with permission.)

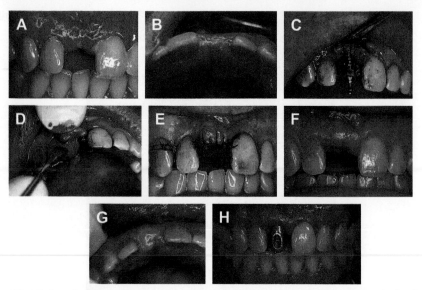

Fig. 14. (*A*) An edentulous space with loss in vertical dimension. (*B*) Occlusal view indicating the loss in buccolingual dimensions; this is a Siebert class III ridge deformity. (*C*) The ridge was expanded and the implant placed. (*D*) A rotated split palatal graft was prepared and rolled over the implant site. (*E*) Suturing of the site. (*F*) Healing after 6 months. (*G*) The occlusal view of the healing after 6 months. (*H*) The gingival zenith at time of abutment placement. (*From* Geurs UC, Vassilopoulos PJ, Reddy MS. Soft tissue considerations in implant site development. Oral Maxillofacial Surg Clin N Am 2010;22(3):397; with permission.)

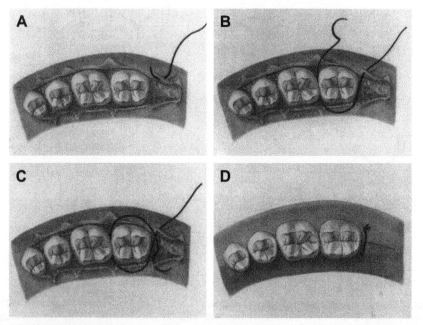

Fig. 15. (*A–D*) Distal wedge suture. This suture is also used to close flaps that are mesial or distal to a lone standing tooth. (*From* Carranza FA. Glickman's clinical periodontology. 7th edition. Philadelphia: WB Saunders; 1990. p. 803; with permission.)

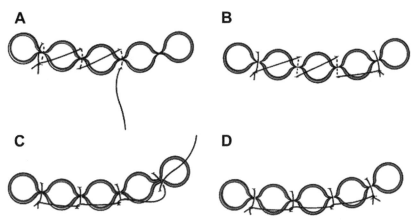

Fig. 16. When multiple sutures are to be placed, the incision can be closed with running or continuous sutures. (A) First, the papilla is closed and the knot tied in the usual way. The long end of the suture is held, and the adjacent papilla is sutured, without the knot being tied but just with the suture being pulled firmly through the tissue. (B) Succeeding papillae are then sutured until the final one is sutured and the final knot is tied. Final appearance is with the suture going across each empty socket. (C) Continuous locking stitch can be made by passing the long end of the suture underneath the loop before it is pulled through the tissue. (D) This stage puts the suture on both deep periosteal and mucosal surfaces directly across the papilla and may aid in more direct apposition of tissues. (From Peterson LJ, editor. Principles of complicated exodontia. In: Contemporary oral and maxillofacial surgery. 3rd edition. Mosby Year Book; 1998. p. 191; with permission.)

Continuous Sling

This technique is the continuous version of the isolated sling technique, and may be used when both buccal and lingual flaps have been reflected. This closure allows both flaps to be repositioned independently because of their anchors or the abutment teeth at either end of the wound (**Fig. 18**).[19,20]

Combination

This technique may include a continuous suture with overlaying vertical or horizontal mattress sutures and/or simple interrupted sutures (**Fig. 19**). The continuous suture is often absorbable with a nonabsorbable or more slowly absorbable suture placed over

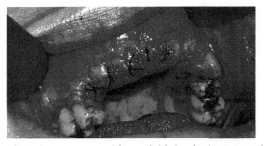

Fig. 17. Continuous chromic gut suture with overlaid simple, interrupted silk sutures in the anterior maxilla.

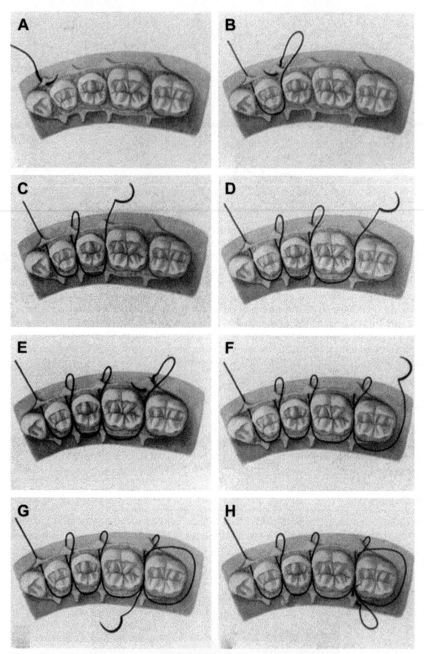

Fig. 18. The continuous, independent sling suture is used to adapt the buccal and lingual flaps without tying the buccal flap to the lingual flap (*A–P*). The teeth are used to suspend each flap against the bone. It is important to anchor the suture on the 2 teeth at the beginning and end of the flap so that the suture does not pull the buccal flap to the lingual flap. (*From* Carranza FA. Glickman's clinical periodontology. 7th edition. Philadelphia: WB Saunders; 1990. p. 806–7; with permission.)

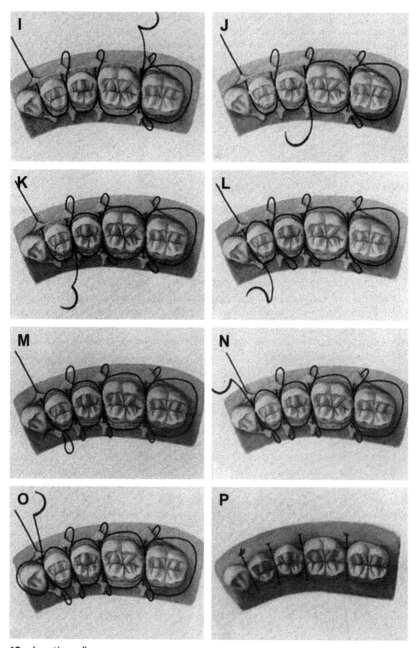

Fig. 18. (*continued*)

the first layer of superficial suturing. This technique helps prevent wound dehiscence if the continuous suture resorbs before initial wound healing has occurred. Dentists often use this technique with larger dentoalveolar defects and cases that require grafting (soft and hard tissue).

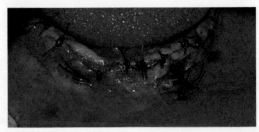

Fig. 19. Combination of absorbable and nonabsorbable simple, interrupted sutures, mattress sutures, and continuous sutures for wound closure in the anterior mandible.

SUMMARY

When suturing is required for wound closure, dentists should be aware of the characteristics of suture material so the most appropriate material can be selected, and the technique used should provide effectiveness and ease. The authors frequently recommend that dentists who routinely perform dentoalveolar surgery, such as the extraction of teeth, should have at least 1 type of absorbable and 1 type of nonabsorbable suture readily available within their operatory supply. Commonly, 3-0 or 4-0 chromic gut suture and 3-0 or 4-0 silk suture can be used successfully to close nearly any type of intraoral wound following dentoalveolar surgery. Familiarity with the concepts presented in this article and continuous practice of the surgical skills presented enhances surgical acumen and allows for improved healing, increased postoperative comfort, and successful surgery.

REFERENCES

1. Macht SD. Sutures and suturing-current concepts. J Oral Surg 1978;36:710–2.
2. Gutman JL, Harrison JW. Surgical endodontics. Saint Louis (MO): Ishiyaku Euro-America; 1994. p. 278–99.
3. Wound closure manual. Somerville (NJ): Ethicon; 2007.
4. Unites States Pharmacopeia (USP). 24th edition. National Formulary. 17th edition. Philadelphia: National Publishing; 1999. p. 1584–6.
5. Knot tying manual. Somerville (NJ): Ethicon; 2007.
6. Romfh RF, Cramer FS. Technique and the use of surgical tools, 2nd edition. Norwalk (CT): Appleton and Lang; 1992. p. 33–124.
7. Herrman JB. Changes in tensile strength and knot security of surgical sutures in vivo. Arch Surg 1973;106:707–10.
8. Greenwald D, Shumway S, Albear P, et al. Mechanical comparison of 10 suture materials before and after in vivo incubation. J Surg Res 1994;56:372–7.
9. Maves TJ, Pechman PS, Gebhart GF, et al. Possible chemical contribution from chromic gut sutures produces disorder of pain sensation like those seen in man. Pain 1993;54:57–69.
10. Wallace WR, Maxwell GR, Cacalaris CJ. Comparison of polyglycolic acid suture to black silk, chromic and plain gut in human oral tissues. J Oral Surg 1970;28:739–46.
11. Lilly GE. Reaction of oral tissues to suture materials. Oral Surg Oral Med Oral Pathol 1968;26:128–33.
12. Lilly GE, Armstrong JH, Salem GE, et al. Reaction of oral tissues to suture materials. Part II. Oral Surg Oral Med Oral Pathol 1968;26:592–9.
13. Lilly GE, Salem JE, Armstrong JH, et al. Reaction of oral tissues to suture materials. Part III. Oral Surg Oral Med Oral Pathol 1969;28:432–8.

14. Lilly GE, Cutcher JL, Jones JC, et al. Reaction of oral tissues to suture materials. Part IV. Oral Surg Oral Med Oral Pathol 1972;33:152–7.
15. DeNardo GA, Brown AN, Trenka-Benthin S, et al. Comparison of seven different suture materials in the feline oral cavity. J Am Anim Hosp Assoc 1996;32:164–72.
16. Selvig KA, Biagiotti GR, Leknes KN, et al. Oral tissue reactions to suture materials. Int J Periodontics Restorative Dent 1998;18:475–87.
17. Pedersen GW. Oral surgery. Philadelphia: WB Saunders; 1998. p. 47–81.
18. Moore UJ. Principles of oral and maxillofacial surgery. Mauldin (MA): Blackwell Science; 2001. p. 77–81.
19. Newman MG, Takei H, Carranza FA, et al. Glickman's clinical periodontology. 10th edition. Philadelphia: WB Saunders; 2006. p. 800–10.
20. Unites States Surgical Corporation, a unit of Covidien (formerly a division of Tyco Healthcare Group, LP). Products by material. Available at: www.syneture.com. Accessed July 21, 2011.

Index

Note: Page numbers of article titles are in **boldface** type.

A

Acetylsalicylic acid (aspirin), 107
Allergic reactions, to local anesthesia, 144
Alloderm: acellular dermal graft, in mucogingival defects, 276–278
Alveolar fracture, as postextraction complication, 81
Alveolar osteitis, as postextraction complication, 82–83
American Heart Association, 2007 antibiotic prophylaxis guidelines, 236–242
American Society of Anesthesiologists, physical status classification, 177, 178
American Society of Anesthesiology, medical conditions and, 6
    physical classification of patients, 7
Analgesia, preemptive, 100–101
Analgesics, oral narcotic, commonly used, 96
      properties of, 97
    postoperative, 101–109
Anesthesia, local, agents, techniques, and complications of, **133–148**
      complications of, 144–146
      relative anatomy and techniques for, 140–144
Anesthetics, injectable, 135–139
    topical, 133–135
      combination of, 134–135
Antibiotic resistance, antibiotic prophylaxis and, 241–242
Antibiotics, review of, and indications for prophylaxis, **235–244**
    used for prophylaxis, 237–239
Anticoagulant therapy, oral, patients fully on, 33
        algorithm for, 37
    oral surgery patients on, **25–41**
Anticoagulants, 30
    conditions requiring, 31–33
Antidepressants/tranquilizers, in temporomandibular disorders, 157
Antiplatelet medications, 29–33
Anxiety control, in dental patient, **1–16**
Arachidonic acid metabolism, pharmacologic interventions in, 99
Articaine, 138

B

Benzocaine, 134
Benzodiazines, 6–9
    overdosage of, reversal of, 9–10
Bleeding, as postextraction complication, 77–78

Dent Clin N Am 56 (2012) 305–312
doi:10.1016/S0011-8532(11)00202-3
0011-8532/12/$ – see front matter © 2012 Elsevier Inc. All rights reserved.

dental.theclinics.com

Bleeding (*continued*)
    intraoperative control of, 19
    postoperative, management of, 21–22
    prevention of, intraoperative considerations for, 19–20
Bone, anatomy of, 209
      and histology of, 209–210
    healing of, 210–211
Bone grafting, alveolar, and reconstruction prior to implacement
    placement, **209–218**
    surgical principles of, 211–212
Bone grafting technique, socket, 297
Bone graft(s), assessments for, 215–217
    interpositional, 217
    types of, 211
Bone harvest sites, 212–215
Bone harvesting, for sinus lift surgery, 222–223
Botox, in temporomandibular disorders, 156–157
Bupivacaine, 139
Butorphanol (Stadol), 105

C

Caine allergy, 140
Cancer chemotherapy, immunosuppression in, antibiotic prophylaxis for, 240–241
Canines, maxillary, impaction of, 186–190
Cardiovascular devices, nonvalvular, antibiotic prophylaxis for, 240–241
Celecoxib (Celebrex), 109
Cellulose, 33
Chart, patient's, handwriting on, 115
Children, dentoalveolar surgery in, **183–207**
    implants in, 203–203, 205
    localized gingival lesions in, 198
    oral sedation in, 10–11
    salivary lesions in, 199–201
Chitosan, 21
Cleidocranial dysplasia, 201–202
Clinical negligence, 114–115
Codeine, 102–103
Connective tissue graft, subepithelial, for mucogingival defects, 271, 272
Continuous sutures, 296, 299, 300–301
COX-2 inhibitors, 109

D

Dental office, risk management in, **113–120**
Dental patient, preoperative evaluation of, 3, 6
    receiving oral sedation, monitoring of, 3
Dentoalveolar surgeon, instrumentation for, 291–294
    needle selection by, 289–290
    suture materials for. See *Suture materials*.
    suture techniques for, 294–302
    suturing principles for, **281–303**

Dentoalveolar surgery, pediatric, **183–207**
Diabetes, insulin-dependent, antibiotic prophylaxis for, 241
Diazepam (Valium), 6
    actions of, 8–9
    contraindications to, 9
Distraction osteogenesis, 217
Doctor-patient relationship, terminating of, 119
Documentation, 115, 116

E

Ectodermal dysplasia, 202–203
Edema, as postextraction complication, 78
Endodontic surgery, **121–132**
    algorithm for, 122, 123
    and concomitant periodontal procedures, 126–127
    biopsy and, 130–131
    of cracked or fractured teeth, 126, 127
    periapical surgical procedures in, 127–129
    preoperative planning for, 121–124
    success of, determination of, 124–126
    surgical access for, 129–130
Epinephrine, 139
Eruption patterns, 183, 184
Erythema multiforme, 50–52, 53
    diagnosis and treatment of, 70
Exodontia, bone removal for, 254–255
    chair position for, 246, 247
    complicated, 248–250
    definition of, 246
    flap design for, 252–254, 255
    indications for, 250–252, 253
    instrumentation for, 261
        and techniques for, 246–248, 249, 250, 251, 252
    postextraction patient instructions in, 259
    sectioning of teeth for, 255–258, 259
    tips and techniques for better outcomes of, **245–266**
Extraction, simple, principle of, 245–248

F

Facial nerve paralysis, due to anesthesia, 145
Fear, dental, prevalence of, 1
        sedation in, 2
Fibrin glue, 35
Follow-up of patient visit, 117–118
Fondaparinux, 29
Frenum, labial, 194, 195
    lingual (ankyloglossia), 194–195, 196, 197
Full joint replacement, antibiotic prophylaxis for, 239–240

G

Gardner syndrome, 203
Gelatin foams, 33
Gelfoam, 20
Gingival autograft, free, 268–271
Gingival hyperplasia, 195–198
Gingival lesions, localized, in children, 198
Gingivostomatitis, primary herpetic, 44–45, 62
Graft harvesting, for free gingival autograft, 269–271

H

HemCon dental dressing, 34
Hemostasis, clotting factors in, 27
    in oral surgery, **17–23**
    normal, 29
Hemostatic agents, 20–21, 34
    for local use, 33–35
Heparin, 28
Herpes lesions, recurrent, 44–45
Herpes simplex viruses, primary and recurrent, diagnosis and treatment of, 60–62
Hydrocodone, 103

I

Ibuprofen, 107–108
Impacted teeth, etiology of, 185
    evaluation of, 185–186
    examples of, 186–192
    extraction of, 192
    incidence of, 184–185
    orthodontic anchorage of, 192
    treatment options in, 186
Implants, pediatric, 203–205
    placement of, alveolar bone grafting and reconstruction prior to, **209–218**
Incisors, impaction of, 191
Infection, as postextraction complication, 78–81
Infective endocarditis, prevention of, 235
    prophylaxis in, guidelines for, 236–242
Informed consent, for oral invasive procedures, 117, 118
    for sinus lift surgery, 221
    in preoperative evaluation, 178–179

K

Ketirikac (Toradol), 108–109

L

Lateral sliding flaps, for mucogingival defects, 273, 274
Lawsuits, reasons for, 113–114
Lichen planus, 47–49
    diagnosis of, 64–65
    treatment of, 66

Lidocaine, 135–136
Lingual nerve injury, due to anesthesia, 146
Lupus erythematosus, 52–54
    diagnosis and treatment of, 70

M

Mallampati classification, 165, 172
Masticatory muscle disorders, recognition and treatment of, 154
Maxillary nerve blocks, 142–144
Maxillary sinuses, anatomy and physiology of, 219–220
Mepivicaine, 136–138
Merperidine (Demerol), 104
Microfibrillar collagen, 34
Midazolam, for children, 10
Molars, impaction of, 191–192
Mucocele, 199, 200
Mucocutaneous lesions, 44–52
    approach to, 43–44
    biopsy in, communication between surgeon and pathologist for, 59–60
        contraindications to, 55–56, 57
        instruments for, 56–59
        techniques of, 52–56
            diagnoses and treatment of, **43–73**
    clinical examination in, 44
Mucogingival defects, alloderm: acellular dermal graft in, 276–278
    cosmetic, repair of, criteria for, 268
        surgical management of, **267–279**
    examination of, 267, 268
    free gingival autograft for, 268–271
        graft harvesting for, 269–271
        technique of, 269, 270
    lateral sliding flaps for, 273, 274
    pedicle grafts/coronally advanced flaps for, 273–276
    pedicle grafts/rotational flaps for, 273
    subepithelial connective tissue graft for, 271, 272
Muscle relaxants, in temporomandibular disorders, 156–157

N

Naproxen (Naprosyn), 108
N_2O, contraindications to, 13
    disadvantages of, 12
    indications for, 13
    metabolism of, 12–13
    pharmocology of, 12
    unregulated, 2–3
    use of, equipment for, 14–15
        history of, 11
        technique for, 13–14
Nonsteroidal antiinflammatory drug class, 106–109
    mechanism of action of, 106–107

O

Odontomas, 193–194
Opioid drug class, 101–106
Oral surgery, acute postoperative pain after, management of, **95–111**
  hemostasis in, **17–23**
  preoperative assessment for, 17–19
Oral surgery patients, on anticoagulant therapy, **25–41**
    assessment of, 25–26
    investigations in, 26–28
  surgical considerations in, 35–36
Organ transplant patients, antibiotic prophylaxis for, 241
Ossifying fibroma, peripheral, 199
Ostene, 33–34
Osteotomy(ies), sandwich, 217
    alveolar ridge split, 217
Ostiomeatal complex, 219, 220
Oxycodone, 103–104

P

Pain, acute, mechanisms of, 95–97
      modulation of, 97–100
  acute postoperative, management of, after oral surgery, **95–111**
  perceived, somatic sensory cortex and, 96–97, 98
Paresthesia, as postextraction complication, 83
Pediatric dentoalveolar surgery, **183–207**
Pedicle grafts/coronally advanced flaps, for mucogingival defects, 273–276
Pedicle grafts/rotational flaps, for mucogingival defects, 273
Pemphigoid, mucous membrane, 49–50
      treatment of, 65–68
Pemphigus vulgaris, 50, 51
  diagnosis of, 68
  treatment of, 68–70
Pentazocine (Talwin Nx), 104–105
Periotome, 258–259
  powered, 259–262, 263
Physics forceps, for tooth extraction, 264–265
Piezosurgery, 262–264
Postextraction, common complication(s) of, alveolar fracture as, 81
      alveolar osteitis as, 82–83
      bleeding as, 77–78
      diagnosis and management of, **75–93**
      displacement of teeth and roots as, 86–87
      edema as, 78
      expected postoperative course and, 76–77
      foreign bodies displacement as, 87–88
      infection as, 78–81
      needle breakage as, 88–89
      paresthesia/anesthesia as, 83
      root fracture as, 81–82
      sinus communications as, 83–85

surgical damage to adjacent structures, 75–76
surgical difficulty and, 76
temporomandibular disorder as, 85–86
tissue emphysema as, 86
trismus as, 85–86
Preanesthesia laboratory guidelines, 174
Premolars, impaction of, 190–191
Prilocaine, 137–138
Pterygomandibular space, anatomy of, 141
Pyogenic granuloma, 198

R

Radiographic studies, 115
Ranula, 199–201
Records, alteration of, 116
Referral of patients, 117
Renal dialysis shunts, antibiotic prophylaxis for, 240–241
Risk management, in dental office, **113–120**

S

Salivary lesions, in children, 199–201
Sedation, administration of, educational requirements for, 4–5
    in dental fear, 2
    oral, achievement of analgesia with, 12
        agents and techniques for, 6–9
        controversies concerning, 11
        dental patient receiving, monitoring of, 3
        pharmacology of, 12
    state laws concerning, 2–3
Sensitization, in modulation of acute pain mechanism, 97–98
Sinus communications, as postextraction complications, 83
Sinus lift procedures, **219–233**
Sinus lift surgery, bone harvesting for, 221–230
    complications of, management of, 231
    indications for, 220, 221
    informed consent for, 221
    postoperative instructions in, 230–231
    preoperative evaluation for, 220
    surgical techniques for, 221–230
Stomatitis, recurrent aphthous, 45–47, 48
        treatment of, 62–64
Supernumerary teeth, 193
Surgical patient, preoperative evaluation of, **163–181**
    airway examination in, 173
    anesthesiologist history and physical for, 165, 170
    beta-blockade and, 173–178
    consent and, 178–179
    for anesthesia, 164
    full stomach, 172–173, 176, 177
    laboratory guidelines for, 168

Surgical (*continued*)
    patient and surgery-specific risks, 171
    perfect plan, 164–165
    risk migration and, 171
Surgical procedures, oral, complications of, 118
Surgicel, 20
Suture materials, 281–282
  absorbable, 284
  biological response to, 283–288
  nonabsorbable, 287
  physical properties of, 282–283
  selection of, considerations for, 288–289
Suture techniques, 31, 34
  for dentoalveolar surgeon, 294–302

T

Tannic acid, 34
Teeth, impacted. See *Impacted teeth.*
Teeth and roots, displacement of, as postextraction complication, 86
Temporomandibular disorders, anatomy relevant to, 150–151
  antidepressants/tranquilizers in, 157
  as postextraction complications, 85–86
  botox in, 156–157
  diagnosis and treatment of, **149–161**
  diagnostic imaging in, 152
  evaluation techniques in, 151–152
  muscle relaxants in, 156
  nonsurgical management of, principles of, 153–157
  pharmacotherapy of, 155–157
  recognition and treatment of, history of, 152–153
  sleep in, 155
Temporomandibular joint, disorders of, surgical management of, 157–159
  dysfunction and pain in, pathophysiology of, 153
  loading of, reduction of, 154–155
Time-out procedure, 116–117
Tissue emphysema, as postextraction complication, 86
Tramadol (Ultram ER, Ryzolt), 105–106
Tranexamic acid, 20–21
Tranexamic acid 4.8% oral rinse, 35
Triazolam (Halcion), 6, 7
  contraindications to, 7–8
Trismus, as postextraction complications, 86

V

Vascular grafts, antibiotic prophylaxis for, 241
Vasoconstriction, 19

W

Warfarin, 28, 29

Moving?

Make sure your subscription moves with you!

To notify us of your new address, find your **Clinics Account Number** (located on your mailing label above your name), and contact customer service at:

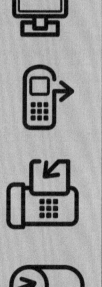

Email: journalscustomerservice-usa@elsevier.com

800-654-2452 (subscribers in the U.S. & Canada)
314-447-8871 (subscribers outside of the U.S. & Canada)

Fax number: 314-447-8029

Elsevier Health Sciences Division
Subscription Customer Service
3251 Riverport Lane
Maryland Heights, MO 63043

*To ensure uninterrupted delivery of your subscription, please notify us at least 4 weeks in advance of move.

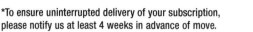

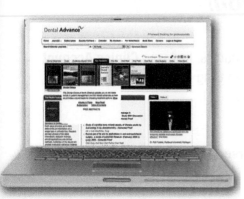
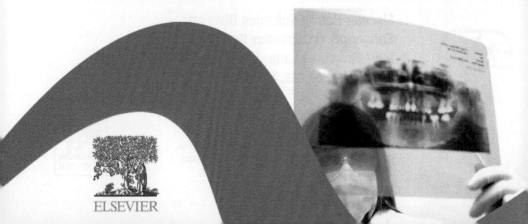

Printed and bound by CPI Group (UK) Ltd, Croydon, CR0 4YY

03/10/2024

01040458-0011